MASTER MEDICINE

Microbiology and Infection

Commissioning Editor: Timothy Horne
Project Development Manager: Barbara Simmons
Project Manager: Frances Affleck
Designers: Judith Wright, George Ajayi

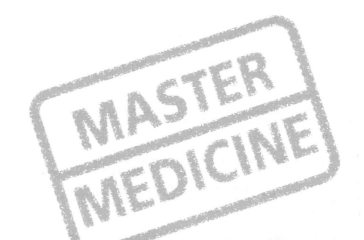

Microbiology and Infection

A clinical core text for integrated curricula with self-assessment

T J J INGLIS

DM FRCPath DTM&H FRCPA

Medical Microbiologist
PathCentre;
Clinical Senior Lecturer
University of Western Australia;
Consultant Microbiologist
Sir Charles Gairdner Hospital
Perth, Western Australia

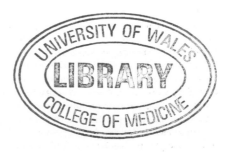

UNIVERSITY OF WALES
LIBRARY
COLLEGE OF MEDICINE

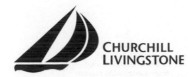

CHURCHILL
LIVINGSTONE

EDINBURGH LONDON NEW YORK OXFORD PHILADELPHIA ST LOUIS SYDNEY TORONTO 2003

CHURCHILL LIVINGSTONE
An imprint of Elsevier Science Limited

First edition 1996
Second edition 2003

ISBN 0443 070954

British Library Cataloguing in Publication Data
A catalogue record for this book is available from the British Library

Library of Congress Cataloging in Publication Data
A catalog record for this book is available from the Library of Congress

Notice
Medical knowledge is constantly changing. Standard safety precautions must be followed, but as new research and clinical experience broaden our knowledge, changes in treatment and drug therapy may become necessary or appropriate. Readers are advised to check the most current product information provided by the manufacturer of each drug to be administered to verify the recommended dose, the method and duration of administration, and contraindications. It is the responsibility of the practitioner, relying on experience and knowledge of the patient, to determine dosages and the best treatment for each individual patient. Neither the Publisher nor the author assumes any liability for any injury and/or damage to persons or property arising from this publication.
The Publisher

The
publisher's
policy is to use
**paper manufactured
from sustainable forests**

Printed in Spain

For Heather

Contents

Section C   Additional information

Using this book

Quick start

If you are new to the field of microbiology and infectious disease you may wonder how you could master such a large subject in so little time. Your task appears all the more difficult if you are aware of the recent explosion of knowledge in this field.

Do not despair! A growing number of medical schools are now reducing the amount of factual information medical students are expected to cope with. Many have changed their undergraduate curriculum by integrating preclinical and clinical subjects. There is also a greater emphasis on clinical problem solving.

This book has been written with the new medical curriculum in mind. The factual detail (particularly concerning the basic biology of microorganisms) has been mercilessly sacrificed in favour of a systems-based approach to clinical problems.

Microbiology and Infection has three main components:

- fundamental concepts in microbiology and infection (Chapters 1–5)
- major clinical syndromes, under headings corresponding to the principal clinical specialties and following the sequence developed in Chapters 1–5 (Chapters 6–19)
- supplementary chapters on bacteriology, virology, parasitology, mycology and entomology (for students following a more traditional medical curriculum) and notes on laboratory tests and antibiotics.

Since different students learn best in different ways, this book has been written to accommodate different learning approaches:

- cover to cover reading (as a basic course in microbiology and infection)
- dipping in at will (chapters have each been written as self-contained units)
- problem-solving and self-assessment, using the questions at the end of Chapters 1–19
- as an outline for more detailed reading.

Whatever approach you take, I hope this book proves to be a useful learning tool and a satisfactory preparation for future clinical practice.

Effective learning

You may have wondered why an approach to learning that was so successful in secondary school doesn't always work in medical school. One of the key differences between your studies at school and your current learning task is that you are now given more responsibility for setting your own learning objectives. While your aims are undoubtedly to pass the exams that punctuate your progress towards qualification as a doctor, you should also aim to develop learning skills that will serve you throughout your medical career. That means taking full responsibility for self-directed learning. The earlier you start, the more likely you are to develop the learning skills you'll need to keep up with changes in medical practice.

We know that students learn in all sorts of different ways, and differ in their learning patterns at different stages in a given course. You may intend to do as little work as you can get away with, or you may do the least that will guarantee to get you through the exams, but the students who gain most are usually those who take a deep and sustained interest in the subject. It will be worth the effort to start out this way, even if good intentions flag a little towards the exam.

It is impossible to write a prescription for success that applies to every student. Moreover, courses differ in their form, content, underlying philosophy and in the quality of the teachers. However, a few tips are worth passing on. Infection, whether taught as microbiology or as infectious diseases, is a very descriptive field. There is a lot of terminology to learn. Your task will be much easier if you try to fit all this new vocabulary into some sort of conceptual framework (e.g. for microorganisms, this might be: classification, identification, diseases, pathogenesis, and antimicrobial agents; whereas for diseases, it might be: epidemiology, pathogenesis, clinical features, laboratory diagnosis, antimicrobial chemotherapy, and prevention. When it comes to recalling what you've learnt, use the framework as a checklist. It's often surprising how much you can remember this way. If you're pursuing a new-style, problem-based integrated course, you'll find it better to organise your learning around clinical problems.

This will make it easier to see the clinical relevance of the subject.

You will also get more out of your course by participating actively. Unfortunately, your teachers can't do your learning for you. Handouts, if given, may help, but they are rarely a satisfactory substitute for personally taken lecture notes. Remember that timetabled teaching sessions are not the only opportunities for effective learning. It is safer to regard lectures, practicals and tutorials as a guide to the breadth and depth of knowledge you are expected to master. Well-organised departments will provide a set of learning objectives and a reading list early in the course. Many medical lecturers will give more detailed learning objectives, either in their handouts or verbally at the start of a lecture. If not, paragraph headings can be used as a rough guide to the teacher's expectations. An active approach to learning doesn't necessarily mean being highly individualistic or over competitive. Many students gain a broader and deeper understanding of the subject by working in small informal groups. This may be particularly helpful when it comes to revision.

The final run up to exams should require little more than a tying up of loose ends, and a filling of learning gaps. An effective way of doing this is to work through a steady stream of self-assessment questions and to keep a daily note of points that need clearing up. In other words, concentrate on what you don't know, and strengthen the links with what you already know. By this time, the value of pigeonholing factual information within a framework should be self-evident.

Panic button (what to do if you left your work till the last minute)

OK, so you left things a little late in the day. Don't panic. All is not lost. You can still do some good work and improve your prospects. But, first of all, don't try to out-work everyone else. Just because someone's working at any time doesn't mean that everyone's working all the time.

What you need to do now is plan your remaining revision time carefully. Plan around achievable objectives, and remember to include eating and sleeping in the equation.

Recognise what you already know. Don't be intimidated by those in your group who claim an encyclopaedic knowledge of the topics to be examined, and remember that some students derive a curious pleasure from adding to the collective pre-exam hysteria.

Next, go through the course plan, lecture list or other guide to what's expected, and decide what areas need to be revised as a matter of priority. Then draw up a list of priority topics to start on. Don't just plod through your notes, reading passively for hours on end. You will spend much of your time flitting from one familiar point to another—material you probably know quite well already. It's far better to do a few self-assessment questions (preferably with worked answers) and follow up the ones you get wrong. This will reinforce your confidence in what you already know and help you target your weak areas more effectively.

Work in short bursts of 30–45 minutes with short breaks in between. Keep a `Don't Know List' for topics that surface as vague recollections, and aim to refresh your memory on these before going to bed. Intensive revision is often stressful, so you may need to do something totally unconnected to help you wind down before going to sleep.

Don't try to cram during the last 24 hours before an exam. Hastily remembered lists learnt under panic conditions can interfere with your ability to efficiently recall previously learnt material. In fact, in the 24 hours before an exam there's little that can be done to alter the outcome, so it's better to concentrate on getting yourself into optimal physical and mental condition for the test. That way you should be able to avoid entering the exam room mentally stale and physically exhausted.

Examiners' secrets

All too often problems in exam technique go no further than the conversation at the examiners' coffee break. Some insight into other students' problems might help improve your chances of satisfying your examiners, and perhaps even pleasing them with the excellence of your performance.

The vast majority of students abandon basic examination disciplines they learnt at secondary school. Learning methods might be different at university, but important principles of exam technique are exactly the same.

You'd be surprised to learn how many fail to (a) read the instructions on the paper CAREFULLY before starting, (b) stick to time on questions, or (c) answer questions accurately.

Many students find the first five minutes of an end of year exam particularly stressful (not a good time to begin an answer). It is wise use of that five minute start-up period to settle down, and to read and re-read the paper. It is surprising how the brain seems to clear after the first rush of adrenaline passes.

When answering **multiple choice** questions be sure you know whether there is negative marking or not. If there is (usually in force for True/False questions) it is wise not to guess. A blank space is safer, and less costly, than a wild guess. Most multiple choice questions test recall of factual information. They will rarely explore paradoxes, ambiguities or esoteric knowledge. If in doubt, go for the less complex interpretation of the question.

Case histories are a newer question format that may vary considerably between centres. At undergraduate level, they will normally be used to test teaching points that are easily related to clinical problems. In a short outline that requires brief (e.g. one word) answers, there will be very little irrelevant information. The clues should all be in the outline if the question has been set well. If pictures or laboratory exhibits are involved, pattern recognition is clearly being tested. A colour atlas (e.g. the Microbiology Colour Guide) may be useful for revision purposes but is not a substitute for practical or demonstration material.

OSCE (objective structured clinical examination). This new question format is introduced in the second edition of this book to reflect some of the changes occurring in medical teaching. Several postgraduate colleges use the OSCE format because it combines an overt clinical relevance with clear, objective marking. In the version of the OSCE used here, the questions take the reader through a series of clinically-related decisions. Answers are either true or false, and under exam conditions may be given negative marks if a wrong answer is given. These questions benefit from a careful read of the case outline. If you don't know the answer immediately, try to imagine what makes best sense in a clinical context. Your other answers may provide some clues, but remember, one or more of these may be wrong.

Short notes questions are a question format best suited to factual knowledge of greater complexity than can be tested by multiple choice. However, they are only rarely used to explore complex concepts or issues currently under debate. The question is usually expressed as a short phrase with a simple instruction. It may help to remember who taught the topic and what points they gave particular emphasis to. Many faculties allow students to answer this type of question in note form. If you can get information down on paper in this way and organise it well without writing in sentences, you may make the job of marking easier for the examiner and help improve your score.

Viva. The oral exam is also new to the second edition of this book, though it has been used in medical schools for many years. Generally oral exams fall into two categories; one for the most able students in medical schools that still run an honours system, and one for other students including those who are being given a chance to prove that they really do know enough to pass despite a poor written exam showing. Despite rumours to the contrary, oral examiners rarely try to trip up examinees with catch questions. They will usually work in pairs, taking turns to ask questions that usually start at the general and progress towards more specific, and difficult. It is good practice to try to begin an answer with a short, quick reply that gives the examiner all or most of what is being asked for. Avoid lengthy sentences, vague explanations or prolonged examples. If the examiner wants more detail, they can always ask for more. If you don't know, it is better to be frank and give the examiner an opportunity to move onto another topic in the time remaining. That way you get credit for what you have been able to talk about. The setting of the viva can be quite intimidating the first time around, so it is good practice to turn up in plenty of time with some idea of the sort of questions that were asked in previous years. If you suffer exam nerves, use a relaxation technique that works best for you.

Essays. Essays are rapidly falling out of fashion due to the difficulty marking them objectively and possibly because educators now recognise a need to test different kinds of knowledge. If you need practice writing essays, you could use the viva questions as essay titles. Alternatively, you could see whether the medical library has a set of past examination papers. Very few students plan their answers, and the result is often a poorly organised stream of information. Five minutes careful planning at the start of a 45-minute question will be time well spent. There are at least two good approaches: start with the relevant checklist (e.g. epidemiology, pathogenesis etc.), or map out a conceptual diagram, linking word bubbles to each other. Whatever approach you use, read the question carefully, marking the command words and noting the topic areas wanted. If it says `explain,' explain. If it asks you to discuss, then discuss (i.e. enter into BOTH sides of the debate). If the question is in two parts, the marks will usually be divided equally, unless otherwise stated, so divide your efforts accordingly. When starting your answer, score through your notes neatly and lay out your answer in clear prose, with paragraph headings where appropriate. This makes it easier for your examiner to mark. Don't overrun on time. Extra time on a subject you know well does not compensate for reduced time on a less familiar subject. Also, many a student has gained marks for points mentioned in a good outline, despite running out of time on the full text version.

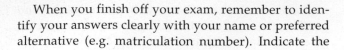

When you finish off your exam, remember to identify your answers clearly with your name or preferred alternative (e.g. matriculation number). Indicate the questions numbers attempted on the cover, if required. It will help your examiners . . . and that should help you.

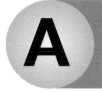

SECTION A Introduction to microbiology and infection

1 Biology of microorganisms

Overview

Microorganisms are classified in groups, the most important of which are the genus and species. Membership of a common group (e.g. genus) implies a certain level of relatedness, or common features. The structural, metabolic, genetic and immunological features of organisms in each successive group are increasingly complex. This chapter also deals with the ecology of microorganisms: where disease-causing species are found and their interactions with the environment.

1.1 Classifying microorganisms

Learning objectives

You should:

- know the main groups of microorganisms
- understand their important structural features
- develop a foundation for understanding the medically significant microorganisms.

Naming microorganisms

All living things have two names, their generic name, e.g. *Staphylococcus*, and their specific or species name, e.g. *aureus*. Either name may contain clues about the organism, the diseases it causes or even its discoverer. Names are usually derived from Latin or Greek and are either <u>underlined</u> or in *italics*. Only the genus is capitalised, and its first letter may be used in an abbreviated version. In addition, a third name may be added to distinguish varieties. A common name derived from historical use may occur. This is often seen with medically important microorganisms, e.g. pneumococcus for *Streptococcus pneumoniae*. So one microorganism may be referred to in several ways:

- *Staphylococcus aureus* (proper name)
- *S. aureus* (proper abbreviated version)
- *Staph. aureus* (colloquial)
- staphylococci (group name)
- *Staphylococcus* sp.

Changing names

The names of microorganisms are under constant review and are frequently subject to change. They can become members of a completely new genus or may be shifted to a previously existing group. Sometimes species or even whole genera are amalgamated. The main reason for this in recent years has been the application of molecular biology techniques such as 16s RNA gene sequencing and DNA hybridisation techniques which measure the genetic relatedness of microbial species. Discrepancies have been ironed out by using multiple complementary methods in a process called **polyphasic taxonomy**. In addition to changing names, microbial taxonomists are now better equipped to give appropriate names to newly discovered microorganisms.

Major categories of microorganism

Microorganisms are usually divided into five groups. The helminth parasites are by no means microscopic but are included because of their ability to infect and cause disease. Viruses are included for the same reason, although they are not living, i.e. are not capable of independent replication. For all practical purposes they behave as living organisms. The main groups are:

- bacteria
- fungi
- helminths
- protozoa
- viruses.

Bacteria

Bacteria are single cell organisms (**prokaryotes**) containing both DNA and RNA but no defined nucleus. They usually have a cell wall and may possess other features such as pili, fimbriae and flagella. They do not have mitochondria or other organelles enclosed by a membrane. Bacteria can be divided into groups based on the staining characteristics in laboratory identification tests and on their shape. Biochemical and genetic characteristics are used to extend this classification.

Staining reactions

The Gram stain is the most widely used staining procedure in medical bacteriology. Many species can be clearly defined as Gram-positive, e.g. streptococci, or Gram-negative, e.g. *Neisseria* sp. Some organisms stain poorly with Gram stain but can be stained with other stains so that they resist decolorisation with strong acid, e.g. the acid-fast bacilli, which include mycobacteria.

Shape

Three fundamental shapes are seen: spherical (coccus), straight rod (bacillus), and curved or spiral rods (Fig. 1). The last group include comma-shaped rods (vibrios) and spirals (spirochaetes, Spirillum and Campylobacter). There is diversity within these groups, e.g. cocci may be arranged in bunches like grapes (staphylococci), in chains (streptococci), in pairs (pneumococci), etc.

Medically important bacteria can be classified as:

- cocci
  — Gram-positive, e.g. staphylococci, streptococci
  — Gram-negative, e.g. *Neisseria* spp.
- bacilli
  — Gram-positive, e.g. clostridia, *Bacillus* spp., *Actinomyces* spp.
  — Gram-negative, e.g. *Escherichia coli, Pseudomonas* spp., *Haemophilus* spp.
  — acid-fast, e.g. mycobacteria
- spiral or curved rods
  — Gram-negative, e.g. vibrios
  — poorly Gram-negative, e.g. spirochaetes.

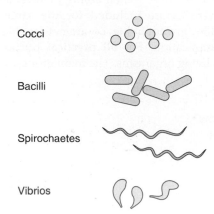

Cocci

Bacilli

Spirochaetes

Vibrios

Fig. 1 Bacterial shapes.

Genetics

Genetic analysis methods can identify pathogens by their nucleic acid contents, e.g. 16s RNA gene sequence.

Biochemistry

Metabolic characteristics can be identified in the laboratory as can requirements for oxygen, temperature range, pH range, carbon and nitrogen sources, etc. These can often be used to distinguish closely related organisms.

Immunology

The antigens present on the surface of pathogens can help to identify or subtype them. Some of the most successful pathogens can change their antigenic character to avoid host defences.

Fungi

Fungi possess DNA and RNA, a defined nucleus and have a cell wall. Fungi have a binomial name; however, because all fungi can reproduce asexually (**anamorphic state**) and most reproduce sexually as well (**teliomorphic state**), some fungi have different names for each state. Clinicians generally use the name of the anamorphic (tissue) state. There are two major types:

- yeasts: small, round, unicellular, e.g. *Candida* spp.
- moulds: grow as filaments (hyphae) that interlace to form a tangled mass (mycelium), e.g. *Mucor* sp., *Trichophyton* sp.

Dimorphic fungi: exist in both forms, usually the yeast form in the body and the filamentous form in the environment, e.g. *Histoplasma* sp., *Sporothrix* sp.

An alternative classification system is based on clinical syndromes:

- superficial mycoses, e.g. dermatophytes (*Trichophyton* sp.)
- subcutaneous mycoses, e.g. *Sporothrix* sp.
- systemic/deep mycoses, e.g. *Histoplasma* sp.

Parasites

The term parasite implies adaptation to life on or in the bodies of higher organisms and can include protozoa (complex unicellular organisms with a defined nucleus and other organelles) and helminths (worms, multicellular organisms). Members of both groups have complex life cycles.

Protozoa

Protozoan parasites include:

- sporozoa, e.g. *Plasmodium* sp., *Toxoplasma gondi, Cryptosporidium* sp.
- rhizopoda, e.g. *Entamoeba* sp., *Naegleria* sp., *Acanthamoeba* sp.

- flagellates:
  — intestinal, e.g. *Trichomonas sp.*, *Giardia lamblia*
  — blood, e.g. *Leishmania* sp., *Trypanosoma* sp.
  — others, e.g. *Pneumocystis carinii*.

Helminths

The parasitic helminths (worms) include:

- cestodes (flatworms or tapeworms), e.g. *Taenia* sp., *Echinococcus* sp.
- nematodes (roundworms), e.g. *Trichinella* sp., *Ascaris* sp.
- trematodes (flukes):
  — tissue, e.g. *Fasciola hepatica*
  — blood, e.g. *Schistosoma* sp.

Viruses

Viruses are very small organisms that contain DNA *or* RNA but not both. They can only grow and propagate inside a living cell. Usually viruses are named according to the disease for which they are responsible (a systematic nomenclature has yet to be accepted). Within the two main classes of DNA and RNA viruses several groups can be recognised:

- single-stranded DNA viruses, e.g. parvoviruses
- double-stranded DNA viruses, e.g. adenoviruses, herpesviruses, papovaviruses, poxviruses
- single-stranded RNA viruses, e.g. bunyaviruses, coronaviruses, orthomyxoviruses, paramyxoviruses, picornaviruses, retroviruses, rhabdoviruses
- double-stranded RNA viruses, e.g. reoviruses
- segmented RNA viruses, e.g. arenaviruses.

1.2 Morphology and physiology of microorganisms

Learning objectives

You should:

- understand the structural features that are important medically and for identification
- know how the metabolism and growth of microorganisms influences their infectivity and their control.

Bacteria

Cell wall

All bacteria, apart from mycoplasmas, possess a cell wall external to the cytoplasmic membrane. The cell wall contains characteristic molecules important to viru-

lence and host antibody production. There are three main types of wall structure, which can be distinguished by their staining ability.

Gram-positive cell wall

The Gram-positive cell wall contains a thick layer of peptidoglycan: a sack-like polymer of *N*-acetyl muramic acid and *N*-acetylglucosamine (Fig. 2). This gives rigidity to the cell and helps the cell to resist changes in osmotic pressure. In the Gram stain, this layer prevents removal of methyl violet stain by organic solvents such as alcohol or acetone. Teichoic acids are also present.

Gram-negative cell wall

In Gram-negative bacteria, the layer of peptidoglycan is much thinner (Fig. 3) and does not prevent removal of stain by organic solvent. External to the peptidoglycan layer is another layer, a specialised outer membrane composed of lipoproteins, and on the outer surface there are lipopolysaccharides. The lipopolysaccharide contains a variable carbohydrate chain comprising repeating saccharide units, which form the **O antigen**. These vary within bacterial species and are recognised by agglutination with specific antisera (**serotypes**). In between these two layers is the **periplasmic space**.

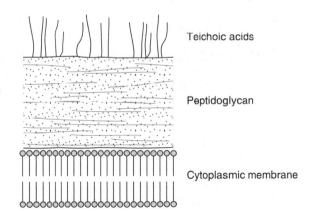

Fig. 2 The Gram-positive cell wall.

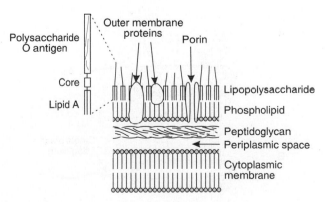

Fig. 3 The Gram-negative cell wall.

Access to the periplasmic space is regulated by the porin molecules illustrated in Figure 3.

Acid-fast bacteria

Acid-fast bacteria are highly impermeable to dyes and organic solvents because of a waxy layer in the cell wall. Special staining procedures are required, such as the Ziehl–Neelsen method.

Cell membrane

In most species, the cell membrane is enclosed by the cell wall; however, mycoplasmas lack a cell wall and have an exposed cell membrane.

Capsule

Some species have a capsule, often composed of polysaccharide, external to the cell wall. This capsule confers resistance to phagocytosis.

Pili and fimbriae

Pili and fimbriae are hair-like structures that protrude from the outer surface of some bacterial species and assist in adhesion to external surfaces (Fig. 4).

Flagella

Flagella are long, thin structures that protrude from the surface of some bacteria and are responsible for producing movement (Fig. 4). Flagella are complex structures capable of rapid changes in the direction of their rotary movement in response to changing environmental conditions.

Spores

Some species surround the bacterial DNA with a thick protective coat to form a spore that can survive extreme physical conditions.

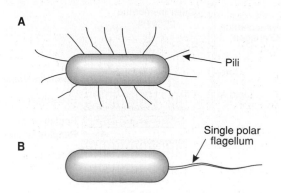

Fig. 4 External pili (A) and a flagellum (B) on a bacterium.

DNA

Bacterial DNA usually takes the form of a single, super-coiled chromosome. It may be accompanied by circular extrachromosomal DNA fragments called plasmids. DNA can be transferred between bacteria by:

- transformation: uptake of naked bacterial DNA across the cell wall
- transduction: DNA fragments transferred by viruses called bacteriophages
- conjugation: DNA transferred between bacteria along a specialised hollow tube ('sex pilus').

Until recently, it has been assumed that genetic diversity in bacteria has arisen mainly from spontaneous mutational change rather than from horizontal gene transfer between related species or genera. However, it is now recognised that large gene sequences can be transferred directly between bacterial species, possibly accounting for the development of chromosomal 'pathogenicity islands'.

Metabolism

A variety of nutrients is needed for growth and division. In the laboratory, they are provided either in liquid (broth) or solid (broth plus agar) form. Also important for growth are:

- temperature
- gaseous atmosphere
- pH.

Most medically important species will grow at or around human body temperature, 37°C, which is the temperature most commonly used to incubate bacteria from clinical specimens. The gaseous environments used include:

- aerobic: oxygen
- anaerobic: lacks oxygen
- microaerophilic: low oxygen
- capnophilic: carbon dioxide.

A few species prefer acidic or alkaline conditions for growth.

Growth

When the nutrients available to bacteria are limited (e.g. a broth bottle), growth follows a series of recognised stages (Fig. 5).

1. Lag phase: no increase in cell number or size
2. Log (also exponential) phase: maximal increase in cell number
3. Stationary phase: no net increase in cell number as a result of substrate limitation or inhibition by metabolite accumulation

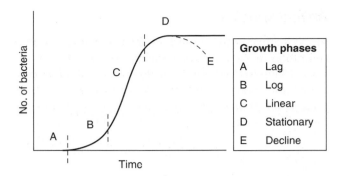

Fig. 5 Bacterial growth curve: lag phase (A), log phase (B), linear phase (C), plateau or stationary phase (D), decline (E).

4. Death phase: net decrease in cell number owing to toxic metabolites or substrate deprivation.

Rate of growth under optimal conditions is expressed in terms of doubling time and ranges from 20 minutes (*E. coli*) to 18 days (*Mycobacterium leprae*).

Viruses

Structure

Viruses are composed of a nucleic acid, either DNA *or* RNA, and a coat of protein subunits (or capsomeres), which together form the nucleocapsid. A lipid envelope and structural proteins are found in some species. Viral particles have helical, icosahedral, or no regular symmetry. Their nucleic acids may be either single or double stranded and most are in a linear molecular form.

Growth

Viruses are obligate intracellular parasites, i.e. they require the metabolic apparatus of a host cell for replication. Many types of virus have a preference or tropism for cells of a particular species or tissue type. Artificially cultivated cells of either primary (finite lifespan) or continuous (immortalised tumour cells) cell type are required for viral culture. Viral growth is usually detected by alterations in the host cells (e.g. change in shape or viability in cell culture) or by antigen recognition (e.g. immunofluorescence).

Fungi

Structure

Fungi have a defined nucleus with both DNA and RNA. They have a complex cell wall that contains sterols. Yeasts are single cell organisms that reproduce by budding, whereas moulds grow by extending filamentous hyphae. They reproduce asexually by releasing spores from specialised hyphae called conidiophores or sporangiophores. Dimorphic fungi grow in both yeast and mould forms.

Growth

Fungi have different nutrients and environmental requirements from bacteria. Most medically important species will grow aerobically on solid media, with a higher carbohydrate content and a lower pH than standard bacteriological agars.

Parasites

The two main groups known to medical microbiologists as parasites are protozoa and helminths. Their complex nutritional requirements and life cycles mean that laboratory culture is only possible in rare cases. However, their microscopic appearance is also more complex and has, therefore, been used to identify them.

Organisms that can cause confusion

Some organisms do not clearly fall into any one group, for example rickettsiae and chlamydiae lead an obligatory intracellular life because of their high degree of specialisation to an intracellular habitat.

Mycoplasmas. Small bacteria that lack a cell wall but can be cultivated on cell-free media (although with exacting nutritional requirements).

Chlamydiae. Small, energy-dependent bacteria that are obligate intracellular parasites and will only grow in cell culture.

Rickettsiae. Small bacteria that are also obligate intracellular parasites. They are transmitted by insect vectors.

Prions. Self-replicating proteins that may have a role in some slow virus diseases.

1.3 The microbial environment

Learning objectives

You should:

- know the typical microbes of different environments
- know the indigenous flora of the human body, the areas colonised and the potential for infection
- understand how the indigenous flora is acquired
- know the medically important species.

Microorganisms are ubiquitous, i.e. they can be found in any environment that supports biological activity. They are to be found in soil, water, air, foods and, particularly, in association with plants, human beings and other animals.

Air

The number of microorganisms found in air depends primarily on air type and on a number of other less important determinants. Airborne microorganisms that may cause respiratory infection include bacteria, fungi and viruses.

Outdoor air will contain bacteria, along with some moulds and spores. Counts depend on soil type, climate (wind, sunshine, rain, humidity, etc.) and population (animal and vegetation).

Indoor air contains organisms that are found in dust, droplets and droplet nuclei. The principal component of house dust is human skin squames, in particularly high concentration on bedding and clothing. Sweeping and draughts stir up dust and increase the airborne organism count.

Water

Surface waters (river, lakes, etc.) contain higher counts of microorganisms than deep waters, which are often free from organisms. Rivers receive the run-off from the land and may also be used for sewage disposal. Surface waters (particularly rivers), therefore, contain:

- natural water organisms, e.g. *Pseudomonas* and *Serratia* spp.
- soil organisms (plant associated), e.g. *Klebsiella, Enterobacter* spp.
- intestinal organisms (from sewage), e.g. *E. coli, Enterococcus faecalis, Clostridium perfringens*.

Water acts as a vehicle for microorganisms that cause a wide range of diseases, such as dysentery, enteric fever, cholera, hepatitis, atypical pneumonia and a range of hospital-acquired infections.

Soil

Soil contains bacteria and smaller numbers of fungi and protozoa. Bacteria are found in highest numbers in the layer penetrated by plants roots (rhizosphere). Many species contribute to atmospheric nitrogen fixation. Cultivated soils may have up to 1000 times the number of bacteria found in poor soils. Pathogenic organisms often found in soil include *Clostridium* and *Actinomyces* spp. Soil exposure is, therefore, important in cases of tetanus, gas gangrene and maduromycosis.

Animal species

Microorganisms are found in particularly high concentration in the immediate vicinity of members of the animal kingdom. Many different bacterial, fungal, protozoal and viral species make up the indigenous flora present on animals. Some of these are shed into the immediate surroundings (e.g. by defaecation), contributing to the microbial flora of soil, water and air. Disease-causing microorganisms from other animal species may be:

- a part of their indigenous flora, e.g. *Pasteurella multocida* (cause of infected dog bites)
- a cause of disease in that species, e.g. *Brucella abortus* (brucellosis in humans, septic abortion in domestic animals)
- involved in host/vector cycle, e.g. *Trypanosoma gambiense* (sleeping sickness).

The indigenous human flora

The indigenous human body flora is the most important source of microorganisms causing human disease. These organisms are normally found in harmless close association with human body surfaces. The tissues, blood and internal body fluids of humans are normally sterile. Occasionally, small numbers of microorganisms gain access to these sites, but defence mechanisms prevent the establishment of infection. Only the body surface has a microbial flora, the composition of which depends on local conditions such as temperature, gaseous atmosphere, nutrient availability, pH, microbial adherence and the presence of other organisms.

Skin

Microorganisms are not evenly spread over the skin surface. Most of the skin is dry, has a high salt concentration and sheds easily. In exposed areas, conditions are suitable for the growth of relatively few species (*Staphylococcus epidermidis*, coryneform bacilli, micrococci and low numbers of *S. aureus*). Numbers are higher in the microenvironment around hair shafts. Glabrous skin, with its apocrine glands, is more suited to the growth of *S. aureus* and the Enterobacteriaceae. Most of these organisms occur in colonies. The majority of organisms in the skin are anaerobic bacteria (e.g. *Propionibacterium acnes*), but these are only found in the relatively anaerobic conditions of the sebaceous glands. The yeast *Pityrosporum ovale* may also colonise skin surfaces. An alteration in skin conditions that increases hydration or damages the surface (e.g. occlusion, high humidity, chronic inflammatory conditions such as eczema and psoriasis) increases colonisation by organisms like *S. aureus*.

Respiratory tract

The upper respiratory tract from nares to nasopharynx is colonised by an extensive bacterial flora. In the anterior nares, the species found are similar to those on the skin of the face. *S. aureus* is present in 25–30% of adults, being present permanently in around half of these and temporarily in the other half. The nasopharynx contains streptococci: both α- and β-haemolytic species. Non-pathogenic *Neisseria* spp., *S. pneumoniae* and *Haemophilus influenzae* are present to a varying extent, partly depending on the person's age and the time of year. Few microorganisms are found below the larynx, and in healthy individuals, the airways smaller than the main bronchi are usually sterile.

Gastrointestinal tract

Mouth

There is a complex indigenous flora in the oral cavity, which differs between the surface of the tongue, mucosa of the lips, cheeks and palate, the tooth surface and gingival crevices. Both α-haemolytic streptococci and non-pathogenic *Neisseria* spp. are found on many surfaces. Less commonly, staphylococci, Enterobacteriaceae, β-haemolytic streptococci and yeasts can be found. *Streptococcus sanguis* (important in the formation of dental caries) is present on the tooth surface shortly after eruption. The more anaerobic conditions of the gingival crevice support the growth of *Bacteroides* sp., fusiforms and actinomycetes.

Stomach

A normally low pH and the secretion of pepsin prevent the growth of most bacterial and yeast species. Spores may survive these conditions and vegetative organisms present in food particles may persist for a while. Impaired gastric acid secretion or neutralisation of gastric acid makes bacterial growth in the stomach contents more likely.

Small intestine

The relatively high motility of the duodenum and jejunum keeps the numbers of microorganisms down to around 10^3 and 10^4/ml, respectively. Impaired intestinal motility causes an increase in numbers.

Large intestine

The slow-moving and relatively anaerobic conditions in the colon favour fermentation and anaerobic growth. Anaerobic bacteria outnumber facultative bacteria by 10 to 1. The single most common species, *Bacteroides fragilis*, is present at 10^9–10^{10}/g faeces, whereas *E. coli* and *E. faecalis* are only present at about 10^5–10^6/g. Other species present in variable but usually smaller numbers include staphylococci, clostridia, pseudomonads and yeasts.

Viruses are often detectable, but it is doubtful that these represent members of the indigenous flora.

Vagina

The vaginal flora varies with age. In childhood, the organisms are mainly aerobic bacteria such as Enterobacteriaceae, staphylococci and yeasts. At puberty, under the influence of oestrogen, vaginal epithelial cells produce glycogen, which encourages the growth of lactobacilli. These metabolise glycogen to lactic acid and create a low pH environment that is hostile to the growth of many other species. Group B β-haemolytic streptococci may also be found colonising the adult vagina. Conditions change on giving birth, when the flora temporarily alters after colonisation by vulval and perineal organisms. At the menopause, reduction in glycogen production causes reversion to a flora similar to that found before puberty, often with an increase in Enterobacteriaceae.

Acquisition of the indigenous flora

In utero, the body surfaces of the fetus are bathed in sterile fluid. Only when the membranes enclosing the baby rupture and it is passed along the mother's birth canal is the baby exposed to large numbers of microorganisms. Within hours, its body surfaces become colonised by organisms from the mother's vagina, skin and respiratory tract. Any other person involved in the care of the newborn infant is likely to contribute to its developing flora. A high proportion of infants born in hospital maternity units have anterior nares colonised by *S. aureus*. The baby's colon is usually colonised within about 6–12 hours of birth. If breast-fed this is mainly with bifidobacteria and if bottle-fed, mainly with Enterobacteriaceae. Once an indigenous flora has been established, it is more difficult for new species to become established in the mouth or lower gastrointestinal tract. This has been called 'colonisation resistance'. However, the indigenous body flora is subject to change throughout life.

Medical importance of the indigenous flora

By definition, members of the indigenous human flora are not harmful in their normal habitat. However, under certain circumstances, they can cause infection, e.g.

- colonic flora: urinary tract infection
- skin flora: surgical wound infection
- oral flora: dental caries, infective endocarditis
- infection in immunocompromised patients.

The alterations in indigenous flora seen when antibiotics are used can cause adverse effects in the patient such as:

- diarrhoea, colitis
- selection of antibiotic resistance
- secondary infection, e.g. candidiasis
- reduced resistance to gastrointestinal infection.

Other adverse effects of the indigenous human flora that can occur include 'blind loop' syndrome and hepatic encephalopathy.

Self-assessment: questions

Multiple choice questions

1. The following are components of the bacterial cell wall:
   a. Peptidoglycan
   b. Capsular polysaccharide
   c. Lipopolysaccharide
   d. Pilus protein
   e. Teichoic acid

2. The following fungi are dimorphic:
   a. *Candida albicans*
   b. *Histoplasma capsulatum*
   c. *Sporothrix schenckii*
   d. *Trichophyton rubrum*
   e. *Mucor* sp.

3. Pair up the following lists:
   a. Single-stranded RNA   i. Arenavirus
   b. Double-stranded RNA   ii. Herpesvirus
   c. Single-stranded DNA   iii. Reovirus
   d. Double-stranded DNA   iv. Parvovirus
   e. Segmented RNA   v. Retrovirus

4. Pair up the correct classifications:
   a. Sporozoan   i. *Entamoeba* sp.
   b. Flagellate   ii. *Ascaris* sp.
   c. Rhizopod   iii. *Plasmodium* sp.
   d. Nematode   iv. *Trypanosoma* sp.

5. Which of the following is a proper name:
   a. Staphylococci
   b. *S. aureus*
   c. *Strep. aureus*
   d. *Staphylococcus aureus*
   e. *Staph. aureus*

6. Where would you expect bacteria from the genus *Clostridium*:
   a. Polluted river water
   b. Farmyard soil
   c. Drinking water
   d. Human faeces
   e. Mountain air

7. The following would cause an increase in numbers of microorganisms in indoor air:
   a. Sweeping
   b. Bright sunshine
   c. Changing bedclothes
   d. Rainfall
   e. Arrival of more people

8. Correctly pair the following:
   a. *Pasteurella multocida*   i. Natural water bacteria
   b. *Pseudomonas* sp.   ii. Bovine septic abortion
   c. *Trypanosoma* sp.   iii. Sleeping sickness
   d. *Brucella abortus*   iv. Infected dog bite

9. Match the organism from the indigenous flora with the most appropriate body site:
   a. *Staphylococcus aureus*   i. Skin
   b. *Bacteroides* sp.   ii. Nose
   c. Alpha-haemolytic streptococci   iii. Mouth
   d. Propionobacteria   iv. Colon

Short notes questions

Write notes on the following:

1. The term 'obligate intracellular parasite'
2. A comparison of the major requirements for laboratory cultivation of bacteria and viruses
3. The major features used in the classification of bacteria
4. The indigenous flora of the human colon
5. The microbiology of water
6. The acquisition of the indigenous human flora

Viva questions

1. How is the genome used to classify microorganisms?
2. What is the medical importance of the normal microbial flora?
3. Attempts have been made to prevent infection by manipulating the normal flora of hospital patients by using antibiotics. Why might this not work and what hazards might the patient be exposed to?

Self-assessment: answers

Multiple choice answers

1. a. **True**. A component of all cell walls.
   b. **False**. Capsular polysaccharide lies external to the cell wall in capsulated bacteria.
   c. **True**. A component of Gram-negative cell wall that has antigenic properties.
   d. **False**. Pilus protein extends in filamentous pili from the cell wall outwards.
   e. **True**.

2. a. **False**. *Candida albicans* is a yeast.
   b. **True**.
   c. **True**.
   d. **False**. *Trichophyton rubrum* is a filamentous fungus.
   e. **False**. *Mucor* sp. is a filamentous fungus.

3. a. and v.
   b. and iii.
   c. and iv.
   d. and ii.
   e. and i.

4. a. and iii.
   b. and iv
   c. and i.
   d. and ii.

5. a. **False**. 'Staphylococci' is a group name.
   b. **True**. *S. aureus* is the approved abbreviated version.
   c. **False**. *Strep. aureus* does not exist.
   d. **True**. *Staphylococcus aureus* is the approved full name.
   e. **False**. *Staph. aureus* is a commonly used unofficial abbreviation of the proper full name.

6. a. **True**.
   b. **True**.
   c. **False**.
   d. **True**.
   e. **False**.

   Presence of *Clostridium* sp. usually reflects recent pollution by human or animal faeces.

7. a. **True**. Stirs up dust containing human skin squames.
   b. **False**. Sunshine may affect the airborne bacterial count but is unlikely to have a major impact on *indoor* air.
   c. **True**. Bedclothes contain human skin squames.
   d. **False**. Rain may affect the airborne bacterial count but is unlikely to have a major impact on *indoor* air.
   e. **True**.

8. a. and iv.
   b. and i.
   c. and iii.
   d. and ii.

9. a. and ii.
   b. and iv.
   c. and iii.
   d. and i.

Short notes answers

1. Explain in terms of absolute requirement for host cell metabolism. Examples should include virus species and *Chlamydia.*
2. Features can be presented in table form and need to include the special features for each group. For bacteria describe cell-free, artificial media with examples. Also mention substrates and growth factors, temperature and atmosphere. For viruses mention primary and secondary cell culture, substrates for cellular metabolism, antibiotics to prevent contamination, temperature and atmospheric conditions.
3. Major features should include morphology/microscopy, metabolic requirements, immunological and genotypic characteristics, with examples of how each can be used in a scheme of classification.
4. You need to mention major species and relative numbers. Also cover acquisition of organisms and causes of variation.
5. Distinguish between surface and deep water. Give examples of natural water, soil and sewage organisms (see prevention of waterborne disease in Ch. 5 for further detail).
6. Cover acquisition both at birth and later in life. Deal with gastrointestinal tract and skin in detail (possibly also mention vaginal changes). A table might help to present major species from different sites.

Viva answers

1. As a final arbiter of microbial taxonomy. Nucleic acid complement divides viruses into those with DNA and those with RNA. Bacteria are increasingly classified according to DNA–DNA hybridisation

and 16s RNA homology. Subtyping of many different microbial species is performed by a range of genotyping procedures.

2. As a potential source of organisms responsible for endogenous, nosocomial infection; as a protection against more pathogenic microbes ('colonisation resistance'); and as a contributor to digestive processes. Development of antibiotic resistance, antibiotic-associated diarrhoea and candidiasis are all worth a specific mention.

3. The question refers to 'selective decontamination' of the gastrointestinal tract with orally administered antibiotics. This approach has been used in neutropenic patients and those receiving intensive care in an effort to prevent nosocomial infection arising from the gastrointestinal flora. The efficacy of selective decontamination is questionable and the possible promotion of antibiotic resistance has been the subject of much discussion.

Pathogenesis of infection

Overview

Given the ubiquitous nature of microorganisms and the many occasions on which they come into contact with humans, it is surprising how infrequently infectious diseases occur. The reason why some organisms can peacefully coexist with humans while others go on to produce disease lies in the nature of the interaction between microbe and host. Much has been learnt in recent years about mechanisms of microbial disease, especially at a molecular level. There is a growing awareness of the active contribution of the mediating environment as a decisive factor in the process of infection. Knowledge of these processes is necessary to understand how to diagnose, treat and prevent infection effectively.

2.1 Stages of infectious disease

Learning objectives

You should:

- know the methods employed by microorganisms that cause infection
- understand infection as a biological process comprising a series of stages.

The process by which microorganisms cause disease involves most or all of the following stages:

1. acquisition
2. colonisation
3. penetration
4. spread
5. damage
6. resolution.

Acquisition of microorganisms

The initial point of contact with a given microbial species is of fundamental importance. Clearly, the indigenous flora is already present on the body surface. Infections acquired from this pool of organisms are said to be 'endogenous', e.g. urinary tract infection. Organisms acquired from external ('exogenous') sources are said to be transmitted. The major routes of transmission are:

- direct contact (including intimate sexual contact), e.g. soft tissue infections, gonorrhoea, genital herpes
- inhalation/droplet infection, e.g. common cold, pneumonia
- ingestion/faecal–oral route, e.g. gastroenteritis
- inoculation or trauma, e.g. tetanus, malaria
- transplacentally, e.g. congenital toxoplasmosis.

Colonisation

Acquisition of a new microbial species may result in nothing more than a brief encounter. To establish itself in its new habitat, the microorganism needs to survive and multiply under local conditions (e.g. of temperature, pH, etc.). It must successfully compete against an established indigenous microbial flora and counter local defence mechanisms. Some species are capable of producing mucolytic enzymes in order to penetrate the layer of overlying mucus on internal body surfaces. Other species have specific adhesins to enable binding with receptor site on human cells (e.g. gonococcal pili attachment to urethral epithelium, and influenza virus adherence to glycoprotein receptors on upper respiratory mucosal cells). Locally active immunoglobulin IgA produced by some mucosal surfaces can be inactivated by bacteria such as *Haemophilus influenzae*, *Streptococcus pneumoniae* and *Neisseria meningitidis*, which produce an IgA protease.

Once established on a body surface, an organism is said to have colonised that site, but not all organisms that colonise will go on to invade and damage host tissues.

Penetration of anatomical barriers

In order to invade living human tissues, a microorganism must breach the relevant surface barrier. In the case of the skin, bacteria probably do not penetrate an intact surface. Infection thus requires a breach in the epithelium, e.g. trauma, surgical wounds, chronic skin disease or insect bites. Some parasites (e.g. schistosomes, the cause of bilharzia) can penetrate intact skin. The respiratory tract is continuously exposed to airborne organisms. However, the upper respiratory tract functions as a inertial filtration system and protects the more delicate lungs from exposure to most inhaled particles. The cough reflex and the mucociliary escalator provide back-up and expel any particles inhaled into the airways. Infective particles (e.g. droplet nuclei, less than 5 μm diameter) may reach the alveoli and establish infection. In the gastrointestinal tract, some disease-causing organisms damage the mucosal surface by releasing cytotoxins (e.g. those causing dysentery), while others (*Salmonella typhi*) are taken up by the M cells overlying gut-associated lymphoid tissue in Peyer's patches. The fetus is not normally exposed to microorganisms in utero. Only a small group of organisms that can cause infection in the mother during pregnancy and that can also traverse the placenta cause intrauterine infection, e.g. toxoplasmosis, rubella, syphilis and cytomegalovirus infection. If an organism is capable of intracellular infection (e.g. tuberculosis, chlamydial disease, viral infection), it must also be capable of cell penetration and survival in an intracellular habitat. At this stage, evasion or subversion of host defences becomes important to microbial survival.

Spread

An invading microorganism may spread by one or more routes: direct extension through surrounding tissues, along tissue planes or via the veins and lymphatic vessels. The vascular route of spread is a particularly effective means of delivering organisms from an initial focus to distant sites around the body. Organisms may play an active part in spread by destroying cells, or even by self-propulsion. As the organisms spread, evasion of host defences becomes increasingly important.

Mechanisms of damage

Microorganisms damage tissues by a variety of mechanisms:

- bulk effect
- toxin mediated

- altered function of host systems
- host response to infection.

Bulk effect

The sheer bulk of organisms may obstruct a hollow organ, e.g. some helminth infections of the intestine.

Toxins

Mediated disease may also be caused by production of microbial substances that damage cells. In bacteria, toxins (Table 1) are usually either proteins released by the organism or a lipopolysaccharide complex located in the cell wall and liberated during cell growth or lysis. A number of toxins have been shown to play an essential role in disease. They include:

- tetanospasmin
- botulinum toxin
- cholera toxin
- diphtheria toxin.

In these infections, the toxin causes the main features of disease. However, toxins do not have to destroy cells to cause damage. They can cause sublethal damage or alter cellular function, thus adding to the disease process in more subtle ways. Many exotoxins have two principal subunits: A (active) and B (binding). The B subunit will determine tissue specificity, while the A subunit causes cellular damage after binding by B and penetration of the cell membrane.

Altered function of organs, tissues or cells

The function of organs, tissues or cells may be altered following microbial invasion. Such changes may be caused by host physiological mechanisms acting to remove the infective agent, e.g. increased bowel motility leading to diarrhoea, or coughing and sneezing.

The host response to infection

The host response usually begins with an inflammatory reaction, which is followed by humoral or cell-mediated immune responses. This may cause damage through swelling, increased fragility of tissues, formation of pus, scarring or necrosis. Chronic intracellular infection may cause formation of fibrous nodules and a state of latency from which acute infection can be re-established at a later stage.

Table 1 Some examples of bacterial toxins

Species	Toxin	Type	Gene location
Clostridium botulinum	Botulinum toxin	Neurotoxin	Bacteriophage
Clostridium tetani	Tetanospasmin	Neurotoxin	Plasmid
Corynebacterium diphtheriae	Diphtheria toxin	A-B ADP ribosylating	Bacteriophage
Escherichia coli	Heat-labile toxin	A-B ADP ribosylating	Plasmid
Vibrio cholerae	Cholera toxin	A-B ADP ribosylating	Chromosome

2.2 Virulence and pathogenicity

Learning objectives

You should:

- know the principal contributors to infection-related tissue damage and the factors that might limit this damage

- understand the balance between the microorganism, the human recipient and the intervening environment in determining the outcome of an infection.

The virulence of an individual species or strain refers to its relative ability to cause disease. A prerequisite of microorganism-induced damage is microbial growth. Microorganisms have evolved a great variety of strategies to enable continued growth in a hostile environment. They compete for substrates, e.g. iron (an important growth-limiting factor) and other trace elements. Many species have defences against phagocytic cells (e.g. the polysaccharide capsule of *S. pneumoniae* or through an antiphagocytic toxin such as staphylococcal leukocidin) and even a capacity to survive inside macrophages (as in *Mycobacterium tuberculosis*). Some organisms change their surface antigenic makeup intermittently to evade the host immune system (e.g. borrelias and trypanosomes).

The genetic control of microbial virulence is complex. In bacteria, the genes coding for toxin production may be on the chromosome, plasmids or even in a bacteriophage. Expression of virulence factors in most cases is a response to an environmental trigger. Recent work with laboratory animals has resulted in the development of a promoter gene trap for the study of bacterial pathogenesis. The system, known as in vitro expression technology (IVET), has led to identification of structural and controllers genes responsible for promoting disease. The products of the structural genes have been classified in six categories: adhesins, invasins and toxins, and cloaking, shielding and scavenging factors. The genetic switching on and off of virulence factor production in response to environmental triggers allows the bacterium to survive mechanical, non-specific and immune defences. Post-transcriptional regulation via sigma factors provides a molecular link between the microbial genome and the organism's physiological response to its immediate environment. Whole groups of proteins can be up- or downregulated as the microbe adapts to its environment. Proteins under a single, unified control mechanism constitute a regulon. Many aspects of bacterial physiology are specific to a particular phase of growth. If also dependent on microbial density, they are said to be subject to quorum sensing, a process in which a group of small-molecular-weight compounds known as acyl homoserine lactones (AHLs) are expressed in a simple system of intercellular communication.

Pathogensis of viral infection

As obligate intracellular parasites, viruses require effective mechanisms of transmission, adherence and penetration to establish infection. Many viruses have specific preferences for certain host tissues (e.g. rhinoviruses for the upper respiratory epithelium and human immunodeficiency virus (HIV) for CD4 T lymphocytes).

Viruses may spread by lysis of the primary infected cell followed by secondary viraemia, or by formation of bridges (syncytia) between cells. Cells need not be destroyed. Viral penetration of the host cell cytoplasmic membrane without cell rupture is a complex process in which the virus may use cell surface molecules to subvert normal membrane and cytoskeletal functions. Viruses can be continually formed at the cell surface or the genome can even be integrated into the host cell's own genome. The long-term survival of viruses within human cells as obligate intracellular parasites places them out of reach of the immune system. Incorporation into the host cell genome gives rise to a state of latency.

Damage is caused by the cytotoxic effects of the virus or by the host immune attack. Later effects may include autoimmune, immune-complex or neoplastic disease.

Pathogenesis of fungal infection

Despite the many species of fungi present in the environment and on the human body surface, fungal disease, particularly life-threatening disease, is relatively rare. Most fungal infections appear to require some breach in host defences before infection can be established.

Yeasts often cause mucosal inflammation following alteration of either vaginal or gastrointestinal flora. Dermatophytic fungi cause a variety of skin conditions but very rarely cause more invasive disease because they are restricted to the skin. There is no good evidence for the involvement of toxins in fungal disease. Most damage is probably caused by host response.

Pathogenesis of parasitic infections

Protozoal and helminth infections have a complex pathogenesis, which is best understood by referring to the parasite's life cycle.

Some protozoal and helminth infections require transmission by a disease vector, often an arthropod. In these infections, the development of disease depends on a three-way relationship between microorganism, vector and human subject. The ecology of the vector or intermediate host is critical to the success of the parasite's maintenance within a human population.

In developed countries, parasitic infections are most common in international travellers, the sexually active, immunocompromised patients and poor people.

The application of novel molecular techniques to medical parasitology is now providing new insight into mechanisms of disease causation.

Opportunist infections

If an organism is adapted to cause disease in an apparently healthy individual, it is clearly a virulent pathogen. If it is normally incapable of causing disease but may do so when the human body is compromised in some way, it is said to be an opportunist.

Opportunist infections are of particular importance in hospital patients and in people whose immune system is depressed by drugs or infection, particularly by HIV.

Infection and the environment

The model mechanism of infection we inherited from Robert Koch places its emphasis on the microbial pathogen; the presumed agent of disease. This emphasis may have been useful in the early days of the germ theory of disease. However, a preoccupation with the microorganism to the exclusion of all other factors misses the wider context of the discoveries made by the early pioneers of microbial disease. Koch provided a rule of thumb to establish the role of a given microorganism as the causal agent of a given disease. Unfortunately, Koch's postulates, as they are known, are only rarely fulfilled, despite attempts to bring them up to date with a molecular biological slant.

The early immunologists recognised the fundamental importance of the response by the infected person in the development of infectious disease. Accepting the contribution of humoral and cellular immunity, tissue reaction and immune compromise to the course of an infection leads to a more sophisticated model of infection as an interactive process with destructive consequences.

Until very recently the environment in which the initial interaction between microbe and host occurs was seen as little more than a passive backdrop to infection, with the possible exception of some vector-borne parasitic infections. The critical role of the environment in mediating the encounter with a potentially infective microorganism, and thereby influencing the outcome, is a new idea.

The emerging picture of infectious disease pathogenesis is one in which the outcome is determined by a three-way tussle between microorganism, human recipient and the intervening environment. The complex cellular and molecular events that determine the final outcome of each encounter are likely to throw more light on the origins of disease. This multilayered picture of infection as a process encompassing molecular events, cellular events, tissue, whole organism, habitat and geography is known as 'biocomplexity'.

Self-assessment: questions

Multiple choice questions

1. Which of the following infections could be described as exogenous:
   a. Gastroenteritis
   b. Urinary tract infection
   c. Pneumonia
   d. Gonorrhoea
   e. Intrauterine infection

2. The following attributes may help a microorganism to colonise a given body surface:
   a. Leukocidin
   b. Pili
   c. IgA protease
   d. Capsular polysaccharide
   e. Mucolytic enzyme production

3. The clinical features of infection may be caused by:
   a. Exotoxin release
   b. Acute inflammation
   c. Altered physiology
   d. Microbial bulk
   e. Microbial death

4. Pair up the type of infection with the factor most relevant to microbial penetration:
   a. Pneumonia   i. Cytotoxin
   b. Soft tissue infection ii. Droplet size
   c. Dysentery   iii. Maternal infection
   d. Intrauterine infection iv. Breach in epithelium

Short notes questions

Write short notes on the following:

1. How microorganisms cause damage in human disease
2. A comparison of pathogenesis of bacterial and viral infections
3. The main routes for transmission of infectious diseases and how microorganisms penetrate the respective anatomical barriers

Viva questions

1. What is the difference between colonisation and infection?
2. Can microorganisms be divided into pathogens and non-pathogens?

Self-assessment: answers

Multiple choice answers

1. a. **True**. By ingestion or the faecal–oral route.
   b. **False**. Urinary tract infection is usually caused by bacteria from the perineal or lower gastrointestinal flora.
   c. **True**. By inhalation or droplet infection.
   d. **True**. Transmission occurs by direct (sexual) contact.
   e. **True**. The fetus is infected by the surrounding environment during birth.

2. a. **False**. Leukocidin is a staphylococcal toxin.
   b. **True**. Adhesins on pili help organisms such as the gonococcus to attach to epithelium.
   c. **True**. This circumvents local IgA production.
   d. **False**. Capsular polysaccharide helps to resist phagocytosis.
   e. **True**. This allows the microbe to penetrate the protective mucous layer.

3. a. **True**. They may damage or kill cells or may alter cell function.
   b. **True**. Damage occurs through swelling, increased fragility of tissues, pus formation or necrosis.
   c. **True**. Such changes may represent a host reaction to remove the infectious agent, e.g. diarrhoea.
   d. **True**. A particular problem with some helminth infections and some systemic fungal infections.
   e. **True**. Pus contains dead microbes and cells.

4. a. and ii.
   b. and iv.
   c. and i.
   d. and iii.

Short notes answers

1. The main topic areas of bulk effect, altered function, toxin-mediated effects and host response should be covered, with examples.
2. Could be tackled as a table. Follow the sequence of acquisition, colonisation, penetration, spread and damage. Give examples of bacteria and viruses.
3. Follow principal routes of transmission and means of penetration, probably best done using a system-based approach.

Viva answers

1. Briefly define the two terms, then give specific examples and *discuss* how confusion of the two terms can cause problems in clinical practice.
2. Some microbes have not yet been shown to cause human infection. Mention the spectrum of virulence from opportunist to those that can be highly lethal in the previously healthy patient. Refer to the balance between patient and microbe and its modification by host defences, antibiotics and environmental factors. Give specific examples of how concepts of pathogenesis have changed recently through developments in molecular and cell biology and now challenge a simplistic pathogen/non-pathogen dichotomy.

3 Diagnosis of infectious diseases

Overview

A diagnosis based on the patient's symptoms and clinical signs may be sufficient to determine the choice of therapy in many branches of medicine. However, in infectious diseases the critical role of the infective agent and the wide range of antimicrobial drugs available make it important to identify the underlying microbial cause. This chapter deals with the major clinical features of infectious diseases and outlines the process used to achieve a specific diagnosis.

3.1 Clinical features of infectious diseases

Learning objectives

You should:

- know how to take a clinical history
- know what features to look for in the clinical examination
- know when follow-up investigations are required.

The clinical features are obtained by taking a clinical history and conducting a careful physical examination of the patient.

Fever

Fever is one of the cardinal features of infection. Normal body temperature (taken with an oral thermometer) is 37°C, varying from 36.0 to 37.8°C. Fever is the result of an abnormal elevation of the set point of the body's own thermostat, located in the thermoregulatory centre of the hypothalamus. Hyperthermia occurs when heat pro-duction by the body exceeds heat loss (resulting in heat stroke, cerebral haemorrhage). Most conditions causing an elevation of temperature in clinical practice are caused by fever. Although fever is an important feature of many infections, it is not always present during infection and may be a feature of some non-infectious diseases. Much has been made of patterns of fever as a guide to specific diagnosis of infectious diseases. Descriptions sometimes used include intermittent, sustained and relapsing fevers. Distinctive fever patterns rarely help in reaching a specific diagnosis. Fever may be absent even in severe infection, particularly at both extremes of age, in uraemia and during glucocortico-steroid therapy.

When the cause of a fever has not been determined after at least 3 weeks of investigation, including one in hospital, it is said to be a pyrexia (i.e. fever) of unknown origin (PUO). Patients who fit the above criteria for PUO require a thorough diagnostic work-up, including a fresh history and clinical examination, baseline and other laboratory investigations. There are many recog-nised causes of PUO, including infectious, neoplastic, collagen vascular and other diseases. Amongst the com-moner infective causes of PUO are tuberculosis and infective endocarditis.

Acute infection

Other non-specific features of acute infection include tachycardia and indicators of the acute-phase response: raised neutrophil count (including neutrophils of increased immaturity), C-reactive protein, erythrocyte sedimentation rate and immunoglobulins. These are all sensitive indices of the extent of acute disease, but they are not specific to infection and do not identify a focus of infection.

Focal features of infection

The local signs of acute infection are usually those of acute inflammation: redness, swelling, heat and pain. There may be an inflammatory exudate, with formation of pus caused by polymorph chemotaxis. Other local signs will be specific to the tissue or organ system involved, for example:

- skin: rash
- heart: new murmur, friction rub
- lungs: cough, respiratory rate.

Chronic infection

In chronic infection, loss of appetite, wasting and lethargy may be present.

Formulating a working diagnosis

The physician will combine these features with epidemiological clues obtained by asking questions about topics such as recent travel, contacts with similar symptoms, pets and type of work. This information will lead to a shortlist of possible diagnoses, of which one will be regarded as the most probable. This is the working diagnosis. From a knowledge of disease syndromes and their microbiology, the physician may then be able to predict the course of the disease and its likely microbial cause.

3.2 Investigative process

Investigative procedures rarely form the entire basis of a diagnosis. More often they confirm the initial working diagnosis or narrow the choice of possible diagnoses. Once the disease has been diagnosed, a rational choice of therapeutic agent can be made. Often it is necessary to start antimicrobial chemotherapy before the causal agent has been identified. This is particularly so in life-threatening conditions, where any delay may have fatal consequences. When anti-infective treatment is started on the basis of a working diagnosis and a 'best guess' choice of therapeutic agent, therapy is said to be presumptive or empirical. The process employed to pin the blame for a given disease on a specific microorganism has its origins in the method Robert Koch used to establish the aetiology of a particular infectious disease (see Ch. 2). These principles, often known as Koch's postulates, require the recovery of the microorganism in pure culture from affected tissues, the reproduction of disease in an experimental animal and isolation of the microorganisms from the diseased animal. Only isolation of a potential disease-causing microorganism has been

retained in routine clinical practice. Inoculation of laboratory animals has largely been replaced by alternatives. The wide range of diagnostic investigations now available to the clinician faced with an undiagnosed infectious disease has made infectious disease medicine more evidence based than it once was. Nevertheless, there are still important knowledge gaps that have yet to be filled by advances in diagnostic technology.

Non-microbiological investigations

Neutrophil count (usually measured as the total nucleated leukocyte count), C-reactive protein and erythrocyte sedimentation rate are not conclusive evidence of infection but may provide a means of measuring the progression of a disease or its response to treatment. Non-specific means of localising focal infection include imaging techniques, such as chest X-ray, computed tomographic scan and isotope scans.

Microbiological investigations

A fundamental part of the process of diagnosing infectious diseases is the identification of the microorganism responsible for the disease in question. This can be done by demonstrating its presence or its specific effects on the body, often referred to as an 'aetiological' diagnosis. Whether infection is bacterial, viral, fungal or parasitic, laboratory confirmation of a given diagnosis often requires more than a single specimen or test. A combination of several specimens may provide a more complete picture of the extent or severity of disease. It may also increase the chance of isolating the causal agent.

Use of the diagnostic laboratory

The diagnostic microbiology laboratory's main function is to help the physician to confirm a clinical diagnosis. Properly used, the laboratory functions as a round-the-clock problem-solving tool, generating information from the specimens sent for analysis (Fig. 6).

Diagnostic microbiology involves a greater variety of specimen types and a larger choice of tests than any

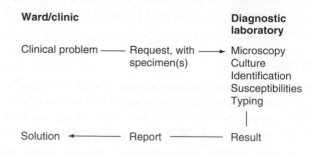

Fig. 6 The role of the laboratory in the diagnosis of infection.

other branch of laboratory medicine. Not all of this work can be automated. The correct selection of diagnostic tests often depends on the provision of detailed information about the patient. Failure to provide the laboratory with all the relevant clinical information may result in the omission of essential tests or the performance of unnecessary tests.

Specimen collection

Specimen collection is probably the single most important determinant of accurate laboratory results.

What sampling site?
The specimen should be taken from the site of suspected infection. If this is normally a sterile body site, an invasive procedure may be required. If the specimen is collected from a hollow organ connected to the body surface or from the surface itself it is likely to be contaminated by the indigenous flora. The best specimen is, therefore, one taken from a normally sterile site, such as blood or cerebrospinal fluid. The limitations of other sites, particularly those with a luxuriant indigenous flora, need to be taken into account during specimen collection and subsequent laboratory processing. A set of blood cultures should be collected whenever direct sampling of the site of infection poses problems in a febrile patient.

What type of specimen?
Body fluids or tissue from normally sterile sites are highly suitable specimens for microbiology. If the quantity is large, viability of microorganisms should be maintained during transport to the laboratory. Formalin must not be added.

Purulent exudate is often sent for processing. Exudate (e.g. from a surgical wound) should be sent in a sterile specimen container. More often, a cotton-tipped swab is sent. This is less satisfactory because the specimen is smaller, easily dries out during transit and may be subject to the antimicrobial effect of cotton fibre.

When to collect specimens
Timing of specimen collection may be crucial. Any specimens for culture should be taken prior to commencing antimicrobial therapy. In some diseases, e.g. enteric fever, different specimens are more likely to result in isolation of the causal agent at different stages in the course of the disease. Serological specimens often require a second sample of serum taken after an interval of several weeks in order to demonstrate a rise in antibody titre. Sometimes, further specimens are collected to check the response to specific treatment. If so, there should be a sufficient interval to allow therapeutic agents to take effect. It is generally better to send specimens during normal laboratory working hours. Out-of-hours pro-cessing should only be done by prior arrangement and should be limited to investigations that have a direct bearing on immediate clinical management.

Specimen container
The container used to transport the specimen to the laboratory should ensure survival of any potential pathogenic organisms anticipated for cultures from that site. It should be leakproof and resistant to crushing. Special swabs or containers may be required for particularly fastidious pathogens (e.g. *Neisseria gonorrhoeae*). The container must be clearly identified, accompanied by a completed request form with all relevant clinical details (also clearly identified) and placed in a self-seal plastic bag.

Safety
Some laboratories require the use of a hazard label on the specimen container if the patient is thought to have an easily transmissible disease (e.g. tuberculosis or hepatitis). Other laboratories apply 'universal' or standard precautions to all specimens of blood, other normally sterile body fluids, tissue and genital secretions; therefore, they may not require a hazard label. Whichever applies, it is important to consider the safety of laboratory staff, who are dependent on the requesting physician for all their information on the patient.

Laboratory specimen reception
When the laboratory receives the specimen, it is entered into the laboratory's records and is sorted by urgency and specimen class. Specimens with insufficient identifying data or inappropriate specimens (e.g. saliva sent in place of sputum) may be discarded at this stage. Samples arriving in leaking containers may also be discarded.

Diagnostic tests

Diagnostic microbiology procedures on a given specimen usually follow the sequence microscopy, culture, identification, through to antimicrobial susceptibility testing. The bulk of the diagnostic microbiology laboratory's workload is general bacteriology.

Diagnostic bacteriology
Where useful, the specimen may be examined by direct microscopy, e.g. Gram stain of purulent sputum, wound exudate or cerebrospinal fluid.

The sample will then be spread onto a selection of solid media. Sterile body fluids and other sites require non-selective media such as blood agar, while samples from sites with an extensive indigenous flora require more selective media (e.g. faeces requires xylose, lysine decarboxylase agar (XLD); gential secretions require agar containing vancomycin, colistin, amphotericin and trimethoprim (VCAT)). An exception is blood for culture, which is inoculated directly into paired liquid media (broth) bottles for aerobic and anaerobic incubation.

The inoculated media will then be incubated in an incubator that delivers the appropriate temperature and gaseous atmosphere, for at least 12 hours. Slow-growing organisms may require much longer (e.g. many anaerobic bacteria require at least 48 hours and mycobacteria may need several weeks).

Media will be examined for bacterial growth after the initial incubation period and regularly thereafter. Possible pathogenic species are examined using simple, rapidly performed tests to give a preliminary identification. If considered significant, further identification tests may be performed, and antimicrobial susceptibility tested. These usually require a further period of incubation.

Antibiotic susceptibility testing

Not all bacteria isolated can be tested against all available antimicrobial agents. The microbiologist has to judge which organisms are likely to be the cause of the presumed infection. A selection of agents that would normally be used to treat an infection with that organism will be tested. In many cases, the choice of suitable agent is already limited. Susceptibility testing often provides the physician with guidance on treatment by further restricting choice.

The most commonly used method of susceptibility testing is based on inhibition of bacterial growth by diffusion of antibiotic from a small paper disk. Six to eight such disks can be placed on a single agar plate (the National Council of Clinical Laboratory Standards, Kirby–Bauer disk diffusion test), see Figure 7, p. 38.

The general recording of antimicrobial susceptibilities of common microbial pathogens allows the plotting of acquired resistance trends and can be used to guide long-term therapeutic strategy.

Reporting of results

The laboratory will usually provide a written report at the end of specimen processing that can then be sent to the requesting physician. The microbiologist may choose to provide a preliminary, often verbal, report at an earlier stage, particularly if the patient's infection is life threatening. Relevant clinical information may alert laboratory staff to the level of priority they should give to the specimen, and the need to produce a result quickly.

Organisms that cannot be cultivated

Many microbial agents of disease cannot be cultivated in the laboratory, may only grow after a prolonged period or may be dangerous to laboratory personnel. These include many viruses, chlamydias, mycoplasmas, rickettsias and mycobacteria. In order to confirm a diagnosis, non-culture-based methods are used.

Serology

The traditional approach to detection of non-cultivatable organisms is to demonstrate an antibody response to the presumed infective agent. This is usually done by measuring the rise in specific antibody in the patient's serum over a time interval. This requires paired serum specimens and may not provide diagnostic information, although it is still useful for the care of the patient. Some infections can be confirmed by detecting specific IgM in a single serum specimen. It may also be possible to detect specific microbial antigens during the acute stage of the disease.

A vast array of serological tests are used in clinical practice. Most are based on one of the following methods: agglutination, direct (DFT) and indirect (IFAT) immunofluorescence, complement fixation (CFT) and enzyme-linked immunoassay (ELISA).

Molecular techniques

The development of the polymerase chain reaction (PCR) to amplify sought-for nucleotide sequences has led to another means of detecting non-cultivatable organisms. PCR-based methods have had considerable impact on the rapid diagnosis of infectious diseases and can be used to investigate outbreaks of community- and hospital-acquired infection. It is possible to use the same approach to detect genes coding for specific viral factors (e.g. toxins) and for antibiotic resistance.

Diagnostic virology

Detection of viruses is not always dependent on serological techniques. Some viral infections can be confirmed by microscopy, using either an electron microscope or direct antigen detection (immunofluorescence). Some viral pathogens can be cultured. The obligate intracellular biology of viruses dictates that they must be grown in virus-free cell monolayers (known as cell culture). After incubation, viral growth is detected by cytotoxic effect, by formation of multicellular syncytia or by use of immunofluorescent antibodies.

Diagnostic mycology

Use is made of microscopy, culture, susceptibility testing and serology in mycology to confirm the presence of fungal infection and to direct its treatment.

Microscopy is useful for direct examination of specimens and for examination of the morphological features of moulds, yeasts and dimorphic fungi. Medically important fungi grow on cell-free media, allowing laboratory manipulation for identification and antifungal susceptibility testing.

Diagnostic parasitology

As most medically important protozoa and helminths cannot be cultivated in the laboratory, confirmation of parasitic infection is dependent on microscopic and serological methods, of which microscopy is the most extensively used. Molecular diagnostic methods (such as PCR) are likely to have less impact in developing countries where these infections are most common.

The appearance of many parasites changes substantially during their life cycle, and the diagnosis often rests on recognition of a particular stage of this cycle (the diagnostic stage) in a clinical specimen. The most frequent specimen types sent for microscopic examination for parasites are blood and faeces, but other body fluids and tissue specimens may be more appropriate in certain diseases.

Therapeutic drugs

Some antibiotics may produce toxic effects when given in excess (e.g. aminoglycosides such as gentamicin). Their use requires careful monitoring with measurement of before-dose and after-dose levels to ensure correct dosage.

Investigation of nosocomial infections

Nosocomial (hospital-acquired) infection may be caused by either the patient's own indigenous flora or organisms from an exogenous source such as hospital staff, other patients or hospital equipment. Subtyping techniques, such as bacteriophage susceptibility, serotype, and molecular typing by pulsed field gel electrophoresis (PFGE) may be required to investigate a possible common source. Recognition of a single type or strain of microorganism common to several patients usually indicates a common-source incident and may help to identify the source. The application of molecular typing methods to hospital or community outbreak investigations and disease surveillance is known as **molecular epidemiology**. Computer analysis of molecular typing results enables analysis of the range of subtypes present in a given collection of isolates belonging to a single species. This determination of the population structure is used to identify clusters of isolates that may suggest a single point of source, a common means of transmission or a single strain with unusual capacity for transmission. Measures to prevent further spread of infection can then be introduced. Longer-term trends in hospital-acquired infection may become apparent from analysis of prospectively collected laboratory data.

Reference laboratories

Some diagnostic tests require special expertise or equipment not normally available in a hospital diagnostic laboratory (e.g. species typing or viral culture). These tests are performed in centres that have specialist expertise, called reference laboratories. Much virology, mycology and parasitology is performed in regional or national reference laboratories. The additional time required to transport specimens to a distant reference facility means that extra care should be taken to select the correct specimen, provide all necessary clinical data and use the correct container and transport media.

Accuracy of diagnostic tests

The physician must have confidence in the accuracy of laboratory results if they are to be used to determine the management of infectious disease. The accuracy of results is checked intermittently by senior laboratory staff (quality control) and by official external bodies (quality assurance). The results can be used to improve laboratory performance or may indicate a need to change the methods used in line with developments in laboratory technology.

Self-assessment: questions

Multiple choice questions

1. Fever occurs:
   a. In some patients with carcinoma
   b. In all patients with acute infection
   c. When the oral temperature is over 37.8°C
   d. When heat production exceeds heat loss
   e. When the thermoregulatory centre set point is raised

2. A specimen for detection of viable microorganisms should be:
   a. Taken from the site of infection
   b. Put into a container with no preservative
   c. Collected after starting specific treatment
   d. Transported in a crush- and leakproof container
   e. Transported to the laboratory without delay

3. Disease-causing microorganisms may not be grown in the diagnostic laboratory because:
   a. Antibiotic therapy has already started
   b. The organisms cannot be grown
   c. They would be a hazard to the laboratory staff
   d. Non-culture-based methods produce faster results
   e. The skills required are not widely available

4. The following methods can be used to establish the source of a hospital infection outbreak:
   a. Plasmid typing
   b. Pyocine typing
   c. Phage typing
   d. Polymerase chain reaction
   e. Microscopic appearance

5. Information that should be sought routinely that helps to make a specific diagnosis includes:
   a. History of recent travel
   b. History of weight loss
   c. Pattern of fever
   d. Exposure to pet animals
   e. Contact with people who have had similar symptoms

Data interpretation

The following laboratory report is for a specimen collected 2 days previously from an adult male patient with persistent fever and a heart murmur.

Blood culture bottle 1

a. *Streptococcus salivarius*
b. *Staphylococcus epidermidis*

Blood culture bottle 2

a. *Streptococcus salivarius*

Antibiotic susceptibilities are shown in Table 2.

Table 2 Susceptibilities of the organisms identified in blood culture

	Streptococcus salivarius	*Staphylococcus epidermidis*
Penicillin	S	R
Erythromycin	S	R
Flucloxacillin		R
Vancomycin	S	S

S, sensitive; R, resistant.

1. What is the likely significance of the different species in this specimen?
2. What further laboratory test would you use to confirm your suspicions?
3. Are there any non-laboratory tests that might help you to reach a diagnosis?
4. What antibiotics would you select from Table 2 to treat this patient? Give your reasons.

Short notes questions

Write short notes on the following:

1. The main features of acute infection
2. The term 'reference laboratory' and its role in diagnostic microbiology
3. What are the key factors that should be considered when comparing molecular typing methods?

Viva questions

1. What procedures occur between a diagnostic specimen's arrival in the clinical microbiology laboratory and the production of a laboratory report?
2. How useful are Koch's postulates in everyday clinical practice?

Self-assessment: answers

Multiple choice answers

1. a. **True**. This is a recognised non-infectious cause.
   b. **False**. Infants, the elderly, uraemic patients and those treated with steroids may not have a febrile response to infection.
   c. **True**. Normal oral temperature is 36.0–37.8°C.
   d. **False**. This is the definition of hyperthermia.
   e. **True**. This is governed in the hypothalamus.

2. a. **True**. If this is a non-sterile site normally, then it may be contaminated by indigenous flora.
   b. **True**.
   c. **False**. Specimens should be collected before starting antibiotic therapy.
   d. **True**. Damaged samples may be discarded by the laboratory as well as being a hazard in transit.
   e. **True**. This is most likely to preserve the sample.

3. a. **True**. Hence the need for a before-therapy sample.
   b. **True**. Some fastidious organisms cannot be grown, e.g. rickettsias.
   c. **True**. Some organisms are too dangerous to grow, e.g. Ebola virus.
   d. **True**. Both enzyme-linked immunosorbent assay (ELISA) and the polymerase chain reaction can be used for rapid diagnosis in some instances, e.g. for *Mycobacterium tuberculosis*.
   e. **True**. Some organisms can only be cultivated in specialist reference laboratories, e.g. some fungi and viruses.

4. a. **True**. Allows 'clonal' strains to be identified.
   b. **True**. Used to type *Pseudomonas aeruginosa*.
   c. **True**. Used to type *Staphylococcus aureus* infections.
   d. **True**. A sensitive means of identifying a single strain, particularly if it is a non-cultivatable organism.
   e. **False**. Microscopy, even with Gram stain, does not differentiate bacteria within species; the basis of any practically useful typing scheme.

5. a. **True**. Travellers are less immune to infections in a new environment and may come into contact with new pathogens (particularly in travel to tropical countries).
   b. **False**. Though a feature of chronic infection, weight loss is not specific to infection.
   c. **False**. Fever pattern occasionally suggests infection with a particular species, but laboratory confirmation is still required.
   d. **True**. Pets carry particular infections, e.g. *Toxoplasma gondii*.
   e. **True**.

Data interpretation answer

1. *S. salivarius* is a viridans group, α-haemolytic streptococcus, a common cause of infective endocarditis. *S. epidermidis* can cause prosthetic valve endocarditis but is more commonly a skin surface species that contaminates blood cultures during the collection procedure.
2. A carefully collected repeat blood culture prior to commencing antibiotics may confirm the significance of the *S. salivarius* isolate. Investigation of infective endocarditis normally includes three sets of blood cultures taken at intervals, over a short period of time.
3. An echocardiogram may confirm the presence of vegetations on a heart valve.
4. Viridans group streptococcal endocarditis is usually treated with intravenous penicillin. Gentamicin is often added to this for its so-called synergistic effect against the causal bacteria. Confirmation that the *Staphylococcus* sp. was a probable skin contaminant would mean that vancomycin would not have to be given unless the patient had a history of allergy to penicillins.

Short notes answers

1. Fever, tachycardia, the acute-phase response and local features should be covered. Probably best as generalised and focal infection.
2. Use specific examples from particular branches of diagnostic microbiology (see main text).
3. Typing methods should be assessed according to discrimination ability, typability, reproducibility, cost and range of applications.

Viva answers

1. Imagine the likely workflow and follow a specific example, e.g. a wound swab. The flow would include logging in, Gram stain, inoculation on a series of culture media, incubation, plate reading, preliminary benchtop tests, definitive identification tests, antibiotic susceptibility testing, recording of results, collation and validation of the report.

2. These have been used historically to argue that a given microbe causes a specific disease. Establishing a causal relationship between a specific microbe and a disease (the aetiology) is particularly difficult at the level of the individual patient. There is rarely sufficient evidence to prove a causal link. Give an example of how a specialist in infectious diseases might use laboratory evidence to narrow the possible range of causes that require antibiotic therapy before a definitive cause can be established.

4 Antimicrobial chemotherapy

Overview

There is a vast choice of therapeutic agents available to treat infectious diseases. In making a choice of agent, the physician has to take into account the likely pathogen, possible adverse effects and the selection of resistant microorganisms. This chapter reviews the mode of action of the principal groups of antimicrobial agents, the basic principles of use in clinical practice and their adverse effects, including antimicrobial resistance.

4.1 How antibiotics work

Learning objectives

You should:

- know the major classes of antimicrobial agent
- know their mode of action.

The basis of antimicrobial chemotherapy is to arrest the growth of the causal pathogen and if possible kill the microorganism without damage to the patient. In order to avoid unwanted toxic effects on human cells, most antimicrobial agents are chosen for their action on microbial constituents not present in mammalian cells. This is referred to as 'selective toxicity'.

There are various potential targets for antimicrobial action (Table 3), the most common of which are:

- cell wall
- cell membrane
- protein synthesis
- nucleic acid synthesis.

Cell wall

The presence of a cell wall in bacteria and its absence in mammalian cells makes it a valuable selective target for antimicrobial agents. Agents that act on cell wall synthesis usually have a low toxicity. Major groups of antibacterial agent in this category are the β-lactams and the glycopeptides.

Antibiotics based on β-lactams interfere with muramic acid polymerisation by inhibiting the transpeptidase that forms the final cross-links between N-acetylmuramic acid and N-acetylglucosamine. The lack of intact murein renders the bacterial cell susceptible to osmotic lysis. The two main groups of β-lactam antibiotic are penicillins and cephalosporins.

Glycopeptide antibiotics, such as vancomycin, also interfere with peptidoglycan assembly but at a different stage to that targeted by β-lactam antibiotics.

Cell membrane

The similarity of microbial cell membranes and mammalian cell membranes means that there are only a few agents that are relatively non-toxic and that target sites on the membrane. They include the polymyxins, and polyene and imidazole antifungals. The polymyxins act like a detergent and disrupt the membrane, causing leakage of cytoplasmic contents. Fungal cell membranes contain sterols, particularly ergosterol. The polyenes (e.g. amphotericin) bind sterol-containing membranes, causing them to leak. The imidazoles prevent ergosterol synthesis, causing direct membrane damage.

Protein synthesis

The process of bacterial protein synthesis is similar to that in mammalian cells. The bacterial ribosome differs from ribosomes in mammalian cells in that it has 30S and 50S subunits. Although there are a number of suitable targets for selective toxicity, there is a greater problem with toxic effects in patients receiving this group of agents. The group includes the aminoglycosides, macrolides, chloramphenicol and tetracyclines.

Table 3 Therapeutic agents: susceptibility and resistance

Therapeutic agent	Target site	Susceptible organisms	Resistance mechanisms
Penicillins, cephalosporins	Muramic acid polymerisation	Gram-positive/ negative bacteria	Altered binding sites, β-lactamases
Glycopeptides	Cell wall	Gram-positive bacteria	
Aminoglycosides	Protein synthesis at the ribosome	Gram-positive/negative bacteria	Modifying enzymes
Macrolides			Mutant binding site
Chloramphenicol			Acetyl transferase
Tetracycline			Efflux mechanism
Sulphonamides, diaminopyrimidines	Folate synthesis	Gram-positive/negative bacteria	Alternative metabolic pathway
Rifamycins	RNA polymerase	Mycobacteria, Gram-positive bacteria	Mutation
Nitroimidazoles	DNA cleavage	Anaerobic bacteria, parasites	–
Quinolones	DNA gyrase	Gram-positive/negative bacteria	Mutant gyrase
Griseofulvin	Mitotic spindle	Fungi	–

Aminoglycosides (e.g. gentamicin) bring protein synthesis to a standstill by blocking reformation of the initiation complex after mRNA has been run off. Macrolides (e.g. erythromycin) bind to the 50S subunit of ribosomal RNA and halt the formation of initiation complexes. Chloramphenicol binds to the 50S subunit and interferes with the linking of amino acids in the growing peptide chain. Tetracyclines bind to the 30S subunit and prevent the binding of transfer RNA, which in turn halts amino acid chain elongation.

Nucleic acids

A number of antimicrobial agents act on the microbial genome. Antibacterials in this category include the quinolones, the sulphonamides and diaminopyrimidines, the rifamycins and the nitroimidazoles. The most useful antiviral agents also act on nucleic acids, as does the antifungal flucytosine.

Sulphonamides are false substrates for folate synthesis, which bacteria require for purine and thymidylic acid synthesis. The diaminopyrimidines (e.g. trimethoprim) also act on folate synthesis at the next step in the metabolic pathway.

Rifamycins (e.g. rifampicin) prevent transcription by inhibiting DNA-dependent RNA polymerase. Nitroimidazoles (e.g. metronidazole) act only after nitroreductases, active at low redox potential, metabolise them to active intermediates that cause DNA strand breakages. The quinolones (e.g. ciprofloxacin) act by preventing the action of DNA gyrases, enzymes bacteria use to produce supercoiling, nicking and resealing of DNA during replication.

Viral replication occurs much more rapidly than replication of the mammalian cell, accounting for the vulnerability of this process to antiviral agents. The most commonly used agents are nucleotide analogues that cause chain termination during transcription (e.g. aciclovir (acycloguanosine), zidovudine, flucytosine,

idoxuridine). One of these, aciclovir, inhibits viral DNA polymerase only after a final phosphorylation step by viral thymidine kinase.

Other target sites

A small number of agents exploit other target sites specific to certain organisms. The antifungal agent griseofulvin interferes with formation of the mitotic spindle. The arsenicals and antimonials used in the treatment of some parasitic infections interfere with glucose metabolism, and quinine inhibits the haem polymerase required to prevent poisoning of the malaria parasite by monomeric haemoglobin. Another group of agents (including amantidine) acts by reducing viral uptake at the point of membrane fusion.

4.2 Principles of antimicrobial therapy

Learning objectives

You should:

- understand how to choose the most suitable antibiotic
- be aware of factors that may make a particular drug unsuitable for a particular patient
- know the adverse effects of these drugs.

The choice and subsequent management of antimicrobial chemotherapy is governed by clinical, microbial and pharmacological considerations.

- Clinical

  1. Does the patient have an infection?
  2. If so, will it benefit from specific antimicrobial therapy?

3. If it will, how urgent is treatment?
4. Are there any focal features?

- Microbiological

  5. What pathogen(s) are likely?
  6. Are there any epidemiological clues?

- Pharmacological

  7. What spectrum, route, dose and dosing frequency are required?
  8. Will the site of infection be reached?
  9. Does anything about the patient limit the choice of agent?
  10. Does treatment need monitoring?
  11. What duration of treatment is required?

If there is still a choice to be made between otherwise equally effective agents when all these issues have been addressed, the cheaper one should be used.

Clinical considerations

1. Does the patient have an infection? Many patients are unnecessarily treated with antimicrobial agents for conditions that are not caused by a microbial agent. The clinical evidence for infection should be reviewed. An adequate history should be sought and the patient properly examined.

2. Will the infection benefit from antimicrobial therapy? In some infectious disease, the patient is unlikely to benefit from antimicrobial therapy (e.g. many upper respiratory tract infections, most cases of gastroenteritis and exanthematous diseases such as measles). Some infectious diseases do not respond to specific therapy (e.g. diarrhoea caused by cryptosporidia).

3. How urgent is treatment? If the patient is seriously ill, antimicrobial therapy will have to begin immediately, before the results of diagnostic microbiology tests are available. The choice of agent will therefore be an educated guess, called 'presumptive therapy', and will have to be reviewed according to clinical progress and laboratory-generated information. Specimens should be collected and dispatched to the laboratory before commencing presumptive therapy. When the condition does not demand immediate treatment, the results of cultures should be awaited before a choice of agent is made.

4. Are there any focal features of infection? The clinical features of the infection may suggest focal involvement of a particular organ system. Recognising the focal features of an infection helps towards a working diagnosis and provides an opportunity for specific diagnostic tests. Some types of focal infection reduce the therapeutic options because of bioavailability issues.

Microbiological considerations

5. What are the likely pathogens? Once the decision to treat the infection has been taken, and the working diagnosis formulated, it is necessary to identify the pathogen(s) involved. This is the purpose of most diagnostic microbiology tests; however, when presumptive therapy is required, the cause of the infection has, by definition, not yet been identified. The likely pathogen(s) must, therefore, be deduced from a knowledge of the syndrome. Some infectious diseases are always caused by one organism, or a small group of similar organisms, in which case the choice of therapeutic agent is relatively easy. Other conditions may be caused by a wide variety of microorganisms, in which case the choice of antimicrobial agent has to cover all the main possibilities. More than one agent may therefore be required.

6. Are there any epidemiological clues? Knowledge of common microbial pathogens and their diseases will help to narrow the therapeutic options. Familiarity with local patterns of antimicrobial resistance will also guide the choice of agent.

Pharmacological considerations

7. What spectrum, route, dose and dosing frequency are required?

Spectrum. A satisfactory antimicrobial agent will be active against the microbial pathogen at the site of infection. Antimicrobial agents, particularly antibacterial agents, may be effective against a range of organisms. This range is called the 'spectrum' of activity. The spectrum of the agent chosen may be extended by adding another agent with a different spectrum of activity.

Route. The route of administration chosen is partly dictated by the severity of disease. The oral route is preferred for convenience, but it may not allow antimicrobial uptake quickly enough or provide sufficient tissue or blood levels. Some agents are either destroyed by gastric acid or cannot be absorbed from the gastrointestinal tract. Some agents can be given as a pro-drug that only becomes active after absorption. Antimicrobial agents are usually given intravenously when the patient is severely ill and in need of rapid treatment. Many of the agents used in this type of clinical situation are not available in oral form.

Dose and dosage frequency. Decisions on dosage are usually based on the results of pharmacokinetic studies completed during the trial stage of drug development. Alterations to dose and frequency may have to be made according to the patient, for example in the elderly or in patients with a concurrent disease such as liver or kidney disease.

8. *Will the site of infection be reached?* The antimicrobial agent must be able to reach the presumed site of infection and reach sufficient concentrations there for long enough to guarantee its effect on the presumed pathogen. Some body sites (e.g. the cerebrospinal fluid in meningitis and bone in osteomyelitis) are not reached by certain antibiotics. This will further reduce the choice of suitable agent.

9. *Does anything about the patient limit the choice of agent?*

Age and Sex. The patient's age and sex may affect choice, dose and dosage frequency of antimicrobial therapy. Modification has to be made to most antibiotic dosage schedules for children, particularly newborns. Some antibiotics should be avoided altogether in children or during pregnancy. These include tetracycline (deposits in teeth and cartilage) and sulphonamides in the newborn (may be the cause of jaundice). The elderly, because of reduced gastric acid secretion, may absorb higher levels of some antibiotics following a dose. They are also more prone to decreased drug excretion because of reduced or senescent renal function and may have poorer drug metabolising activity in the liver.

Concurrent disease. The underlying condition of the patient will also affect dosage and choice of therapy. Patients with impaired renal function may require either dose and frequency adjustment or avoidance of renally cleared compounds. This particularly applies to aminoglycosides (e.g. gentamicin) and glycopeptides (e.g. vancomycin). In both these groups, optimal therapeutic levels are close to toxic levels. In order to avoid dose-related toxic effects, the serum levels of such agents should be measured intermittently during treatment. Aminoglycosides, glycopeptides and flucytosine are the most common antimicrobial agents subjected to routine therapeutic drug monitoring. Monitoring of penicillins or cephalosporins is only very rarely required. The need to adjust the dose or dosage frequency is an opportunity to re-examine the need for treatment with that agent.

Past medical history. Any history of possible allergic or other adverse reaction to an antimicrobial agent should result in caution over choice of agent. Allergic reaction may be precipitated by other antimicrobials in the same group. However, it is usually possible to choose a satisfactory agent from another group.

10. *Does treatment need monitoring?* The more serious infections, particularly life-threatening conditions, require careful monitoring to ensure that the patient responds to the antimicrobial therapy and, in the case of some agents, to avoid toxic side effects. Response to treatment is usually judged from changes in the clinical features of infections, and an alteration in the measurable components of the 'acute-phase response' (e.g. leucocyte count and C-reactive protein). There is usually a delay between commencing specific antimicrobial therapy and clinical improvement. The reasons for failure to respond to specific therapy include a non-infective cause; treatment started too late; wrong agent, route or dose; or antibiotic resistance. Failure to respond, or the discovery that organisms thought to cause the infection are resistant to antibiotics currently in use, should result in an immediate change of therapy. It is also worth reconsidering the diagnosis, especially if more diagnostic information is available.

11. *What duration of treatment is required?* The issue of duration of antimicrobial therapy is difficult, and simple generalisations cannot be made. For many life-threatening or other serious infections, there are guidelines drawn up by specialists in that field. But there is still considerable variation in the response to therapy despite the best choice of agent. When treating infections in seriously ill patients, it is wise to avoid the most rigid of protocols and to review progress periodically. When there is a sustained improvement in the patient's condition, it may be possible to convert therapy from an intravenous to an oral agent ('step-down' therapy). Some infections require weeks or even months of antibiotic therapy after initial clinical improvement to prevent relapse (e.g. tuberculosis).

Combinations of agents

Antimicrobial agents are often used in combination with one or more additional agents. The most common reason for this is to increase the spectrum of antimicrobial activity during presumptive therapy of serious infection. If this is done, the physician should drop as many of the additional agents as possible when diagnostic microbiology results become available. In rare circumstances where antimicrobial resistance can develop during therapy, combination of agents is used to attempt to prevent treatment failure (e.g. tuberculosis, staphylococcal infection). Another reason is to achieve a combined effect on the likely pathogen. In most cases, two antibiotics working at different target sites in the same organism achieves an additive effect. In rare circumstances, the combined effect is greater than the individual effects added together (referred to as 'synergy', probably only of clinical significance in enterococcal endocarditis). Sometimes, the manufacturers of antimicrobial agents market formulations containing a fixed combination of agents, though not always for scientifically justifiable reasons. The use of such agents is not to be recommended.

Antimicrobial prophylaxis

The prevention of infection by prescribing antimicrobial agents is called 'antibiotic prophylaxis'. This topic is deal with under the prevention and control of infectious disease (Ch. 6).

Adverse effects of antimicrobial therapy

Toxic reactions

Toxic reactions are usually, but not always, dose dependent and some are irreversible. They do not rely on the patient's immune system. Of the antibacterial agents in regular use, aminoglycosides and glycopeptides have the lowest threshold of toxicity. Many antiviral, systemic antifungal and antiprotozoal agents have significant toxic effects.

Allergic reactions

The β-lactam antibiotics cause toxic reactions less often but are a more common cause of allergic phenomena, varying from short-lived rashes to severe anaphylaxis. More common than β-lactam allergy is the development of a fine, measles-like rash during treatment with compounds in the ampicillin group. This is not a true allergic reaction and does not imply cross-reactivity to other β-lactam agents. A carefully taken history of previous drug reactions should distinguish between the two. The history can be confirmed by skin tests with dilute solutions of antibiotic. Around 10% patients with allergy to the penicillin family of antibiotics also have allergy to the cephalosporins.

Patients with a history of antibiotic allergy can usually be treated with an agent from another group of antimicrobial drugs. On the rare occasion where this is not possible, the patient can be desensitised by administering gradually increasing doses of the agent under medical supervision.

Ecological effects

Despite the fact that the ecological consequences of antimicrobial therapy are the most commonly observed adverse reactions, they are often ignored. Alterations in the indigenous bacterial and fungal flora are easily demonstrated during antibacterial therapy. In general, the broader the spectrum of antibacterial activity, the higher the dose and the longer the duration of treatment, the greater this effect will be. After the prolonged periods of intravenous, broad-spectrum antibiotic treatment received by many hospital patients, resistant species survive preferentially. Intrinsically resistant species already present (e.g. yeasts) are thus given an ecological advantage and exploit the new situation. Antibiotic therapy is one of the commoner causes of 'thrush' or candidiasis, caused by overgrowth of the yeast *Candida albicans*. The patient is also prone to colonisation by strains of bacteria that have acquired resistance to the relevant antimicrobial drugs; these strains are particularly common in hospital practice. Hospitals are therefore amongst the most effective breeding grounds for drug-resistant organisms. The consequences of antimicrobial resistance include treatment failure, infection control problems and increasing drug costs.

Overgrowth of minority organisms from the indigenous flora can cause disease. This is why candidiasis is so common following antibacterial treatment. It is also the reason for antibiotic-associated diarrhoea. In fact, antimicrobial therapy is the most common cause of diarrhoea in hospital patients. A severe form of diarrhoea in antibiotic-treated patients is **pseudomembranous colitis**, which may be a life-threatening condition. This is associated with overgrowth of toxin-producing *Clostridium difficile*. Hospital outbreaks have been reported in which there has been patient-to-patient spread of *C. difficile*.

4.3 Laboratory tests for antimicrobial agents

Learning objectives

You should:

● know how to use laboratory tests to guide choice of agent

● understand how and when to monitor therapy with tests.

The clinical diagnostic laboratory has a prominent role to play in guiding the choice of and monitoring therapy with antimicrobial agents.

Susceptibility testing

Microorganisms that can be cultivated in the clinical laboratory can also be tested for their susceptibility to antimicrobial agents. Although there are some species that have a predictable susceptibility pattern, this group is diminishing as time passes because of the continual occurrence of new forms of antimicrobial resistance. In practice, most medically important bacteria and some fungi are tested for antimicrobial susceptibility. Ideally, every strain isolated from a clinical specimen and thought to be the cause of infection would have its precise level of susceptibility determined.

The method used to determine this value is based on growing the test organism at diminishing concentrations of test antibiotic. The lowest concentration at which organisms do not produce visible growth is called the minimum inhibitory concentration (MIC). It would be very laborious to perform MIC tests with every relevant antibiotic against every potential pathogen isolated.

A more easily performed method of determining antimicrobial susceptibility is to grow a lawn of the test organism on an agar plate on which paper disks have been placed containing known quantities of test antibiotics (disk diffusion test). Several agents can be tested on the same plate in this way (Fig. 7). After incubation, a zone of inhibition where no growth occurs is found around disks containing an antibiotic to which the organism is sensitive because of diffusion of antibiotic into the agar. A reduced zone or no zone at all signifies resistance. The MIC test can be reserved for situations where the precise level of susceptibility is important, such as in infective endocarditis and in neutropenic patients.

If an MIC test is performed, the level at which all bacteria have been killed can be determined by inoculating each dilution of each test tube onto an agar plate. The lowest concentration at which bacterial growth does not occur is called the minimum bactericidal level (MBC). If there is a wide margin between MIC and MBC, the organism is said to be 'tolerant' of the antimicrobial agent in question.

The computerisation of many diagnostic laboratories has enabled the accumulation of antimicrobial susceptibility data from clinical isolates. This forms a valuable epidemiological database that can be used to guide local physicians in their choice of antimicrobial agents for specific conditions and may also provide early warning of new types of antimicrobial resistance.

Therapeutic drug monitoring

It is necessary to measure the levels of certain antimicrobial agents periodically to ensure that the serum level does not fall below a minimum therapeutic threshold or rise into the toxic range. The most commonly tested agents are the aminoglycosides (e.g. gentamicin), the glycopeptides (e.g. vancomycin) and flucytosine. In each case, the agent is measured in serum from blood collected immediately before and at a specified period after administration of a dose. The results can be used to adjust dose or dosage frequency to achieve the optimum serum level; if very high levels in the toxic range are detected, the drug should be stopped until levels are within acceptable therapeutic limits.

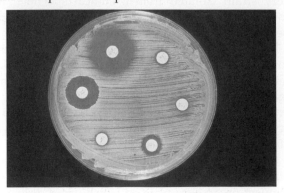

Fig. 7 The disk diffusion test for antimicrobial susceptibility.

4.4 Antimicrobial drug resistance

Mechanisms of resistance

Learning objectives

You should:

- understand the characteristics that allow microbes to avoid drug actions
- know how resistance is acquired
- know the strategies used to minimise the development of resistance.

Resistance to antimicrobial agents may be either intrinsic or acquired. Intrinsic resistance is when the organisms lacks the target site for the agent or has other features that *always* render it resistant to the agent. Acquired resistance refers to organisms that were previously susceptible to the agent in question. It is the latter form of resistance that causes greater concern, because of its potential for reducing the range of previously useful antimicrobial agents available. Its greatest importance is in the treatment of bacterial infections.

Resistance may also be either phenotypic or genotypic. Phenotypic resistance is not genetically determined. There are two types, the first being L-form bacteria, which lack a cell wall but survive in an isosmolar environment despite continued exposure to antibiotics. The other type are called persisters because they represent a small fraction of the initial bacterial population that persist after the start of antimicrobial therapy. In patients with normal host defences, persisters are successfully eradicated.

Genotypic resistance is determined by resistance factors carried in the chromosome or on extrachromosomal genetic material called plasmids. Plasmids can replicate independently of the bacterial chromosome, and smaller plasmids may be present in large numbers in any one bacterium.

There may be a reassortment of genes on the plasmid and on the chromosome. Recombination ensures more efficient adaptation to a rapidly changing antimicrobial environment. Sequences of genes that have the ability to recombine with both the chromosome and any plasmids are called transposons. The accumulation of resistance factors on a transposon may result in chromosomally coded antimicrobial resistance being transferred first to a plasmid and then to other species.

There are four principal mechanisms of acquired resistance (see Table 3) to antibacterial agents:

- enzyme mediated
- altered target site
- altered transport
- altered metabolic pathway.

Enzyme-mediated resistance

The production of enzymes that inactivate antibacterial agents is one of the most common mechanisms of acquired antimicrobial resistance. Enzymes have been described that inactivate the b-lactam agents, aminoglycosides and chloramphenicol.

Enzymes that inactivate the β-lactam antibiotics are called β-lactamases. They hydrolyse the β-lactam ring and include enzymes that inactivate compounds in either the penicillin group, the cephalosporin group, or both. In Gram-positive bacteria, β-lactamases are released into the surrounding medium. Gram-negative bacteria tend to produce smaller quantities in the periplasmic space, where high concentrations are achieved. The presence of porins in the outer cell wall of Gram-negative bacteria guarantees that small amounts of β-lactam agents reach the periplasmic space and the waiting β-lactamase. These enzymes may be produced continually, in which case they are called constitutive, or their production may be switched on in the presence of the antibiotic—these are inducible. The β-lactamases may be either chromosomal or plasmid in origin. Aminoglycosides are inactivated by three groups of bacterial enzymes: acetyl transferases, adenyl transferases and nucleotidyl transferases. These are often plasmid mediated and are found in Gram-negative bacilli.

The enzyme responsible for inactivating chloramphenicol is chloramphenicol acetyl transferase.

Altered target site

Alterations in the point where antibiotics bind to the bacterium or exert their main action are also important means of conferring resistance. Examples include changes in the penicillin-binding proteins of *Staphylococcus aureus*, which confer resistance to a range of β-lactam agents including methicillin (such strains are called methicillin-resistant *S. aureus* or MRSA). There is a form of chromosomal resistance to the quinolone agents (e.g. ciprofloxacin) caused by the production of mutant DNA gyrase.

Altered transport

Some antimicrobial agents are dependent on bacterial active transport systems in order to reach the target site inside the organism. In the case of the aminoglycosides, part of the reason for acquired resistance is a decreased uptake of the agent. In some species, tetracycline resistance is caused by increased active transport out of the organism.

Altered metabolic pathway

Antimicrobial agents that act on metabolic pathways are prone to resistance developing as a result of mutations favouring alternative pathways. An example is trimethoprim resistance, which may be plasmid mediated.

Transmission of antimicrobial resistance

The initial event that produces antimicrobial resistance is usually some form of mutation. Despite the rate of microbial replication, extensive exposure to antimicrobial selection pressure and the consequent opportunities for development of resistant mutants, new types of acquired resistance are surprisingly rare. The reason why acquired antimicrobial resistance is so widespread is the ability of bacteria to transfer resistance factors between strains and species (Fig. 8), with subsequent spread between patients, e.g. in hospitals.

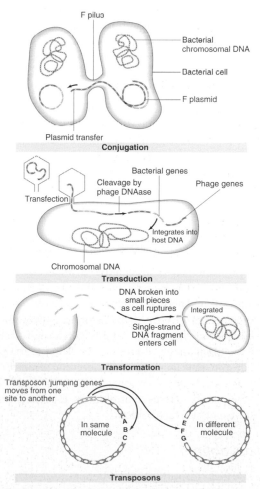

Fig. 8 Mechanisms by which resistance is transferred between microorganisms.

Conjugation

Another means of transferring resistance is by a process called conjugation in which the cytoplasm of two bacteria becomes linked via a specialised pilus, along which plasmids can be transferred. Gram-negative bacteria can exchange genetic material between species in this way.

Transduction

In Gram-positive bacteria, the genes coding for antimicrobial resistance are transferred by a bacteriophage vector in a process called transduction.

Transformation

More rarely, naked DNA released during lysis of the organism may be taken up by intact organisms. This is called transformation and is much less efficient as a means of transferring genetic material.

Control of antimicrobial resistance

There is now widespread concern at the loss of whole groups of formerly useful antimicrobial agents as a result of acquired antimicrobial resistance. Attempts have been made to reduce the problem of resistance, but only rarely has a genuine reduction been achieved. Nevertheless, some precautions can increase the time it takes for new forms of acquired resistance to become widespread.

The principle that underlies most control strategies is to achieve a reduction in the pressure to select resistance. This can be done by:

- avoiding unnecessary excessive duration and use
- avoiding topical agents
- avoiding fixed combinations.

Unnecessary use and excessive duration

The responsible physician can avoid unnecessary use of antimicrobial agents by following the approach to choice of agents outlined above. The physician should also aim to use single agents where possible, with the narrowest spectrum appropriate for the likely pathogen. Prophylactic use of antimicrobial agents should be restricted to the period of maximum risk in patients undergoing procedures in which prophylaxis is of proven benefit (see Ch. 5). Excessively long courses of antibiotics, especially for prophylaxis must also be avoided.

Topical agents

The skin is an important site where antimicrobial activity can develop and from which resistant strains are easily disseminated. The use of topical antimicrobial agents is only rarely justified. Infections involving superficial structures are better treated systemically, with the exception of conjunctival infection. Non-absorbable antimicrobial agents delivered into the gastrointestinal tract are another form of topical antimicrobial use that may promote antimicrobial resistance.

Fixed combinations

Some antimicrobial agents are available as a fixed ratio combination with another agent, supposedly for the convenience of the patient and prescribing physician. The differing pharmacokinetics of different agents means that the ratio of the components of a formulation may not be maintained in all target tissues. Moreover, the use of a fixed combination prevents the physician from ceasing treatment with the unnecessary component when the results of diagnostic test are returned. In addition, components of some fixed combinations may increase the risk of toxic and other adverse effects (e.g. sulphamethoxazole in co-trimoxazole).

Pharmaceutical companies

It should be remembered that the major pharmaceutical companies invest enormous resources in the development and manufacture of antimicrobial agents. Patent regulations mean that they have to achieve a return on their investment within 15 years or less. The activities of the pharmaceutical industry are therefore not always sympathetic to the principle of reducing antibiotic selection pressure.

Advertising has led many physicians to the erroneous belief that newer, more and broader-spectrum antimicrobial agents are better. Some have unwisely abandoned the principle of relying on diagnostic tests to fine-tune the choice of chemotherapy in serious infections, in favour of so-called 'broad-spectrum cover'. Medical practitioners should avoid making a virtue of diagnostic indecision, particularly where antimicrobial resistance may be the consequence.

The clinicians, the pharmacy and laboratory departments should all be involved in attempts to bring antimicrobial resistance under control. The pharmacy and microbiology laboratory, in particular, can provide useful surveillance data.

Many countries permit the use of industrial quantities of antibiotics as growth promoters for livestock or in the fish farming industry. It is thought that the use of some agents including quinolone and glycopeptide antibiotics have led to the emergence of resistant strains of bacteria in the gastrointestinal flora of those animals. The risk posed to the human population as a result of this practice is difficult to measure and therefore controversial. A growing list of countries has placed restrictions on the use of antibiotics in agriculture.

Self-assessment: questions

Multiple choice questions

1. Which of the following statements are correct:
   a. Chloramphenicol inhibits cell wall synthesis
   b. Trimethoprim is a nucleotide analogue
   c. Amantidine inhibits cell fusion with viral particles
   d. Cephalosporins inhibit peptidoglycan cross-linkage
   e. Polyenes interfere with protein synthesis

2. When treating a given bacterial infection, choice of antimicrobial agent may be limited by:
   a. The probable pathogen
   b. Absence of known resistance
   c. Renal failure
   d. Site of infection
   e. Pregnancy

3. Therapeutic drug monitoring:
   a. Is required during gentamicin therapy
   b. Is usually performed by bioassay
   c. Requires only a post-dose level
   d. Is usually performed during intravenous penicillin therapy
   e. Is needed when using vancomycin

4. The following infections do not usually require specific antimicrobial therapy:
   a. Gastroenteritis
   b. Pneumonia
   c. Pharyngitis
   d. The common cold
   e. Measles

5. Categorise the antimicrobial agent according to the most appropriate form of resistance:
   a. Benzylpenicillin   i. Enzyme mediated
   b. Gentamicin   ii. Altered target site
   c. Ciprofloxacin   iii. Altered transport
   d. Erythromycin   iv. Altered metabolic pathway

Short notes questions

Write short notes on the following:

1. The mode of action and the mechanisms of resistance to the β-lactam antibiotics
2. The methods used by diagnostic microbiology laboratories to test antimicrobial susceptibility of common bacterial isolates
3. The principal adverse effects of using antimicrobial agents
4. The role of agriculture in promoting antibiotic resistance

Viva questions

1. What types of acquired antibiotic resistance are likely to have the greatest effect on antibiotic prescribing?
2. Given the increasing problem of antibiotic resistance, what potential targets might be explored for novel antibacterial agents?

Self-assessment: answers

Multiple choice answers

1. a. **False**. Chloramphenicol inhibits protein synthesis.
   b. **False**. Trimethoprim inhibits folate synthesis.
   c. **True**. This prevents entry of the virus into the cell.
   d. **True**. They inhibit the transpeptidase that forms the final cross-links between *N*-acetylmuramic acid and *N*-acetylglucosamine.
   e. **False**. The polyenes act on sterols in the fungal cell membrane.

2. a. **True**. Some infectious diseases are always caused by one or a few species.
   b. **False**. It is antimicrobial resistance that *limits* choice.
   c. **True**. Renally cleared drugs may need to be avoided.
   d. **True**. Some sites such as cerebrospinal fluid or bone are not reached by some drugs (although disease can alter this).
   e. **True**. Some drugs cross the placenta and can affect the fetus. The first trimester is a period when drugs should only be used with particular care for clear reasons.

3. a. **True**. Both to avoid toxic effects and to ensure adequate serum peak and trough concentrations.
   b. **False**. Therapeutic drug monitoring is usually performed by rapid immunoassay.
   c. **False**. It requires pre- and post-dose serum levels.
   d. **False**. Penicillin therapy requires monitoring only very rarely.
   e. **True**. To ensure toxic levels are not reached.

4. a. **True**. The patient is unlikely to benefit from antimicrobial therapy.
   b. **False**. Acute pneumonia requires presumptive therapy with agents chosen based on the symptoms.
   c. **True**. It is most often viral. Streptococcal pharyngitis is treated because although therapy may not alter the course of the primary pharyngeal infection it reduces the risk of serious sequelae such as rheumatic heart disease.
   d. **True**. This is a viral infection.
   e. **True**. This is a viral exanthem and does not respond to therapy.

5. a. and i.
   b. and i.
   c. and ii.
   d. and ii.

Short notes answers

1. Cover the process of inhibiting peptidoglycan cross-linkage. Then describe hydrolysis of the β-lactam ring. Outline categories of β-lactamases and their properties. Remember to mention penicillin-binding proteins and methicillin resistance.
2. Describe disk diffusion tests with and without control. Explain minimum inhibitory and bactericidal concentrations. Mention limitations of both approaches.
3. Remember to cover toxic, allergic and ecological effects. The answer could be broken down into effects on the patient and on the microorganism, and the consequences of each.
4. The role of agriculture in antibiotic resistance is controversial. Outline links with specific examples (e.g. glycopeptide-resistant enterococci) but explain why pinning the blame on industry is difficult.

Viva answers

1. The continued spread of methicillin resistance in *Staphylococcus aureus*, the emergence of vancomycin intermediate susceptibility *S. aureus* and vancomycin-resistant enterococci are all worth a mention, as is multiresistance in Gram-negative bacilli (from ESBLs and aminoglycoside-modifying enzymes). These all reduce therapeutic options in hospital practice. But in global terms, resistant *Mycobacterium tuberculosis*, resistant *Salmonella typhi*, penicillin-resistant *Neisseria gonorrhoeae* and chloroquine-resistant *Plasmodium falciparum* are likely to cause greater problems with antibiotic selection.
2. Minor modifications to the existing range of agents active against cell wall or protein synthesis are unlikely to expand the current therapeutic armamentarium dramatically. There are many unique aspects of bacterial biology worth further attention from pharmaceutical developers, but probably intercellular signalling compounds, programmed cell death inhibitors and stress–starvation response regulators are likely targets. There is a pressing need for agents effective against bacteria in biofilm mode (e.g. in device-associated infections) or those with permeability-mediated broad-spectrum resistance.

5 Prevention and control of infectious diseases

Overview

Our ability to prevent infectious disease antedates the germ theory of disease and the advent of antimicrobial chemotherapy. The introduction of effective therapy for infections with a previously high mortality has reduced the concern to prevent these diseases. However, increasing resistance to antimicrobial agents and the recognition of new pathogens and diseases that do not respond to currently available agents has led to a renewed interest in prevention, the principal methods available and their application in an epidemic setting.

5.1 Prevention and control

Learning objectives

You should:

- understand the difference between control and prevention
- understand the pathogenesis of infectious disease
- know the strategies to prevent infection
- know when to use chemoprophylaxis.

Professional preoccupation with therapeutic intervention has led to ignorance and confusion over the prevention of infectious diseases. Prevention is often regarded as the responsibility of specialists with a particular interest in the field and is looked upon by some physicians as inferior to therapeutic medicine. The discovery and development of antimicrobial agents during the 1940s, 1950s and 1960s led some to predict the imminent elimination of infectious diseases. That prediction has proved

to be little more than wishful thinking. New microbial pathogens have been discovered in recent years, not all of which can be eliminated by currently available agents, human immunodeficiency virus (HIV) being just one notable example (see Ch. 20). The relentless pace with which microbes adapt to new antimicrobial agents continuously erodes the choice of agents available to treat common infections and, in some cases (such as multidrug-resistant tuberculosis or drug-resistant malaria), may make the disease untreatable with conventional therapy. The many limitations of therapeutic intervention have led to a renewed interest in preventive methods. Significant progress has been made in this area as a result of recent developments in epidemiological methods.

Pathogenesis and prevention

The methods used to prevent communicable diseases in the past developed slowly through an empirical trial-and-error process. Today, the design of preventive strategies is based on a more deliberate process that relies on a detailed understanding of the pathogenesis of infection. For practical purposes this process (see Ch. 2) can be divided into three stages.

1. Exposure to infective agent
2. Establishment of clinical disease
3. Secondary dissemination of infective agent.

Preventing exposure

The initial acquisition of microorganisms responsible for infectious disease can be prevented by strategies aimed either at the individual or at the whole community. Community-wide activities are the responsibility of community and public health workers and include removal of the source, interruption of transmission (e.g. insect vector control) and, when neither of these is possible, isolation.

Preventing establishment of disease

If it is impractical or too late to prevent exposure to a microbial pathogen, it may still be possible to start pre-emptive treatment in time to avoid the consequences of infection (e.g. prophylaxis of bacterial endocarditis).

This is really prevention of morbidity and mortality and is better described as disease control.

Preventing the spread of disease

Preventive interventions at the point where the microbial pathogen leaves the body of an infectious patient are unlikely to benefit the index patient but will stop the spread of disease to contacts. The safe disposal of contaminated waste from patients is an important part of isolation practice. Not all infectious diseases are communicable (e.g. many hospital-acquired infections, meningococcal septicaemia), in which case they will not be prevented by blocking secondary spread.

Strategies to prevent infection

Public health measures

Antimicrobial agents have not been the most effective means of combating infections in whole populations. Rather, it has been clean drinking water, reliable sewage disposal and vector control that have had the greatest impact on infectious disease. The widespread application of vaccination programmes has contributed further to the declining incidence of specific infections in most developed counties.

Safe drinking water

Sewage is usually disposed of by discharge into natural water bodies such as rivers and the sea. Separation of sewage and drinking water is probably the single most effective means of preventing enteric infection. Drinking water is usually purified and rendered suitable for human consumption by a combination of filtration and chlorination. There are statutory regulations for drinking water standards in many countries. The provision of a safe potable water supply is a major priority for the rest of the world's population.

Safe food chain

Infections contracted from animals (zoonotic infections) can be prevented at source by avoiding contact with the animal concerned. However, this is not possible for agricultural workers, veterinary surgeons and pet owners, who may be at risk of infection. The rest of the population may be at increased risk of infection if the food supply becomes contaminated. The creation of herds free from diseases such as tuberculosis and brucellosis removes an important source of zoonotic infection, but protection of food between the point of initial production and consumption (the entire food chain) is required to prevent food-borne infection. This means using methods to avoid spoilage during processing and packaging and safe preparation, cooking and storage techniques. There are many methods to preserve food safely, including cold storage, canning, bottling and the use of preservative agents such as salt or sugar. The shift away from consumption of recently prepared fresh foodstuffs to packaged, convenience foods transported from distant places, with few preservatives, presents a range of opportunities for food-borne pathogens. Increased reliance on rapidly prepared foods from 'fast food' outlets may also place the consumer at risk of food-borne infection, because cooking times are often inadequate to successfully destroy gastrointestinal pathogens.

Action against vectors of disease

Many diseases are transmitted by either living or inanimate vectors. Inanimate objects can be cleaned (see below), whereas living vectors present a different kind of target for preventive intervention. Insects play a particularly important role in the transmission of infectious disease in warmer climates. Eradicating an insect vector or preventing contact with the human subject can be effective ways of preventing infection (e.g. mosquito netting and malaria).

Private hygiene

Although public and community health involves the supervision and surveillance of disease prevention strategies in the community, it is ultimately the responsibility of members of that community to make a strategy work. For example, operators of water purification and sewage-treatment works, farmers and catering assistants all help to prevent infection. Effective prevention requires the education of every individual in basic preventive methods, e.g. personal lavatory hygiene, food preparation and storage techniques, and prudent sexual behaviour.

Once an infection has gained access to a community, the preventive approaches described above are no longer adequate. Additional public health measures aim to contain the problem by separation or isolation (sometimes called quarantine). Patients with communicable diseases are often cared for in physical isolation from susceptible, uninfected individuals for the duration of the disease. The term 'isolation' has been replaced by the concept of standard and additional infection control measures. Additional measures differ according to the type of infection risk, while standard precautions are those that apply in all clinical settings. Standard precautions encompass all the hygiene measures that should be a part of the routine care of any patient, e.g. proper hand washes after each contact with a patient. There is little value in continuing additional infection control measures after a patient has ceased to be an infection hazard, or when the infection has already become established in the community.

Vaccination

Harnessing the human immune system to combat infection antedates the germ theory of disease. The use of vaccinia virus (similar to the cause of cowpox) to prevent smallpox became widespread long before pox viruses were discovered and implicated as a cause of human infection. Insights into the pathogenesis of communicable diseases provided by early exponents of the germ theory led to immune-based strategies both to prevent and to treat disease (immunoprophylaxis and immunotherapy, respectively). Many countries have a detailed vaccination schedule listing which vaccinations should be given, when and in what circumstances.

Types of vaccine

Vaccines such as the Sabin polio vaccine use live virus to provoke a protective immune reaction. This is achieved by intentionally exposing the subject to a modified strain of the virus, in this case that has lost its pathogenic capability: a *live*, attenuated vaccine. Other examples are measles virus and the BCG (bacille Calmette Guérin) strain of *Mycobacterium tuberculosis*. Live vaccines are usually very effective immunogens, producing long-lasting protective immunity.

Not all disease-producing microorganisms can be attenuated to a safe, non-pathogenic strain. Some vaccines are produced by killing the microorganism in question. These vaccines (e.g. pertussis, tetanus and diphtheria) are often not as immunogenic and may require several doses given at intervals to produce protective immunity. Further doses may have to be given much later because the protective effect wanes with time. Developments in molecular biology have thrown further light on the specific microbial components responsible for disease. In some cases, it has been possible to use genetic engineering to mass produce microbial components that stimulate protective immunity without causing disease (e.g. hepatitis B vaccine). These are referred to as *subunit vaccines*.

Ideally, immunisation should take place before exposure to the infective agent in order to allow the development of protective immunity. However, some exposures inevitably take place in the absence of effective acquired immunity. Purified antibodies (*immune antiserum*) are available to give to individuals thought to be at high risk of specific diseases following exposure. These include infection with hepatitis B, rabies, tetanus and varicella.

Vaccination programmes

The scheme of vaccination followed in most developed countries includes vaccines against:

- polio
- diphtheria
- pertussis
- tetanus
- rubella.

The following are used in some countries or more selectively:

- mumps
- measles
- hepatitis B
- *Haemophilus influenzae*
- tuberculosis.

There are wide variations in the content and form of vaccination programmes as a result of differences in disease pattern and health-care spending. Generally, vaccines will be used if they can be delivered to the principal at-risk population using available financial and human resources. They should be considered for use if there are good prospects for preventing a significant proportion of the infections that cause death, serious incapacitating illness or have a serious socioeconomic impact.

Chemoprophylaxis

Antimicrobial agents can be used in a preventive sense for chemoprophylaxis. Chemoprophylaxis does not normally deal with infection at source or at the transmission stage but interferes with the invasion of sterile tissues and secondary spread. The agent chosen for prophylaxis should preferably be directed against a single microbial pathogen. Where a variety of species is expected, prophylaxis should be directed against the most common microbial pathogen expected. Ideally, the chosen agent will be active against the expected pathogen, non-toxic and cheap.

The desire to use prophylactic antimicrobial agents routinely in large numbers of patients has led to the development of many different prophylaxis protocols. A particular protocol should only be used in the group of patients for which it was intended and should be based on the results of properly conducted clinical trials. Most regimens have the following features:

- the antimicrobial agent given reaches peak concentration in the relevant tissues during the period of greatest risk, i.e. during the surgical procedure
- the prophylactic regimen is continued for no more than 24 hours after the procedure
- the prophylactic agents are not used for the treatment of subsequent infection or other infections in the same group of patients.

In surgical practice, many regimens involve only a single dose given with the premedication or at the time of induction of anaesthesia. The two principal reasons surgical patients require chemoprophylaxis are:

- a high risk of perioperative microbial spillage because of a procedure involving a heavily contaminated mucosal surface (e.g. colonic surgery)
- insertion of a sterile prosthetic device, which reduces the size of the bacterial inoculum required to establish deep infection (e.g. prosthetic heart valve, hip replacement).

Patients with infection prior to surgery (e.g. a deep abscess or compound fracture) need to start effective antimicrobial chemotherapy before the operation begins. This is not prophylaxis and should not be stopped immediately after the procedure.

5.2 Preventing infection in hospital

Learning objectives

You should:

- be aware of the risk of infection in a hospital setting
- know of strategies to minimise the risk of hospital infection.

Hospitals contain a higher concentration of patients with infection and a high concentration of compromised individuals at risk of infection. Hospital workers, there-

fore, have a particular responsibility to safeguard the immediate environment of their patients from potential microbial hazards.

Hand hygiene

It has long been recognised that the hands of doctors and nurses are very effective vehicles for the transmission of infection between patients in hospital (Fig. 9). Simple hand-hygiene techniques are among the most effective methods for preventing hospital-acquired infection. It is therefore surprising that less than half of all health-care workers wash their hands between patient contact, and that medical staff have been repeatedly shown to have the worst record of all groups of health-care workers.

There are two main types of hand-washing technique: the surgical scrub (involving a systematic cleansing of all surfaces of the wrists and hands with disinfectant for several minutes, prior to drying with a sterile towel and donning sterile gloves) and the standard wash (involving a 10–20 second wash of all hand surfaces with disinfectant, followed by thorough drying). The surgical scrub is performed prior to handling any sterile tissue or equipment; the standard hospital hand wash should be performed before and after any physical contact with the patient or his/her body fluids. A single failure to observe personal hand-washing practice may undo the combined efforts of other staff over many days.

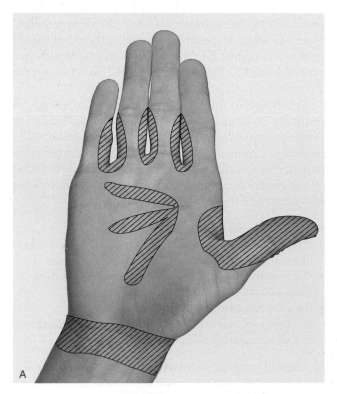
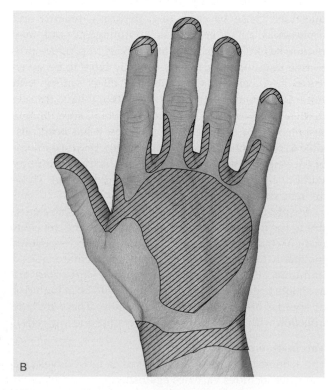

Fig. 9 The palmar (A) and dorsal (B) surfaces of the hand showing areas particularly prone to harbouring microorganisms.

Patient's body surfaces

Transmission of potentially infective material from heavily colonised sites, such as surgical wounds and mucosal surfaces, can be prevented by avoiding physical contact. This can be achieved simply by covering the relevant part (e.g. surgical wound dressing). Higher standards of professional and personal hygiene must be practised by nursing and medical staff caring for an incapacitated patient, because he or she will be unable to maintain an adequate standard of personal hygiene. The patient's faeces and body fluids must be considered to be potentially infective and handled with caution.

Disinfection

Disinfection involves removal of disease-causing microorganisms by chemical or physical means (Table 4). It reduces the possibility of infection by killing microorganisms. The extent of decontamination depends on the duration of exposure of the contaminating organisms to lethal levels of disinfectant (a constant fraction of organisms are killed per unit time, so the fall in numbers is logarithmic).

Chemical disinfectants

In most cases, disinfectants are too toxic to use for systemic antimicrobial chemotherapy. However, they are useful for removing microorganisms from external body surfaces and the inanimate environment . Disinfectants that are not harmful to body surfaces can be used as antiseptics. Although there is a large selection of disinfectants, it is only necessary to know about those in common use.

Chlorhexidine and povidone iodine are commonly used for both hospital hand hygiene (scrub and hand wash) and in preparation of skin incision sites. Chlorhexidine is a diphenyl disinfectant, active against a wide range of microorganisms. Its activity against some bacterial species persists on skin after use. Povidone iodine is an iodophor compound, i.e. it releases active iodine, which is a potent antimicrobial agent. It is more active and probably less allergenic than liquid iodine. Alcohols are often used either alone or with other agents as surface disinfectants. Isopropyl alcohol in aqueous solution is the most effective one in common use. When used for skin disinfection, the surface should be allowed to dry for maximum effect. Aldehyde compounds are effective against all bacteria, fungi, viruses and bacterial spores. They are too toxic to use directly on human tissues but are often used to decontaminate fragile equipment (as glutaraldehyde solution, or formaldehyde vapour). Another important group that is too toxic to use on human tissues is the phenolic disinfectants. These also have broad antimicrobial activity and may be used in hospital wards for contaminated spillages.

Pasteurisation

Heat can be used to disinfect fluids in a process called pasteurisation. This requires heating the fluid to a temperature below 100°C at which vegetative bacteria can be killed. The duration of heating depends on the temperature used: 63°C for 30 minutes, or 71°C for 30 seconds. Pasteurisation is also used to reduce the risk of transmitting infection via cow's milk.

Sterilisation

Sterilisation:

- involves the total removal of all live microorganisms
- is not achieved by most chemical disinfectants.

Provision of sterile surgical equipment is one of the key advances that allows modern surgical practice. Most hospitals with an acute surgical service have their own department specialising in sterilisation and packing of operating theatre and other surgical equipment; this is called the Central or Theatre Sterile Supply Department (CSSD/TSSD). Amongst the most common processes used to achieve sterility are heat-based methods that denature microbial proteins. Dry heat is relatively ineffective unless very high temperatures are reached for prolonged periods. The method is only suitable for glassware and a few other items. Moist heat is the method employed in autoclaves, which use steam under pressure to obtain temperatures higher than 100°C. Steam ensures adequate penetration of a porous load. The reduction of pressure caused by condensation of steam on an inert surface causes a further local influx of steam, which in turn ensures efficient distribution of heat throughout the autoclave load. Autoclave performance is checked by measuring the temperature inside the chamber and by using

Table 4 The uses of common disinfectants

Use	Agent	Type	Cautions
Hand hygiene, body surfaces	Chlorhexidine	Diphenyl	–
	Povidone iodine	Iodophor	Allergy risk
	Isopropyl alcohol	Alcohol	Diathermy hazard
Medical equipment	Glutaraldehyde	Aldehyde	Respiratory irritant
Hospital, clinic environment	Phenol solution	Phenol	Avoid skin contact
	Hypochlorite	Halogen	Corrosive to metal

heat-sensitive tape that undergoes a permanent colour change when the desired temperature has been reached. Much higher temperatures, possibly with repeat sterilisation cycles or prior treatment with sodium hydroxide solution may be required to disinfect reusable operating equipment thought to have been contaminated with the prion agents of human spongiform encephalopathies (e.g. Creutzfeldt–Jakob disease).

Other physical processes used to achieve sterility include ultraviolet and ionising radiation, and filtration with a membrane of sufficiently small pore size.

5.3 Outbreaks and epidemics

Learning objectives

You should:

- know how to recognise an epidemic
- know how to respond to epidemics in hospitals and the community.

Regular, inaccurate use of the terms 'epidemic' and 'outbreak' by health-care professionals has rendered both these words useless as accurate descriptors of infectious disease events in human populations. In order to be precise about a recognised cluster, we now have to refer to clusters occurring in time and space. A suspected outbreak reported in the local newspaper thus more accurately described an apparent time–space cluster. This is a bit of a mouthful but distinguishes a professionally recognised epidemiological event from an outbreak of journalism. An epidemic is said to occur when a given communicable disease is present in a particular group at a higher than normal rate. If the same disease is continuously present with little variation in rate, it is said to be **endemic**. The occurrence of an epidemic implies that the existing preventive measures are inadequate and is often taken to indicate a need for further action. In general, the following approach should be taken:

1. Accurate diagnosis
2. Identification of the microbial cause
3. Confirmation of an epidemic, with preliminary surveillance data: this involves collecting information on the time of onset, personal details of each case and the geographical location
4. Production of a working hypothesis as to the likely cause, source and means of transmission
5. Intervention, aimed to remove the source and interrupt transmission
6. Surveillance, in order to measure the effect of actions taken and to indicate any need to modify those actions.

It is useful to plot the frequency histogram of cases against time. This should reveal an 'epidemic curve' and may also provide clues as to the incubation period for the infection (if not already known) and the presence of secondary spread (sometimes referred to as 'propagation').

Community case cluster

When an epidemic occurs in a community, public health physicians will normally coordinate the response. Any of the control or preventive methods described below might be employed singly or in combination. For instance, measures may be taken against a source in the environment, vector control may be stepped up, cases treated and isolated, members of the surrounding community vaccinated and chemoprophylaxis given to high-risk groups. When the epidemic has been brought under control, underlying factors that contributed to its onset should be addressed. These might include water supply, sewage disposal or overcrowded accommodation.

Arrangements vary from country to country. Generally a key individual liaises with other health-care workers and official bodies (e.g. in Australia, the Director of the Public Health Unit; in the UK, the Consultant for Communicable Disease Control). The same individual is often responsible for surveillance of infectious diseases in the community. They collate and evaluate data from medical practitioners (e.g. cases that are officially 'notifiable diseases') and pass them on for inclusion in regional and international surveillance databases.

Hospital case cluster

If a series of infections cluster in time and space in a hospital setting, a different group of people is involved. This is usually the Infection Control Team. In many countries, this comprises a doctor (usually a medical microbiologist or an infectious disease physician) and a nurse with specialist training in hospital infection control. Their function is to contain and prevent infection in hospital patients. In the USA, infection control is usually practised by a hospital epidemiologist with training in infectious diseases and a team of infection control nurses. Emphasis is placed on continuous surveillance of hospital-acquired, or nosocomial, infections.

The inaccurate use of the terms 'outbreak' and 'epidemic' by the popular media to dramatise events may add confusion to an already demanding situation. There is often intense media interest in hospital outbreaks. The appointment of a properly briefed spokesperson with experience of handling the media is an important aspect of the overall management of a significant nosocomial infection problem.

Self-assessment: questions

Multiple choice questions

1. The following methods are likely to prevent exposure to infection:
   a. Isolation of index cases
   b. Transfer of passive immunity
   c. Eradication of source
   d. Vector control
   e. Chemoprophylaxis

2. The following are preventive means of combating infection (which has had the greatest impact?):
   a. Chemoprophylaxis
   b. Mass vaccination
   c. Antimicrobial chemotherapy
   d. Purification of drinking water
   e. Pasteurisation of milk

3. Match up the disease with the category of vaccine used to prevent it:
   a. Measles   i. Live attenuated
   b. Hepatitis B   ii. Killed whole cell
   c. Polio   iii. Subunit
   d. Tuberculosis

4. Surgical chemoprophylaxis should:
   a. Cover all possible infective agents
   b. Deliver peak antibiotic levels during the operation
   c. Continue for at least 24 hours after the end of the operation
   d. Employ drugs used in the treatment of postoperative septicaemia
   e. Be used when a patient has a known infection at the time of operation.

5. The following antiseptics can be used to disinfect skin surfaces:
   a. Phenol
   b. Chlorhexidine
   c. Glutaraldehyde
   d. Povidone iodine
   e. Aqueous isopropyl alcohol

Short notes questions

Write notes on the following:

1. The point at which food may become contaminated by disease-causing microorganisms and the methods used to prevent this from happening
2. What is meant by 'isolation' in the context of infectious diseases
3. Physical methods of decontamination used in clinical practice, how they work and what are their principal applications
4. Disinfection of surgical equipment in the light of variant Creutzfeldt–Jakob disease (vCJD)

Viva questions

1. What has been the single most effective measure to prevent infection?
2. If you suspected there was an outbreak of staphylococcal wound infection in your hospital, what would you do?

Self-assessment: answers

Multiple choice answers

1. a. **True**. This does not help the index patients but does help to contain the disease.
   b. **False**. Passive immunity is achieved by giving immunoglobulin and is mainly used for postexposure immunoprophylaxis.
   c. **True**. This is particularly important for water contamination.
   d. **True**. Insect vectors are major problems in many countries.
   e. **False**. It provides temporary protection against antigens that have gained entry to human tissues. Chemoprophylaxis also prevents the establishment of infection but is not useful in prevention of initial exposure.

2. a. **True**. However, it should be used only in specific situations.
   b. **True**. This produces 'herd' immunity and reduces the infective sources in a community.
   c. **False**. Chemotherapy is by definition *not* a means of prevention.
   d. **True**. Vector control has the greatest impact.
   e. **True**. It kills bacteria such as those of tuberculosis and typhoid.

3. a. and i.
   b. and iii.
   c. and i.
   d. and i.

4. a. **False**. Only the most likely pathogens should be the target of a prophylactic regimen.
   b. **True**.
   c. **False**. There is evidence to show that continuing prophylaxis for more than a few hours after the end of the operation does not increase the preventive effect.
   d. **False**. The therapeutic agents chosen to treat serious postoperative infections such as septicaemia should *not* include those incorporated in prophylactic regimens.
   e. **False**. Established infection at the time of operation requires full, appropriate chemotherapy. It is often better to delay the operation if possible until the infection has been effectively treated.

5. a. **False**. Phenol is too toxic to use for skin disinfection but is used for decontamination of inanimate surfaces in hospital.

   b. **True**. It is used for both hand hygiene and preparation of skin incision sites.
   c. **False**. Glutaraldehyde is too toxic to use for skin disinfection but is used for decontamination of inanimate surfaces in hospital.
   d. **True**. See b.
   e. **True**. The skin should be allowed to dry for maximum effect.

Short notes answers

1. The answer should reveal an understanding of the sequence of food production from raw material to the point of consumption. A systematic approach, perhaps illustrated with a flow diagram, would help to avoid omission of major preventive methods.
2. Explain in terms of interrupting transmission. Describe different types of isolation, what they aim to achieve and how they might be applied in clinical practice.
3. Could be answered succinctly in tabular form. Dry heat, moist heat (autoclaving, pasteurisation), ultraviolet and gamma radiation, and filtration should all be mentioned.
4. vCJD requires additional measures. Equipment used for neurosurgical and other high-risk procedures in patients with CJD will need to be destroyed. Other measures include careful cleaning of instruments after use, before autoclaving at a higher than usual temperature, equipment tracking, and more careful preoperative patient screening.

Viva answers

1. In the general community, the provision of a clean potable water supply separated from human sewage. Vaccination and improvements in general nutrition have also made a significant contribution. Specific medical interventions have been disappointing in their own right in terms of their impact on the health of populations. In hospital practice, a high level of hand hygiene is probably the single most important and effective preventive measure. Sterilisation of operating theatre equipment and the widespread use of disinfectants and antiseptics have also had widespread preventive benefit.
2. Define the problem with as much information as is already available. Descriptive epidemiology: infected patient time, location, procedure, surgical

team, etc. Bacteriology: detailed identification, antibiotic susceptibility patterns. Develop a working hypothesis with infection control team, introduce preliminary interventions and organise molecular typing. These case clusters often turn out to be pseudo-outbreaks caused by ascertainment bias. Bacterial typing will help you to discriminate between unrelated bacterial strains of the same species. Finally, introduce definitive control methods and educational support for the clinical unit.

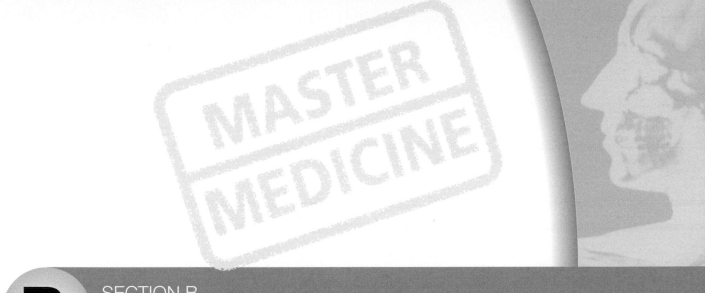

6 Infections of the skin and soft tissues

Overview

The skin is the principal barrier between human tissues and the external environment. Penetration of that barrier by microorganisms may lead to infection of the skin and underlying soft tissues. This results in a variety of diseases whose features depend on the microbial species, the tissue response and the location. Although the skin may show signs of infection at distant sites, this chapter will only deal with primary infections of the skin and soft tissues.

6.1 Pathogenesis

Learning objectives

You should:

- understand the role of the skin as a physical barrier to infection
- know what factors make skin vulnerable to infection.

The growth of microorganisms on normal skin is restricted by a combination of factors, including dryness, high salt concentration, the inhibitory effect of the pre-existing microbial flora and shedding of skin squames. Microbial penetration of the skin is prevented under normal conditions by the integrity of the epidermis, particularly the stratum corneum. It is probable that skin and soft tissue infections cannot take place without a break in the epidermis, even if only on a microscopic scale. The risk of infection is also raised by the presence of moisture (as in hot, humid climates), by a foreign body or by necrotic tissue.

6.2 Diagnosis

Learning objectives

You should:

- know the signs and symptoms of skin and soft tissue infections
- know what investigations can be used.

Clinical features

The superficial location of skin and soft tissue infections leads to early detection of clinical signs, which include redness, swelling and an inflammatory exudate. Other features such as scaling, desquamation and blister formation may be specific to particular infections. Recognition of these features may narrow the range of microorganisms being sought. Lesions can also be described by their location, number, rate of change or associated systemic features such as fever, tachycardia or shock.

Laboratory tests

The most common type of specimen collected from patients with this type of infection is inflammatory exudate. Exudate sent to the laboratory on a dry, cotton-tipped swab is less satisfactory than material collected into a transport container designed to support continued survival of fastidious bacterial species. Lesions thought to be bacterial in origin, without exudate or broken skin, require needle aspiration of tissue fluid. The needle used for this purpose should be regarded as a potential infection hazard for health-care workers. 'Pus swabs' are also unsuitable for detection of superficial fungal infections. Fungal infection is best diagnosed by sending skin scrapings or nail clippings to the laboratory in purpose-made paper containers. Blood cultures should be obtained from the patients with fever or other features of systemic infection.

A microscopic examination of Gram-stained inflammatory exudate should be requested. In bacterial infection, this should confirm the presence of inflammatory cells and may provide early information on the bacterial pathogens involved. The specimen will be cultured on selective and non-selective media, which are incubated overnight. If anaerobic infection is a possibility, the cultures will be incubated in either an anaerobic gas jar or an anaerobic cabinet. Early culture results, with preliminary identification based on simple bench-top tests, should be available after 18–24 hours, but less common bacterial pathogens and anaerobic species may take at least 48 hours to grow. Definitive identification and antibiotic-susceptibility testing often takes a further 24 hours. Specimens that are difficult to repeat may have to be incubated in enrichment medium, e.g. cooked meat anaerobic broth. The laboratory may release important preliminary results if further work has yet to be done before the final report can be issued.

Specimens for fungal diagnosis may provide clinically useful information quickly after microscopy. Potassium hydroxide is used to digest skin squames, hair or nail material and leave fungal hyphae intact. The initial, presumptive laboratory diagnosis can then be confirmed by culture using specialised mycological media. Specimens of tissue fluid from skin lesions are occasionally sent for electron microscopy, viral culture or immunofluorescence when a viral pathogen is suspected. Electron microscopy is not available in smaller hospitals but can yield a same-day diagnosis in specific conditions.

6.3 Management

Learning objectives

You should:

- know the principles governing choice of chemotherapy
- be aware of techniques that help to prevent skin and soft tissue infections.

Chemotherapy

The range of agents available for antimicrobial chemotherapy of soft tissue infections is considerable. Choice of agent will, therefore, depend on clinical and laboratory diagnosis. Some superficial infections (e.g. furuncles) do not usually require antimicrobial therapy and therapy should be avoided to prevent selection of

antibiotic resistance. When infection occurs in deeper soft tissues, antimicrobial agents are usually required. Since *Staphylococcus aureus* is particularly common, an antistaphylococcal antibiotic is often used as part of presumptive therapy. Deep, penetrating wounds, and those with necrotic or foreign material present, are potential sites for infection with anaerobic bacteria and require an appropriate anti-anaerobic agent. Presumptive antibiotic therapy may have to be modified when the results of laboratory investigations are returned because of the wide range of potential pathogens and the prevalence of resistance to commonly used antibiotics. However, not all microbial species isolated from soft tissues are necessarily the cause of infection, particularly when a body surface was sampled.

Prevention

Some soft tissue infections can be prevented, especially those involving superficial sites. Simple wound toilet with antiseptic and maintenance of a clean dry surface (with a dressing if necessary) helps to prevent infection while the wound is vulnerable. A number of strategies employed during surgical procedures rely on the same principles to prevent surgical wound infection (Ch. 17). Anaerobic bacterial infection following traumatic soft tissue injury can in part be prevented by removal of devitalised tissues and foreign material. Tetanus prophylaxis should also be given, depending on past history of immunisation (see below).

6.4 Diseases and syndromes

Learning objectives

You should:

- know the major infections of the skin and underlying soft tissues
- know the factors contributing to their occurrence
- know the basis of their clinical management.

Infectious diseases primarily affecting the skin and soft tissues (Fig. 10) can be grouped as:

- superficial, spreading
- localised to skin appendages
- primarily in deeper soft tissues
- associated with occupational, environmental or geographical exposure.

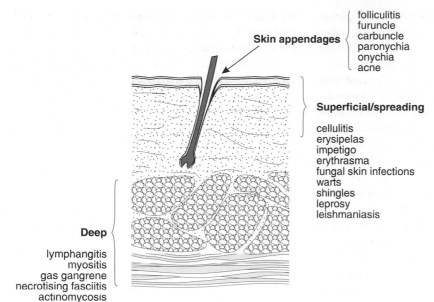

Skin appendages
- folliculitis
- furuncle
- carbuncle
- paronychia
- onychia
- acne

Superficial/spreading

cellulitis
erysipelas
impetigo
erythrasma
fungal skin infections
warts
shingles
leprosy
leishmaniasis

Deep
lymphangitis
myositis
gas gangrene
necrotising fasciitis
actinomycosis

Fig. 10 Skin and soft tissue infections.

Spreading, superficial infections

These conditions (Table 5) are usually caused by bacteria or fungi.

Cellulitis

Cellulitis may occur as a complication of wounds, skin disease, ulcers or burns. The bacteria that cause the infection gain access via breaks in the keratinised epidermis. The features of cellulitis are:

- redness
- swelling
- exudate.

The edge of the lesion is usually gradual, in distinction to erysipelas (see below). Regional lymph nodes may be enlarged or there may be signs of systemic infection, such as fever and tachycardia.

The most common type of specimen sent for laboratory investigation is the 'pus swab', but needle aspiration of tissue fluid from the advancing edge of the lesion is better, when available.

Choice of presumptive antibiotic therapy may be helped by Gram stain results. The most common bacterial cause of cellulitis is *S. aureus*. In unvaccinated children in the preschool age group, cellulitis may be caused by *Haemophilus influenzae*. Presumptive treatment of cellulitis in adults should be a penicillinase-resistant antibiotic such as flucloxacillin; in children treatment should include ampicillin or an alternative agent effective against *Haemophilus* spp.

Wound infection

Cellulitis often complicates wounds caused by trauma, surgery or following bites. Bacteria enter normally sterile tissues at the time of penetration or after a short delay. The presence of dead tissue, haematoma or a foreign

Table 5 Superficial spreading skin infections

Infection	Features
Bacterial	
Cellulitis: wound infection, infected burns, infected ulcers	Acute, spreading infection of the skin and subcutaneous tissues
Erysipelas	Infection of skin with *Streptococcus pyogenes*; may involve the lymphatics
Impetigo	Acute infection of the superficial epidermis that occurs mainly in children
Erythrasma	Itchy lesion that appears as a reddish-brown patch, usually in the groins or armpits/axillae
Fungal	
Ringworm/tinea	Inflamed patches with a quieter centre
Cutaneous candidiasis	Bright red lesions with small satellite pustules; white patches in the mouth
Pityriasis (tinea versicolor)	Fine macular–papular lesions giving skin a rough appearance
Viral	
Warts	Firm horny papules
Shingles	Painful vesiculating lesions distributed over one or more dermatomes

body, such as dirt or suture material, reduces the inoculum required to initiate infection. *S. aureus* remains the most common bacterial pathogen, but anaerobic bacteria may infect deep penetrating wounds or wounds contaminated by earth. *Streptococcus pyogenes* is also isolated occasionally. *Pasteurella multocida* infection frequently complicates injuries resulting from dog or cat bites and is susceptible to penicillin. Wounds sustained after contact with human teeth (bite or 'knuckle sandwich') carry a high risk of infection with anaerobic and other bacteria from the oral flora.

These infections can be very difficult to treat and require careful surgical and antibiotic management, even when the wound appears trivial.

Infected burns

Burns are a form of trauma that leave the skin at increased risk of infection, particularly with *S. aureus* and *Pseudomonas aeruginosa*. Exudate from the burn surface also provides a suitable environment for microbial growth. Infection is responsible for around 50% of the mortality following burns and is a major concern in any burns unit. The eschar is prone to bacterial colonisation. The signs of infection include the eschar turning green or separating rapidly. Manipulation of the burn increases the risk of bacteraemia and systemic infection.

Culture of material from the burn surface is of limited value. However, a rising bacterial count in sequential quantitative cultures of burn biopsy indicates a poor prognosis.

Parenteral antibiotics do not penetrate the eschar effectively and are therefore reserved for treatment of systemic infection in these patients. Topical agents are used extensively in burn units to delay the onset of burn colonisation (e.g. silver nitrate or mefanide acetate). Treatment may also require surgical deroofing of the burn.

Infected ulcers

Decubitus and varicose ulcers provide a breach in the skin and a moist surface prone to colonisation by the indigenous microbial flora of the skin and lower gastrointestinal tract. This may in turn cause cellulitis, septic thrombophlebitis and subsequent bacteraemia. The usual species implicated include staphylococci, streptococci, Enterobacteriaceae, *Ps. aeruginosa* and anaerobic bacteria.

Specimens of exudate from this type of lesion usually contain a mixture of colonising bacteria.

Antibiotic therapy should be used only in patients with evidence of spreading or systemic infection. Otherwise, topical antiseptic agents should be used.

Erysipelas

Erysipelas can be distinguished from cellulitis by its appearance. The area of redness is usually on the face or legs in areas of prior ulceration, abrasion or lymphatic damage. The lesion has a distinct raised edge caused by obstructed dermal lymphatics. Fever is common and septicaemia occurs in around 5% of patients.

Laboratory confirmation of the diagnosis is difficult, but needle aspiration of tissue fluid followed by culture may confirm the diagnosis. The condition is caused by *S. pyogenes* (group A streptococci).

Treatment is best with an oral penicillin, unless the patient has a fever, in which case intravenous benzylpenicillin should be used.

Impetigo

The lesions of impetigo are painless, progressing from confluent vesicles and pustules to dried out yellow crusts. Impetigo occurs more commonly in hot, humid weather and poor, crowded housing conditions.

The bacterial cause of infection can be confirmed by culturing exudate from under the crusts. Specimens taken by swabbing the crusts are not representative. The most common cause is *S. pyogenes* (group A streptococci), but *S. aureus* may be a secondary invader.

Treatment is best with oral or intramuscular penicillin. Topical antibiotics are less effective.

Bullous impetigo

Bullous impetigo is a similar condition, where the vesicles form large blisters (bullae) that burst to leave a moist, red surface with thin crusts. Fever is uncommon. Bullous impetigo occurs mainly in newborns and infants. It is caused by *S. aureus*.

Treatment is with a penicillinase-resistant antibiotic such as flucloxacillin.

Staphylococcal scalded skin syndrome

Staphylococcal scalded skin syndrome is a similar condition caused by particular strains of *S. aureus*, it affects older preschool children. Fever is more common and there is a rash similar to scarlatina.

Erythrasma

The lesion in erythrasma has a clearly defined edge that is not raised. It is caused by *Corynebacterium minutissimum* and should be distinguished from tinea versicolor. This can be done by clinical examination under ultraviolet light. Erythrasma fluoresces coral pink. Treatment is with erythromycin.

Fungal skin infections

Fungal and bacterial skin infections can be distinguished by clinical examination and simple laboratory investigations. To diagnose a fungal infection, specimens should be collected by scraping the edge of the lesion gently with a special round-bladed knife. Scrapings should be placed in a black paper container and sent to the laboratory for microscopy. Microscopic preparation involves digestion of the keratin in the specimen with potassium hydroxide solution to expose any fungal bodies present. Identification to genus and species level requires fungal culture, which takes longer than bacterial culture. Fungal skin infections include ringworm/tinea, cutaneous candidiasis and pityriasis.

Ringworm/tinea

The ringworm/tinea group of conditions are caused by dermatophytic fungi. Ringworm is so-named because it was once erroneously thought to be caused by the presence of worms in the skin. Lesions take the form of an inflamed patch with a raised edge and a quieter centre (hence the 'ring'). The various types of ringworm are named after the body region where they appear rather than the species of fungus:

- tinea capitis: scalp
- tinea corporis: body
- tinea cruris: groin
- tinea pedis: feet (athlete's foot).

Extensive dermatophyte infections that do not respond to conventional treatment regimens occur in patients with the acquired immunodeficiency syndrome (AIDS) or AIDS-related syndrome.

Diagnosis is by skin scraping and fungal culture. The species isolated does not correspond to the location of the lesion and there are also geographical variations in species isolated. Generally, they belong to the following genera: *Trichophyton*, *Microsporon* and *Epidermophyton*.

Milder dermatophyte infections may be self-limiting or can be treatable with a topical antifungal. When oral treatment is required, the imidazoles (e.g. miconazole) or griseofulvin may be employed. Topical agents containing steroids should be avoided.

Cutaneous candidiasis

The yeasts, particularly *Candida albicans*, cause a variety of superficial infections of moist epidermal surfaces. These infections are associated with moist surfaces subject to regular friction: most commonly the submammary folds in obese women and the groins and buttocks of babies (napkin dermatitis). In both cases, satellite lesions can be observed at a distance from the primary lesion.

Laboratory confirmation of the diagnosis is by microscopy of a saline-mounted preparation of exudate and fungal culture on Sabouraud's medium.

Treatment is with an imidazole (e.g. miconazole) or oral nystatin. Drying may help the affected area of skin recover more quickly.

Pityriasis (tinea versicolor)

Pityriasis is also known as tinea versicolor and results in extensive areas of fine, macular–papular lesions, which give the skin a rough texture. In light skins, it prevents the development of suntan, while in dark skins it may cause depigmentation. The condition is caused by an organism with several names, *Malassezia furfur*, *Pityriasis orbiculare* or *Pityriasis ovale* (one species), which has also been implicated in the development of dandruff.

Diagnosis is mainly clinical, supplemented by microscopy of a potassium hydroxide preparation.

Treatment is with selenium sulphide or Whitfield's ointment.

Viral skin infections

Warts

Warts are caused by an infection with the human papillomavirus, a small DNA virus that results in epithelial overgrowth after a period of latent viral infection of cells in the basal layer of the epidermis. Initial penetration by the virus probably occurs via mucous membranes or areas of minor skin trauma. Warts are self-limiting and do not require specific treatment in individuals with a normal cellular immune system. However, the infection may be much more extensive in patients with AIDS because of the patient's compromised cellular immune response. Infection at the squamocolumnar junction of the uterine cervix may result in the development of cervical dysplasia and, in a very small percentage of cases, cervical carcinoma. Viral transmission during intimate sexual contact can be prevented by avoiding intercourse with partners who have genital warts and (to some extent) by using contraceptives.

Shingles

Shingles usually occurs on the thorax or abdomen and occasionally occurs on the face or other parts of the body. It is caused by reactivation of varicella-zoster virus, a member of the herpes group of viruses, which can lie dormant in sensory ganglia following primary infection (chickenpox). Reactivation triggers are poorly understood but correspond to physiological stress, e.g. pneumococcal pneumonia. The condition is usually self-limiting and does not respond very well to any form of antiviral therapy. Symptomatic relief is difficult because the pain is neural in origin. Severe forms of shingles that may be very long-lasting are seen in patients with AIDS. The lesions should be covered to prevent dissemination of viral particles. Chickenpox can be contracted following contact with shingles, but shingles is not contracted directly as a result of contact with chickenpox.

Infections of the skin appendages

The various appendages of the skin can act as points of entry for infective agents and therefore as foci for infection. The hair, nails and sebaceous glands, in particular, are recognised as the location of a number of common infections (Table 6).

Folliculitis

Folliculitis is usually caused by *S. aureus* and occurs in areas of hairy skin, particularly in men in the beard area. Multiple papules form with pustules corresponding to hair follicles.

A variant of the condition—hot tub folliculitis—occurs after immersion in warm water contaminated with high counts of *Ps. aeruginosa*. This source is suggested by the distribution, e.g. the lesions are restricted to the area not covered by the patient's swimming costume. Folliculitis is usually self-limiting, but individual lesions may progress to become deep inflammatory nodules, known as **boils**.

Furuncle (boil)

Furuncles normally begin with a nidus of infection around a hair follicle caused by *S. aureus*. Furuncles tend to occur in areas of hairy skin subject to heavy perspiration or friction.

The condition is self-limiting and does not require antibiotic treatment, but local application of moist heat may encourage drainage of pus and more rapid resolution. Recurrent episodes of boil formation occur in some individuals. The risk of recurrence can be reduced by improved skin care and bodily hygiene. If this fails, it may be necessary to resort to dressings and a short course of oral antistaphylococcal antibiotics.

Carbuncle

A carbuncle is a rare but serious complication of boils that tends to occur in diabetics and patients receiving steroid therapy. A carbuncle is a collection of abscesses in the skin that coalesce to form a confluent area with multiple drainage points. It occurs on the nape of the neck, the back and the thighs. *S. aureus* is the most commonly isolated pathogen. Spread to adjacent structures and the systemic circulation may follow.

The condition is managed by combination of moist heat (to encourage drainage to the surface), antistaphylococcal antibiotics and surgical drainage.

Paronychia

Paronychia is usually caused by *Candida* spp. Diagnosis is by microscopy and culture of pus drained from the nailfold. Drainage and drying out of the hand may be sufficient, but occasionally antifungal therapy with an imidazole or nystatin may be required.

Onychia

Onychia is evident when there is distortion and discoloration of the nail substance. It most often affects nails that have already been damaged, commonly the big toenail. Diagnosis is by microscopy and culture of nail clippings. The condition may be difficult to eradicate and requires prolonged antifungal treatment (several months in the case of a big toenail) with griseofulvin or one of the newer antifungals.

Acne

Increased production of secretions by the sebaceous glands occurring at puberty results in blockage of some glands, with comedones or 'blackheads'. Infection of the blocked glands results in the formation of vesicles, which may progress to pustules. A Gram-positive, anaerobic rod, *Propionobacterium acnes*, contributes to the process, but its isolation is not required for diagnosis, which is largely clinical.

Mild disease does not require specific treatment, but the rarer severe forms of the condition may benefit from tetracycline or retinoin.

Infections in deeper structures

Infections of deeper structures include a number of life-threatening conditions usually resulting from trauma to soft tissues (Table 7). Tetanus is included with these infections because it is a potentially life-threatening complication of trauma.

Table 6 Infections of the skin appendages

Infection	Features
Folliculitis	Papules from focal infection of hair follicles
Furuncle	Focus of acute pyogenic inflammation in the skin, with the appearance of an angry pustular lump
Carbuncle	Collection of abscesses that coalesce to form a confluent area with multiple drainage points
Paronychia	Nailfold infection that occurs in people whose hands are frequently immersed in water, e.g. barmaids
Onychia	Infection of the nailbed causing distortion/discoloration of the nail
Acne	Vesicles and pustules from infection of sebaceous glands; common in teenagers and young adults

Table 7 Infections in deeper soft tissues

Infection	Features
Lymphangitis	
Acute	Thin red streaks in skin and enlarged regional lymph nodes from infection of peripheral lymphatics
Chronic	Nodules on line of lymphatic vessels; enlargement of area drained by vessels can occur (elephantiasis)
Actinomycosis	Deep suppurative foci with purulent exudate containing yellow flecks and chronic inflammation with sinus tracks
Myositis	Infection of muscle, which feels hard; fever and pain occur
Gas gangrene	Occurs in anaerobic conditions, with pain in muscle and subsequent systemic features of fever, anxiety and pallor; tissues break down with fluid-filled bullae on adjacent skin
Tetanus	Tetanic spasms of muscles following infection of a penetrating soft tissue injury
Necrotising fasciitis	Infection of subcutaneous soft tissues with spread along tissue planes, particularly deep fascia; overlying skin breaks down to form bullae
Anaerobic deep soft tissue infections	Progressive destructive lesions caused by a mix of anaerobic and aerobic bacteria

Lymphangitis

Lymphangitis is an acute or chronic infection of the peripheral lymphatic vessels.

Acute lymphangitis

Acute lymphangitis can be recognised by the combination of thin red streaks in the skin and enlarged regional lymph nodes. A primary wound is often present nearby. The most common bacterial pathogen is *S. pyogenes* (β-haemolytic streptococcus, group A). Systemic spread with septicaemia may follow. The infection may also lead to blockage of the lymphatic vessels and subsequent lymphoedema.

Diagnosis is largely clinical, but blood cultures should be taken if the patient has a fever.

The treatment of choice is intramuscular or intravenous penicillin. Swollen extremities should be elevated to assist drainage of tissue fluid.

Chronic lymphangitis

Chronic lymphangitis is caused by a range of different organisms, including the fungus *Sporothrix schenckii* and the nematodes *Wuchereria bancroftii* and *Brugia malayi*. Sporothrix infection (sporotrichosis) follows minor trauma caused by plants (e.g. rose thorn) and leads to a string of subcutaneous nodules corresponding to the lymphatic vessels. Diagnosis can be confirmed by microscopy of any exudate and by fungal culture. Treatment is with potassium iodide solution or itraconazole. *Wuchereria* and *Brugia* spp. cause obstruction of the vessels, resulting in enlargement of the limbs, breasts or scrotum. These infections occur in parts of Africa and Asia and are transmitted via the bites of certain culicine mosquito species. The massive enlargement seen in untreated, chronic cases is known as elephantiasis. Patients with this condition are prone to recurrent bouts of acute streptococcal lymphangitis that exacerbates lymphatic damage. The parasite responsible for the disease may be identified in its earlier stages by microscopic examination of thin blood smears in which the diagnostic stage, microfilaria, can be seen. The optimal time for specimen collection depends on the species of parasite prevalent in the area.

Treatment is with diethylcarbamazine and is more likely to be effective in the earlier stage of the disease. Prevention is by avoiding contact with mosquitoes and by vector control.

Actinomycosis

Actinomycosis is a deep suppurating infection caused by *Actinomyces* spp. Suppurative foci may form in the cervicofacial region, thorax or abdomen following minor trauma or surgical procedures. There is chronic inflammation, with formation of sinus tracks and a purulent exudate containing yellow flecks ('sulphur granules'). The condition is caused by branching, filamentous Gram-positive bacilli of the actinomyces group; most commonly *Actinomyces israelii*.

Diagnosis is by Gram stain of purulent exudate. Actinomycetes require an anaerobic or microaerophilic environment for growth and so time to isolation may be prolonged.

Treatment is with penicillin.

Women using certain types of intrauterine contraceptive device are prone to pelvic actinomycosis. When actinomycete-like organisms are demonstrated following cervical smear, removal of the device is usually sufficient, but penicillin treatment may be required in a small minority.

Myositis

Myositis is an infection of the muscle bulk most often caused by *S. aureus*. Fever and pain are present. If accessible, the muscle feels hard and 'woody'.

Pus should be drained and sent for microscopy and culture if a focal collection can be identified.

Presumptive antibiotic therapy should include an anti-staphylococcal agent and should be given intravenously.

Gas gangrene (clostridial myonecrosis)

Gas gangrene is an infection that involves the muscles and adjacent soft tissues and is caused by toxin-producing anaerobic bacteria of the genus *Clostridium* (usually *C. perfringens*). Infection occurs in the presence of devitalised or ischaemic muscle, i.e. following penetrating trauma or in peripheral vascular disease. The first clinical feature is often pain in the muscle. The patient becomes anxious, pallid and moderately febrile. Later the skin overlying the affected muscles becomes dusky bronze, forms fluid-filled bullae and breaks down. As the patient deteriorates, shock and renal failure set in.

The serous exudate from blistered or broken skin should be sent for immediate Gram stain. This may reveal chunky Gram-positive bacilli, but spores are usually absent in clinical specimens. The 24–48 hour delay to identification of the organism and demonstration of toxin production (lecithinase, by Nagler method) is too long to be helpful in management of the patient. X-rays of affected tissues may be more helpful since they may demonstrate outlining of muscle compartments by gas resulting from bacterial metabolism.

Management

Prompt management is necessary to avoid loss of life and requires a combination of surgical resection of necrotic tissues, antibiotics (intravenous benzylpenicillin) and hyperbaric oxygen (to improve tissue oxygenation). Even with optimal management, the mortality is high. Some cases of gas gangrene can be prevented by careful wound toilet and debridement of traumatic wounds. Avoiding primary closure of battle injuries has been shown to help to prevent gas gangrene.

Tetanus

Tetanus is a paralytic condition caused by exposure to toxin produced by *Clostridium tetani*. Tetanus is neither a true infection nor a disease primarily involving the skin or soft tissues but is a potentially life-threatening complication of soft tissue trauma. (Tetanus also occurs in neonates in some developing countries where traditional birth attendants smear the umbilical stump with earth or dung.)

Tetanus usually follows penetrating soft tissue injury in agricultural, gardening or road traffic accidents where the wound becomes contaminated with *Clostridium tetani*, a Gram-positive, spore-forming, anaerobic bacillus. *C. tetani* produces a toxin called **tetanospasmin** in the relatively anaerobic conditions at the bottom of a penetrating wound containing dirt or necrotic debris. The toxin is then taken up by motor neurones and blocks the action of presynaptic inhibitory neurotransmitters, including glycine and γ-aminobutyric acid (GABA), causing an exaggerated response to motor stimuli. The patient with tetanus suffers from tetanic spasm of affected muscle groups, including facial and respiratory muscles. Progressive tetany of muscles may lead to respiratory failure and a need for mechanical ventilation. In severe disease, the interval between injury (exposure) and onset is short and the frequency of muscle spasm is high.

The laboratory has little part to play in the diagnosis of tetanus.

Prevention

Although antibiotics (intravenous penicillin) and anti-toxin (human tetanus immunoglobulin, TIg) are given to patients with tetanus, they have little effect on the course of the disease. Treatment is mainly supportive until respiratory function returns to normal. The emphasis is therefore on *tetanus prevention*, which has been achieved in many countries by combining thorough active management of soft tissue trauma (removal of foreign material and devitalised tissue) with immunoprophylaxis. Immunisation is carried out with a formalin-denatured *C. tetani* toxin (toxoid) in three doses, starting several months after birth and ending about 3–6 months later. As immunity is not lifelong, booster doses of toxoid should be given at 10-year intervals. This programme is supplemented by vaccination after an injury as follows:

- clean, minor wound: booster toxoid unless three or more doses in the last 10 years, no immunoglobulin
- other wounds: toxoid booster if two doses or less in the last 10 years or a course more than 10 years ago; immunoglobulin if one dose of toxoid or less or uncertain history.

Necrotising fasciitis

Necrotising fasciitis is an infection of the subcutaneous soft tissues involving the superficial and deep fascia.

It is usually caused by *S. pyogenes* (group A, β-haemolytic streptococci) but may also involve other bacteria. Infection spreads along soft tissue planes, particularly the deep fascia of the lower limbs. The overlying skin breaks down to form bullae, and there may be a foul-smelling exudate. The condition is more frequent in patients with peripheral vascular disease or diabetes mellitus.

Laboratory diagnosis is by microscopy and culture of necrotic material or exudate from the affected area. Blood cultures are often positive.

A combination of ampicillin, gentamicin and metronidazole given intravenously is used for presumptive treatment. Surgical exposure of the affected fascial planes and incision to the fascia is often required.

Anaerobic deep soft tissue infections

There is disagreement over the precise classification of anaerobic deep soft tissue infections: a group of conditions usually caused by a mixture of anaerobic and aerobic bacteria. This combination may act synergistically to cause progressive, destructive lesions.

Specimens should be transported to the laboratory rapidly in an anaerobic container. The laboratory should be warned that a synergistic infection is suspected, otherwise a mixed bacterial growth obtained from cultures may be regarded as insignificant.

Treatment with a single antibiotic agent may be inadequate. A combination of agents, such as ampicillin, gentamicin and metronidazole, should be used, guided by the results of a Gram stain of inflammatory exudate.

Infections associated with occupation, environment or geography

Certain infections only commonly occur under exposure to a specific environment (Table 8). This may be occupational or related to geographical areas: the latter group are less clearly defined with increasing numbers of international travellers.

Leprosy (Hansen's disease)

Leprosy is distributed worldwide, especially in Africa, India and Asia and is caused by *Mycobacterium leprae*. It is probably spread by droplet transmission. A spectrum of disease exists from the common tuberculoid (TT) form to the lepromatous (LL) form. In between, three overlapping intermediate stages, BT, BB and BL, are recognised. The principal clinical features of the two extreme forms are:

TT:

- single or few, asymmetrical nodules
- hypopigmentation
- anaesthesia
- adjacent nerve thickening
- lepromin test positive.

LL:

- symmetrical macules
- papules or plaques
- extensive skin involvement
- enlarged earlobes and facial tissues
- nasal discharge
- lepromin test negative.

Diagnosis is mainly clinical, with confirmation by skin scrape/smear or biopsy, followed by acid-fast stain for mycobacteria.

Management

The mainstay of treatment is dapsone, a long-acting sulphonamide, but increasing resistance requires the addition of rifampicin. All types of leprosy other than TT also require clofazimine. Reactions are common during treatment, but there is disagreement over their classification. They include **erythema nodosum leprosum** (ENL) and a cell-mediated immune reaction. They can be severe and even life threatening. Prevention and control is by a combination of treatment, contact tracing, prevention of droplet spread and general improvements in the standard of living. BCG may provide some protection against leprosy.

Cutaneous anthrax

Anthrax is a zoonotic disease, and cutaneous anthrax follows occupational exposure: usually agricultural

Table 8 Infections associated with specific occupation, environment or geography

Infection	Association	Features
Leprosy	G/E	Mycobacterial infection of skin and adjacent tissues; course and features determined by host response
Cutaneous anthrax	O	Initially an itchy papule that subsequently breaks down to form an ulcer, surrounded by vesicles; eventually a dark eschar forms at the ulcer base
Erysipeloid	O	Lesion looks like erysipelas, a red, raised plaque-like patch of inflamed skin with a definite edge, but is caused by a different bacterial pathogen
Fish tank granuloma	E	Suppurative or granulomatous skin lesion that occurs following minor trauma in fish tanks or swimming pools
Orf	O	Large nodular lesion that forms on the extremities
Cutaneous diphtheria	G/E	Chronic skin ulcer with a dirty grey membranous base
Tropical ulcer	G	Painful chronic skin ulcers
Cutaneous leishmaniasis	G	Persistent ulcers or sores on face or extremities; lesions depend on the species of parasite

O, occupation; E, environment; G, geographical area.

workers or handlers of animal products such as wool, hides and goat hair. The occurrence of cutaneous anthrax in mail handlers in the USA was attributed to a deliberate biohazard release and was part of a larger anthrax incident that caused several deaths from pulmonary anthrax infection. The condition is caused by a spore-forming, Gram-positive bacillus, *Bacillus anthracis*.

Diagnosis is confirmed by microscopy and culture or by nucleic acid amplification.

Treatment is with intravenous benzylpenicillin and prevention is by control of disease in animals. Humans at high risk can be vaccinated.

Erysipeloid

Erysipeloid occurs most often on the hands of butchers and fishery workers. The lesion is painful and there is often pain or stiffness in an adjacent joint. It is caused by *Erysipelothrix rhusiopathiae*, non-spore-forming Gram-positive bacillus.

Diagnosis is by microscopy and culture of tissue fluid from the lesion or biopsy.

Treatment is with penicillin, but the lesion is often self-limiting.

Fish tank granuloma

Fish tank granuloma is a suppurative or granulomatous lesion occurring at a site of trauma. It is caused by *Mycobacterium marinum*, one of the 'atypical' mycobacteria with a lower optimal temperature range and occurs, therefore, in association with swimming pools and fish tanks.

Diagnosis is by acid-fast stain of exudate or curettings from the lesion. Culture for mycobacteria is required to confirm the identity of any acid-fast bacilli seen.

The condition requires treatment with antituberculosis agents, e.g. rifampicin and ethambutol.

Orf

Orf is caused by a poxvirus that infects farm workers during close contact with lambs. Large nodular lesions occur on the extremities. Large, oval poxvirus particles can be seen on electron microscopy.

The condition resolves spontaneously without specific treatment.

Cutaneous diphtheria

Cutaneous diphtheria presents as a chronic skin ulcer with a dirty grey membranous base. It is most common in tropical climates and among the poor and homeless. It is caused by *Corynebacterium diphtheriae*, but *S. aureus* and group A streptococci are often involved as secondary invaders.

These ulcers do not respond to antitoxin therapy but may act as a reservoir for classical diphtheria.

Tropical ulcer

Tropical ulcers are painful, chronic skin ulcer with raised edges that occur in people living in the tropics. They occur mainly on the lower leg. A variety of bacterial species have been implicated, including non-cultivatable spirochaetes, *Borrelia vincenti* and fusiform bacteria. Diagnosis is clinical.

Treatment is with a combination of wet dressings, penicillin and, once clean, a non-adherent paraffin dressing.

Tropical ulcers should be differentiated from Buruli ulcer, which also occurs in the tropics. The latter are necrotising skin ulcers caused by *Mycobacterium ulcerans*, in which many acid-fast bacilli can be found. Treatment of Buruli ulcers is difficult because of resistance to antimycobacterial agents.

Cutaneous leishmaniasis

Cutaneous leishmaniasis is a parasitic infection caused by protozoa of the genus *Leishmania* that are transmitted by the bite of female sandflies. In cutaneous leishmaniasis, lesions depend on the particular organism, the geographical location, the primary reservoir and the host response (cellular immunity). In parts of Africa and the Middle East, the most common form of the disease is a persistent, raised-edged lesion, usually on the face or extremities. Mucocutaneous leishmaniasis (including the aggressive variant 'espundia') is found in South America.

Diagnosis is by demonstration of *Leishmania* sp. in a skin biopsy.

Treatment is with a pentavalent antimonial agent. Prevention, by avoiding contact with sandflies or by control of wild rodent reservoirs, has had limited success. A vaccine containing *Leishmania* sp. from cutaneous lesions is used in some countries.

6.5 Organisms

A checklist of the organisms discussed in this chapter is given in Box 1. Further information is given on the pages indicated.

Box 1 Organisms infecting the skin and soft tissues

Bacteria	see page	Fungi	see page
Staphylococcus aureus	243	*Trichophyton* spp.	269
Streptococcus pyogenes	244	*Microsporum* spp.	269
Pseudomonas aeruginosa	249–50	*Epidermophyton* sp.	269
Clostridium perfringens	247	*Pityrosporum ovale*	270
Clostridium tetani	247	*Candida albicans*	269
Bacillus anthracis	246	*Sporothrix schenckii*	270
Corynebacterium diphtheriae	246–7		
Corynebacterium minutissimum	–	**Viruses**	
Propionibacterium acnes	–	Human papillomavirus	258
Pasteurella multocida	252	Varicella-zoster virus	257
Haemophilus influenzae	251	Orf virus	258
Erysipelothrix rhusiopathiae	246	Poxvirus	258
Actinomyces israelii	247	**Parasites**	
Mycobacterium ulcerans	254	*Leishmania* spp.	265
Mycobacterium marinum	254	*Wuchereria, Brugia* spp.	266
Mycobacterium leprae	253		

Self-assessment: questions

Multiple choice questions

1. The following factors limit bacterial growth on the skin surface:
   a. Moisture
   b. Shedding of skin squames
   c. Salt content
   d. Surface occlusion
   e. Indigenous flora

2. A swab of exudate is suitable for laboratory diagnosis of infections with the following organisms:
   a. *Staphylococcus aureus*
   b. Varicella-zoster virus
   c. *Pityrosporum ovale*
   d. *Clostridium tetani*
   e. *Erysipelothrix rhusiopathiae*

3. Cellulitis:
   a. Is an infection limited to the most superficial layer of skin
   b. Is often caused by *Staphylococcus aureus*
   c. Does not require a prior break in the skin surface
   d. May lead to septicaemia
   e. Is usually characterised by a sharply defined edge

4. Tetanus can be prevented by:
   a. Active immunisation in infancy
   b. Immunisation following trauma
   c. Careful wound toilet
   d. Tetanus immunoglobulin
   e. Parenteral penicillin

5. Impetigo:
   a. Is usually caused by *Staphylococcus aureus*
   b. Is most common in young adults
   c. Can be recognised by the presence of crusting, exudative lesions
   d. Does not involve the dermis
   e. Often results in septicaemia

6. Obligate anaerobic bacteria:
   a. Cause gas gangrene
   b. Cause ecthyma
   c. May cause destructive deep soft tissue infections with aerobic bacteria
   d. May not survive transport to the laboratory
   e. Are unlikely to cause infections of deep, penetrating wounds

7. Pair up the infection with the corresponding risk group:
   a. Cutaneous anthrax   i. Butchers
   b. Erysipeloid   ii. Veterinary surgeons
   c. Buruli ulcer   iii. African subsistence farmers
   d. Orf   iv. Wool sorters

Case history questions

History 1

A 75-year-old woman with a venous stasis ulcer had reddening around the ulcer margin. She complained of severe itching in the region of the ulcer, which was being regularly dressed with an antibiotic-containing dressing. Cultures of exudate from the ulcer surface grew *Enterobacter* sp., which was resistant to gentamicin. The patient was apyrexial.

1. Why might the ulcer be inflamed?
2. What reason can you give for the gentamicin resistance?
3. What topical agent might be used to good effect?

History 2

A 42-year-old butcher complained of a bluish-red patch on his forearm where he had previously sustained a minor graze whilst manhandling pork carcasses in his shop.

1. What is the condition most likely to be?
2. What organism causes it?
3. How would you confirm the diagnosis?

Data interpretation

A young man from southeast Asia developed a depigmented nodular patch on his arm. On examination, the affected skin was anaesthetic and there was palpable thickening of the nearby ulnar nerve. A skin scraping and split skin smear was performed over the lesion. The results were as follows:

- skin scraping: preliminary report showed no fungal elements

- split skin smear: no acid-fast bacilli seen (results of culture for mycobacteria would be reported in a supplementary report).

1. What tropical infection do these features suggest?
2. Does the negative skin smear rule out the diagnosis?
3. What other skin test could confirm the most likely diagnosis?
4. Are culture results likely to help with the diagnosis?
5. How do these results help with your choice of antibiotics?

Objective structured clinical examination (OSCE)

A 73-year-old man who had been febrile for 2 days developed pain over the surface of his right calf. He was known to the vascular surgery service because of his peripheral arterial disease, which was linked to a smoking habit. Examination of the painful calf revealed a dusky blue area with a small central area of skin breakdown, and a much wider area of fluctuation and tenderness. Peripheral pulses were weak in both feet. Radiographs of both lower legs suggested separation of tissue planes in the right leg. An urgent surgical procedure was performed. You are asked the following:

1. Do these features point to a diagnosis of cellulitis of the right calf?
2. Are the wide margin of tenderness and the X-ray changes features of the same pathophysiological process?
3. Can deep vein thrombosis (DVT) be ruled out without further investigation?
4. Would the surgical procedure have both diagnostic and curative value?
5. Should antibiotic therapy include an agent active against group A streptococci?

Short notes questions

Write short notes on the following:

1. The major factors that lead to wound infection
2. Why tetanus should be considered in the context of soft tissue infection
3. The common fungal skin infections
4. Gas gangrene

Viva question

How do soft tissue infections differ in the tropics from those in more temperate regions?

Self-assessment: answers

Multiple choice answers

1. a. **False**. Moisture increases microbial growth on the skin.
   b. **True**. Prevents a build up of bacteria.
   c. **True**. Inhibits the growth of many species.
   d. **False**. Occlusion increases surface moisture.
   e. **True**. Inhibit the growth of invaders.

2. a. **True**.
   b. **False**. Shingles, caused by varicella-zoster virus, is diagnosed clinically.
   c. **False**. An exudate is not a predominant feature of infection with *Pityrosporum* spp.
   d. **False**. The laboratory plays little part in the diagnosis of tetanus, a disease caused by the action of a toxin.
   e. **False**. An exudate is not a predominant feature of infection with *Erysipelothrix* spp.

3. a. **False**. Cellulitis involves the dermis and may extend to adjacent tissues.
   b. **True**. In unvaccinated preschool children, *Haemophilus influenzae* may be involved.
   c. **False**. It requires a break in the keratinised epidermis.
   d. **True**. Infection of regional lymph nodes and systemic spread can occur.
   e. **False**. A sharply defined edge is a characteristic of erysipelas.

4. a. **True**. Boosters are required at 10-year intervals.
   b. **True**. A booster is given.
   c. **True**. This removes the milieu in which *Clostridium tetani* can grow.
   d. **False**. Human tetanus immunoglobulin is given during treatment of tetanus to prevent further toxin binding. It does not have a place in tetanus prophylaxis programmes.
   e. **False**. Penicillin is given during treatment of tetanus to prevent further toxin production. It does not have a place in tetanus prophylaxis programmes.

5. a. **False**. Impetigo is most often caused by *Streptococcus pyogenes*, the group A β-haemolytic streptococcus. *Staphylococcus aureus* is the cause of bullous impetigo and is often a secondary invader in classical impetigo.
   b. **False**. It is most common in children.
   c. **True**.

d. **True**. It affects the superficial epidermis.
   e. **False**.

6. a. **True**. Infection therefore requires an anaerobic environment such as devitalised or ischaemic tissue.
   b. **False**. Ecthyma is caused by streptococci (or *Pseudomonas aeruginosa* in the case of ecthyma gangrenosum).
   c. **True**.
   d. **True**. Management must be commenced rapidly. X-ray to show gas production may be more helpful.
   e. **False**. Penetrating wounds are *more* liable to infection with obligate anaerobic bacteria.

7. a. and iv.
   b. and i.
   c. and iii.
   d. and ii.

Case history answers

History 1

1. Hypersensitivity, cellulitis.
2. Selection of resistance caused by the use of a topical antibiotic.
3. Antiseptic, e.g. povidone iodine.

History 2

1. Erysipeloid.
2. *Erysipelothrix rhusiopathiae*.
3. Aspiration of tissue fluid from lesion, Gram stain and culture for non-spore-forming, Gram-positive bacilli.

Data interpretation answer

1. These are the features of leprosy (Hansen's disease).
2. No. There may be very few acid-fast bacilli in tuberculous leprosy lesions.
3. A lepromin test is often positive in this type of leprosy.
4. No. *Mycobacterium leprae* cannot be cultured in the diagnostic laboratory.
5. These results suggest that the patient has TT leprosy, which is usually treated with dapsone alone. Other types usually require the addition of clofazimine.

OSCE answer

1. No. The clinical features and setting point to necrotising fasciitis rather than a more superficial cellulitis.
2. Yes. Both are consistent with a progressive destruction of deep tissue planes, which undermines the more superficial layers, as seen in necrotising fasciitis.
3. No. Although less likely, DVT should be excluded by ultrasound examination.
4. Yes. Early surgical intervention is indicated in suspected necrotising fasciitis to confirm the diagnosis and to arrest progression of tissue destruction by laying open the lesion and debriding necrotic tissues.
5. Yes. Group A β-haemolytic streptococci (*Streptococcus pyogenes*) are commonly isolated from the lesion or blood cultures from patients with necrotising fasciitis. However, the condition may occur as part of a more generalised group A streptococcal sepsis. High-dose benzylpenicillin is often used, sometimes in combination with clindamycin. However, more broad-spectrum antibiotic cover is required in patients with polymicrobial necrotising fasciitis or infection caused by a single bacterial species other than group A streptococci.

Short notes answers

1. Cover microbial and host factors. Use examples from traumatic, surgical, burn and bite wounds.
2. It is a complication of soft tissue trauma. The life-threatening condition results from a toxin produced by *Clostridium tetani*. Put emphasis on prevention. Describe modern approach to post-trauma tetanus prophylaxis.
3. Cover dermatophyte infections, cutaneous candidiasis and pityriasis.
4. Cover bacteria, pathogenesis, epidemiology, diagnosis, treatment and prevention.

Viva answer

Many soft tissue infections are more common in warm climates because of a combination of heat, insect vectors and hygiene. Some conditions (e.g. tropical ulcer and leprosy) are only found in warm climates. You could pick a representative bacterial, fungal and parasitic infection to illustrate your answer.

Overview

This chapter deals with infections of structures that constitute the upper and lower respiratory tract. The general population commonly experiences upper respiratory tract infections, which are often seen in general practice. Lower respiratory tract infections are less common but are more likely to cause serious illness and death. Diagnosis and specific chemotherapy of respiratory tract infections present a particular challenge to both the clinician and the laboratory staff. Successful preventive strategies are available for several respiratory infections.

7.1 Pathogenesis

Learning objectives

You should:

- understand the mechanisms by which respiratory infections occur
- know how pathogens overcome host defences
- understand what factors increase vulnerability to respiratory infections.

The principal function of the respiratory tract is gas exchange. It is therefore constantly exposed to the gaseous environment, including particulate organic material, such as bacteria, viruses and spores (Ch. 3). Although the entire respiratory tract is constantly exposed to air, the majority of particles are filtered out in the nasal hairs and by inertial impaction with mucus-covered surfaces in the posterior nasopharynx (Fig. 11). The epiglottis, its closure reflex and the cough reflex all reduce the risk of microorganisms reaching the lower respiratory tract. Particles small enough to reach the trachea and bronchi stick to the respiratory mucus lining their walls and are propelled towards the oropharynx by the action of cilia (the 'mucociliary escalator'). Antimicrobial factors present in respiratory secretions further disable inhaled microorganisms. They include lysozyme, lactoferrin and secretory IgA.

Particles in the size range 5–10 µm may penetrate further into the lungs and even reach the alveolar air spaces. Here, alveolar macrophages are available to phagocytose potential pathogens, and if these are overwhelmed neutrophils can be recruited via the inflammatory response. The defences of the respiratory tract are a reflection of its vulnerability to microbial attack. Acquisition of microbial pathogens is

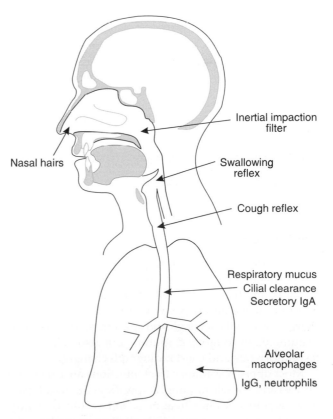

Inertial impaction filter

Nasal hairs

Swallowing reflex

Cough reflex

Respiratory mucus
Cilial clearance
Secretory IgA

Alveolar macrophages
IgG, neutrophils

Fig. 11 Defences of the respiratory tract.

primarily by inhalation, but aspiration and mucosal and haematogenous spread also occur. Individuals with healthy lungs rarely have any bacteria beyond the carina.

Respiratory pathogens have developed a range of strategies to overcome host defences. Influenza virus, for example, has specific surface antigens that adhere to mucosal epithelial cells. The virus also undergoes periodic genetic reassortment resulting in expression of novel adhesins to which the general population has no effective immunity. *Streptococcus pneumoniae* and *Haemophilus influenzae* both produce an enzyme (IgA protease) capable of disabling mucosal IgA. Both these species, other capsulated bacteria and mycobacteria are all resistant to phagocytosis. Penetration of local tissues is usually required before damage occurs, although viruses causing the common cold appear to be an exception. In some lower respiratory tract infections, the host response is the principal cause of damage.

Human behaviour can also increase the risk of respiratory infection. Tobacco smoking has this effect by reducing the efficiency of cilial function and by causing the production of more viscous respiratory secretions. Tracheal intubation for prolonged periods in the critically ill bypasses the upper respiratory tract and provides a conduit for microbial access directly into the lungs.

7.2 Diagnosis

Learning objectives

You should:

- know which features indicate that a specific area of the respiratory tract is infected
- know how to assess respiratory compromise
- know how to identify the pathogen.

Clinical features

The features of different respiratory tract infections largely depend on the structures where inflammation is localised and the extent to which function is altered. So, infection of the nasopharynx will result in a nasal discharge, bronchitis in cough and sputum production, and pneumonia in cough and sputum, but also in increased respiratory rate and chest radiograph changes.

Most upper respiratory tract infections are caused by viruses and are self-limiting. A specific aetiological diagnosis would not alter treatment and would be costly. The role of the physician is limited to reassuring the

patient and recognising the more serious bacterial infections that require specific antimicrobial chemotherapy or more extensive supportive treatment.

Lower respiratory tract infection should always be taken seriously since it is more likely to cause serious morbidity or even death.

Laboratory tests

History, physical examination, X-rays and laboratory investigations focus on two issues: the degree of respiratory compromise and the identity of the causal pathogen. Since a wide range of candidate pathogens may have to be considered, the number of likely candidates should be reduced as far as possible by searching for clues in the history, examination and preliminary results. A history of tobacco consumption, recent travel, occupation, pets, and contacts with similar symptoms should be sought.

Diagnostic specimens can be obtained from the respiratory tract with deceptive ease, but their value is often limited by contamination by the indigenous flora of the oral cavity. To prevent contamination of lower respiratory tract specimens, the upper respiratory tract must be bypassed. Chest X-rays are a fundamental part of evaluation of lower respiratory tract infections and provide evidence of the distribution and extent of disease more reliably than signs elicited by auscultation. Postero-anterior views are most commonly used, but a lateral view can provide valuable additional information.

Blood gas analysis should be performed if there is any suspicion of acute respiratory compromise. The key indicators of disease severity in pneumonia are raised respiratory rate (> 30 beats/min), hypoxia, hypercapnia, bilateral or recently enlarging radiographic opacities, shock, renal failure and confusion.

7.3 Management

Learning objectives

You should:

- know when chemotherapy is indicated
- know how to choose the most suitable drug
- know how to prevent infection and the spread of infections.

Chemotherapy

The antimicrobial therapy of respiratory tract infection depends not only on the likely microbial cause of infection but also on the primary site involved and the severity of disease. The commoner upper respiratory tract infections are rarely life threatening and in many cases are self-limiting. It is therefore possible to manage many of these infections without specific chemotherapy, thereby avoiding all the possible adverse effects. However, even apparently trivial infections such as pharyngitis may require specific antibiotic treatment in some cases. The problem is in knowing who and when to treat with antimicrobial agents.

Lower respiratory infections are less of a problem in this respect, since infection is much more likely to cause significant morbidity and mortality. Antibiotics should be used as early as possible in the course of infection. The problem here is in knowing which of a wide range to choose. It is often necessary to make a 'best guess' or presumptive choice in severely ill patients, based on the most likely microbial agent. The initial choice of chemotherapy may have to be substantially modified in the light of laboratory results. Patients with pneumonia who are ill enough to require hospitalisation usually require parenteral antibiotics. A syndrome-based choice of therapy has become the preferred approach, since antibiotic choice and decisions on the need for hospital admission and active supportive care do not have to wait for a laboratory-based aetiological diagnosis.

Prevention

The ease with which respiratory infections can be spread and their associated morbidity has led to the development of specific preventive approaches. Influenza can be prevented by immunisation with a live attenuated vaccine. The changes in epidemic strains of influenza virus necessitate periodic changes in vaccine composition and revaccination of high-risk groups such as the elderly and patients with cardiac or renal failure. Pneumococcal infection can also be prevented by vaccination. Like influenza, changes in prevailing infective strains (capsular polysaccharide types) require alterations in the composition of the polyvalent vaccine. Again, vaccination is restricted to high-risk groups. Infection with *Mycobacterium tuberculosis* can be prevented by vaccination with a live-attenuated strain (BCG; bacillus Calmette–Guérin), although protection against pulmonary infection may be only partial in some populations. In hospitals, the spread of respiratory infection from known cases of influenza and pneumonia can be prevented by infection control procedures. These are referred to as 'additional precautions' and include nursing the patient in a separate side ward, away from other patients and non-immune staff. Filter-type masks and aprons are also worn by staff and other visitors. At a personal level, covering the mouth when coughing or sneezing is a simple but effective means of preventing the spread of respiratory pathogens.

7.4 Diseases and syndromes

Learning objectives

You should:

- know the major infections of the respiratory tract
- know the factors contributing to their occurrence
- understand the basis of their clinical management.

The main infectious diseases of the respiratory tract are listed in Table 9.

Pharyngitis

Pharyngitis is an inflammation of the throat, resulting in pain on swallowing and swollen, red pharyngeal mucosa. It is most often caused by a respiratory virus (rhinovirus, coronavirus, adenovirus, influenza virus, parainfluenza viruses, respiratory syncytial virus), Epstein–Barr virus or coxsackievirus.

Aetiological clues include:

- conjunctivitis: adenovirus
- constitutional symptoms (lethargy and malaise) and tonsillar exudate: Epstein–Barr virus
- posterior palatal ulcers: coxsackievirus
- abrupt onset, 'doughnut' pharyngeal lesions and beefy uvula: *Streptococcus pyogenes* (group A streptococcus)
- grey pharyngeal pseudomembrane in unvaccinated subject: *Corynebacterium diphtheriae*.

Bacterial pharyngitis
Bacterial pharyngitis is less common and its single most frequent cause is *S. pyogenes*. Other rare bacterial causes include *Neisseria gonorrhoeae, Mycoplasma pneumoniae, C. diphtheriae* and *Arcanobacterium haemolyticum*. Peak incidence is between autumn and spring in temperate climates, and during the rainy season in the tropics. Transmission is more rapid among groups sharing crowded living quarters and is by droplet spread or direct transmission.

Viral pharyngitis
Viral pharyngitis is a self-limiting condition that does not usually require a specific aetiological diagnosis.

Table 9 Infectious diseases of the respiratory tract

Infection	Features
Pharyngitis	Acute inflammation of the throat, resulting in pain on swallowing and swollen, red pharyngeal mucosa
Common cold	Self-limiting rhinitis, causing nasal discharge, nasal obstruction, discomfort and sneezing
Influenza	Acute, usually self-limiting, viral infection with respiratory and systemic features
Otitis media	Acute inflammation of the middle ear
Otitis externa	Inflammation of the external auditory meatus
Acute sinusitis	Inflammation of the maxillary, frontal, ethmoid or sphenoidal sinuses
Laryngitis	Inflammation of the larynx, with hoarseness and loss of voice
Bronchitis	Cough and sputum production; can be acute or chronic
Pneumonia	
Acute, community-acquired	Occurs prior to or immediately after hospital admission; cough, chest signs and fever
Acute, hospital-acquired	Occurs in vulnerable patients in hospital; onset gradual and symptoms unreliable for diagnosis
Chronic	Insiduous onset, prolonged course; usually diagnosed by radiological findings
In AIDS	See Ch. 18
Pulmonary tuberculosis	Coughing and sneezing occur, fever, night sweats, weight loss and coughing blood; chest X-ray demonstrates lung changes
Empyema	Accumulation of purulent fluid in the pleural space
Croup	See Ch. 16
Epiglottis	See Ch. 16
Bronchiolitis	See Ch. 16

Diagnosis

When Epstein–Barr virus infection (**infectious mononucleosis**) is suspected, full blood count, blood film and Paul–Bunnell test for heterophile antibodies should be requested. This is not sensitive in Asians; in this group IgM to viral capsid antigen should be sought. The investigation most frequently requested for pharyngitis is detection of *S. pyogenes*. This species is detected either by culture on blood agar and subsequent latex agglutination reaction for group-specific polysaccharide, or by direct antigen detection. Neither method can distinguish oropharyngeal colonisation from true infection, but only culture allows antibiotic susceptibility testing. Suspicion of infection with *N. gonorrhoea*, *Mycoplasma* spp., *Arcanobacterium* sp. or *Corynebacterium* spp. should be communicated to the laboratory so that specialist, non-routine culture media can be used.

Treatment

An oral penicillin or erythromycin is used to treat streptococcal pharyngitis. Treatment may not alter the course of the primary pharyngeal infection, but it should reduce the risk of major non-infective sequelae such as rheumatic heart disease, poststreptococcal glomerulonephritis and Sydenham's chorea. The need for antibiotic treatment of streptococcal pharyngitis has been questioned in developed countries, since the non-infective sequelae of streptococcal infection are all rare; but the recent increase in streptococcal infection in Europe and North America may change this view.

The other complications of streptococcal pharyngitis include scarlet fever (less common than in the past in developed countries), streptococcal toxic shock syndrome (both caused by toxin) and **quinsy** (paratonsillar abscess). In quinsy, there may be secondary infection with oral anaerobic bacteria, but these are often penicillin sensitive. Drainage of purulent foci is required.

Common cold

The common cold is a frequent occurrence, especially in young children and their parents during the autumn–spring period. The condition is caused mainly by rhinoviruses. The size of the rhinoviral group, and the causal role of other respiratory viruses in a minority of common colds, has prevented the development of an effective vaccine. There is a nasal discharge, nasal obstruction and sneezing. Pharyngitis and cough may be present, but fever and myalgia are both rare features. There is no reason to use antimicrobial agents, and treatment should be restricted to alleviation of symptoms.

Influenza

Epidemic and endemic influenza occurs, caused by influenza virus groups A–C. Some of the features of a common cold may be present, but systemic and respiratory symptoms are more pronounced. Fever, lethargy and myalgia are all common. The influenza virus is an RNA virus with a segmented genome. Two major surface antigens are used in typing epidemic strains: haemagglutinin and neuraminidase. The different types of influenza virus noted in successive epidemics are the result of genetic reassortment which causes an antigenic shift. Minor changes in antigenic makeup occur between epidemics. These are referred to as antigenic drift. Antigenic shift results in influenza epidemics because it renders pre-existing specific immunity to influenza virus antigens obsolete. High mortality rates have been recorded during influenza epidemics as a result of cardio-respiratory failure or secondary bacterial pneumonia (caused by *Staphylococcus aureus* or *S. pneumoniae*).

Diagnosis

Diagnosis is usually clinical, with serology reserved for epidemiological studies and pandemic surveillance.

Treatment

Treatment is aimed at symptomatic relief and at complications if they occur. However, amantidine treatment may be of benefit if commenced early during infection with epidemic type A strains.

New treatments for influenza infection, such as the neuraminidase inhibitor oseltamivir, may reduce the duration of symptoms in a proportion of patients.

A vaccine is available, but it is only effective against previously isolated strains. The vaccine is therefore offered to those at high risk of complications, i.e. the elderly, those with cardiac or respiratory disease, those with renal failure, the inhabitants of residential institutions and those in high-risk occupations (e.g. health care).

Otitis media

Otitis media is an acute inflammation of the middle ear. It is most frequent in the younger child, whose eustachian tube is shorter and more horizontal. It is also more prone to blockage by hypertrophic lymphoid tissue at the proximal end, as a result of prior respiratory tract infection. Purulent fluid accumulates behind a tense, red tympanic membrane and may discharge externally after rupture of the membrane. Infection is most often caused by *S. pneumoniae* or *H. influenzae*. Fever and local pain are common features. Common complications include secretory otitis media and impaired hearing. Much rarer complications are meningitis and mastoiditis.

Diagnosis

Diagnosis is mainly clinical. Auroscopic examination of both tympanic membranes should be performed. Aetiological diagnosis is possible only if purulent exudate from the middle ear is cultured, either following discharge via the eardrum or following tympanocentesis.

Treatment

Antimicrobial treatment is with an antibacterial agent (e.g. oral ampicillin or erythromycin for 7–10 days). Some authorities recommend decongestant therapy as an alternative in uncomplicated acute otitis media.

Otitis externa

Inflammation of the external auditory meatus is most often caused by the hyphae-forming fungus *Aspergillus niger*.

Diagnosis is by culture of fungus from exudate.

Aural toilet and treatment with a topical agent such as aluminium acetate may be sufficient. Topical antibiotic preparations should be avoided. A rare, sometimes life-threatening variant, called malignant otitis externa, occurs in diabetics and is caused by *Pseudomonas aeruginosa*. Therapy with agents effective against *Pseudomonas* spp. should be used.

Acute sinusitis

Infection of the axillary, frontal, ethmoid or sphenoidal sinuses with bacteria from the nasopharynx follows impaired drainage of sinus secretions as a result of a prior upper respiratory tract infection or similar cause. The bacteria most commonly implicated are *S. pneumoniae* and *H. influenzae*. Infection causes the sinus to fill up with mucopus, which alters the resonance of the voice and causes a feeling of local discomfort.

Diagnosis

Diagnosis is mainly from the symptoms, but special radiographic views may show filling of a maxillary sinus. Representative bacteriological specimens are difficult to obtain.

Treatment

Treatment is with decongestants to improve drainage. Surgical procedures may be required in more severe or persistent cases. Some authorities argue that oral antibiotics (e.g. ampicillin or erythromycin) should be used in addition.

Laryngitis

Laryngitis is caused by one of the 'respiratory' viruses and is a self-limiting condition of hoarseness and loss of voice. It may also be a feature of a common cold or influenza. No specific therapy is required.

Bronchitis

There are three related conditions: acute bronchitis (in the strict sense), tracheobronchitis and acute exacerbation of chronic bronchitis.

Acute bronchitis. This condition involves a cough, sputum production (which is usually white to cream in colour) but no radiographic changes on chest X-ray. Infection is with *M. pneumoniae*.

Tracheobronchitis. Here, acute bouts of coughing are not accompanied by significant sputum production. Infection is caused by influenza virus, and features of systemic infection such as fever and myalgia may be present.

Acute exacerbation of chronic bronchitis. A chronic productive cough changes to become productive of larger quantities of newly purulent sputum. This may be the result of infection with one of the respiratory viruses, *S. pneumoniae* or *H. influenzae*.

Diagnosis
In practice, there is considerable overlap between these three conditions. Sputum culture is of limited diagnostic value. Some authorities recommend culture only when there is no response to treatment after 48 hours.

Treatment
Some patients will benefit from a few days' treatment with an antibacterial agent (e.g. oral ampicillin or erythromycin), but many patients will not experience any benefit from therapy.

Patients at risk of cardiac or respiratory failure should be vaccinated against pneumococcal infection and influenza.

Pneumonia: acute, community-acquired

Acute pneumonia has its onset either prior to or immediately after admission to hospital. It is one of the most common infectious causes of death worldwide. Patients with acute pneumonia usually have a cough, chest signs and fever. The cough may or may not be productive of purulent sputum. Chest signs are variable and prone to subjective interpretation. They may indicate areas of consolidation, fluid in the air spaces or even the presence of an effusion or cavity. The most important consequence of acute pneumonia is impairment of respiratory function, which should be assessed as a first priority. The identity of the likely infective agent will determine choice of antimicrobial therapy. A careful history, thorough examination and appropriate chest X-rays should provide some clues to the likely causative agent.

Four main clinico-pathological patterns of acute pneumonia are recognised:

- lobar pneumonia
  —pulmonary consolidation demarcated by border of segment or lobe

  —most often caused by *S. pneumoniae*
  —also caused by *S. aureus*, *S. pyogenes* (group A streptococcus) and *Legionella pneumophila*
- bronchopneumonia
  —patchy consolidation around the larger airways
  —caused by *S. pneumoniae*, *H. influenzae*, *S. aureus* and *L. pneumophila*
- interstitial pneumonia
  —fine areas of interstitial infiltration in lung fields
  —usually no sputum production at presentation
  —caused by *Legionella* sp., *Mycoplasma* spp. or virus
  —initial treatment is with erythromycin
- aspiration pneumonia
  —follows aspiration of oral or gastric contents
  —damage usually caused by chemical or mechanical insult
  —chest X-ray changes either in lower right lobe or, if supine, apex of right lower lobe
  —bacterial damage caused by oral streptococci or anaerobes.

Aetiological clues
The causative organism can be suggested by the type of symptom observed (Table 10).

Diagnosis
The choice of presumptive therapy may be narrowed by sputum Gram stain results. Culture and antibiotic susceptibility results take too long to affect the initial choice of treatment but may be reason for subsequent modification, particularly if the response to initial therapy has been poor. Sputum specimens should be obtained with the minimum of contamination by oral flora. A deep cough sputum specimen collected first thing in the morning is best. This should be preceded by a gargle with sterile water. A physiotherapist may help if the patient has difficulty producing a specimen. A rigid, screw-top container should be used, and the patient instructed how to avoid contamination of its outer surface.

Specimen contamination by the oral flora can be avoided altogether by more invasive methods that

Table 10 Features of pneumonia caused by different bacteria

Organism	Symptoms
Streptococcus pneumoniae	Sudden onset pleuritic pain, fever, rusty sputum, cold sores
Klebsiella pneumoniae	Thick, viscous red sputum, alcoholic patient
Staphylococcus aureus	Pneumonia following influenza
Streptococcus pneumoniae	Pneumonia in the chronic bronchitic
Haemophilus influenzae	Pneumonia in the chronic bronchitic
Mycoplasma pneumoniae	Non-productive cough, pharyngitis in young adult with family contacts; ambulant despite positive chest X-ray
Legionella pneumophila	Non-productive cough, confusion, diarrhoea, middle-aged male, smoker, exposure to air conditioning or hotel shower
Mycobacterium tuberculosis	Upper lobe consolidation, hilar lymphadenopathy, vagrant or alcoholic
Chlamydia psittaci	Close contact with parrot or similar type of bird

bypass the mouth. These include transtracheal aspiration, bronchoscopy with protected specimen collection device and transbronchial or transthoracic biopsy. All these techniques require time, skill and special equipment and may cause unwanted side effects. Blood culture should be performed if the patient has a fever.

Preliminary result based on Gram stain can be provided in minutes after the laboratory receives the specimen. If the smear is full of neutrophil polymorphs and a single type of organism (e.g. Gram-positive diplococcus), the result may make a timely contribution to clinical decision-making. Large quantities of saliva or the presence of buccal epithelial cells in the smear suggest that it is unsuitable for further bacteriological evaluation. It is important to alert the diagnostic laboratory to the possibility of *Mycoplasma*, *Legionella* or *Mycobacterium* spp. because these organisms all require non-routine procedures for detection. Some laboratories offer direct or indirect immunofluorescent detection of *Legionella* and *Chlamydia* spp. Legionella and mycoplasmas can be cultured, but there is a low rate of detection compared with serological methods. However, the delay necessary for a second serum titre makes the information obtained of less use in patient management.

Treatment
Presumptive therapy of acute pneumonia is often chosen on a 'best guess' basis and now follows a syndrome-based approach that does not depend on being able to name the microbial cause of infection before choosing the most suitable antimicrobial agents. It is rarely practical to cover all possible pathogens with a presumptive chemotherapeutic regimen. Agents should be chosen for their action against the most likely pathogens and given by the route and dose that guarantees maximum antimicrobial effect. In practice, this usually means by the intravenous route. Response to presumptive therapy should be monitored carefully. However, the response may not be immediate, and some patients die from acute pneumonia despite optimal antimicrobial therapy. It may, therefore, be difficult to decide whether a particular antibiotic has had the desired effect or not. Radiographic improvement may lag behind clinical response by several days.

Prevention
Pneumococcal pneumonia can be prevented by vaccinating with a polyvalent vaccine to capsular polysaccharides. Protection is only partial because of changes that occur in the relative prevalence of particular pneumococcal capsular types (around 84 at present). Vaccination is, therefore, limited to those at greatest risk: the elderly, those with chest or heart disease, chronic renal failure and prior to splenectomy.

Legionella infection can be prevented by public health measures to reduce the risk of exposure by biociding or heating water sources likely to act as a source of contaminated aerosols, e.g. evaporative condensers and air-conditioning cooling towers.

Pneumonia: acute, hospital-acquired

Pneumonia is the third most common hospital-acquired (nosocomial) infection but the most common one to cause death. It affects smokers, patients with prior chest disease or following operations (especially thoracic and upper abdominal), and ventilated critically ill patients. The last group has the highest relative risk.

Nosocomial pneumonia is most often caused by *P. aeruginosa*, *S. aureus* and the Enterobacteriaceae. Rarely Legionellas or respiratory viruses are implicated. There is a particular association between *S. aureus* pneumonia and traumatic head injury.

The mechanically ventilated patient is prone to colonisation of the lungs by bacteria from the stomach and mouth. These organisms enter the trachea along the outside of the tracheal tube. Occasionally, bacteria from the mechanical ventilator and other respiratory support devices get into the lungs via the lumen of the tracheal tube.

Diagnosis
Onset of nosocomial pneumonia is typically more gradual than community-acquired infection. In the critically ill, the usual signs of pneumonia—purulent sputum, fever, raised leucocyte count and radiographic infiltrates—may each signify the presence of non-infective processes. Clinical diagnosis is therefore unreliable, and bacteriological examination of tracheal secretions will only demonstrate the extension of upper respiratory tract bacterial flora into the trachea. Protected collection techniques (e.g. bronchoalveolar lavage with a protected bronchoscopy catheter) are the preferred method for collection of satisfactory bacteriological specimens in untreated patients.

Management
Antimicrobial chemotherapy must be tailored to the needs and susceptibility patterns of the hospital or unit in question. Regular epidemiological review of laboratory results should be used to plan presumptive therapy. Many patients who develop nosocomial pneumonia are already debilitated and may not respond to optimal antimicrobial therapy. A number of preventive strategies have therefore been developed. As yet, no preventive strategy offers complete protection against nosocomial pneumonia, and antibiotic prophylaxis has been the most disappointing.

Pneumonia: chronic

Chronic pneumonia has a more insidious onset and prolonged course than acute pneumonia. There is no single symptom complex, so the diagnosis is often based on radiological findings. Fever is variable but, where present, may be accompanied by night sweats and shaking attacks (rigors). Features of chronic sepsis such as weight loss and anorexia may also be present. Cough may be productive of purulent sputum, occasionally bloodstained (haemoptysis).

Not all causes of chronic pneumonia are infective. Other causes include neoplasms and connective tissue disease. The most common infective cause is pulmonary tuberculosis. Other infective causes include atypical mycobacteria, other bacteria and fungi.

Diagnosis

A careful history and clinical examination are important. Investigation should include a full workup for acute pneumonia. Sputum examination should be accompanied by a request for acid-fast stain (Ziehl–Neelsen or auramine–phenol), silver stain and cytology. This will help to exclude mycobacteria, fungi and neoplasms. The chronicity of the condition should allow completion of diagnostic tests before commencing specific antimicrobial chemotherapy. Since some conditions may require months of chemotherapy, it is important to do everything possible to obtain a specific diagnosis before committing the patient to a prolonged course of treatment.

Pulmonary tuberculosis

While chronic pneumonia is a common presentation of *M. tuberculosis*, there are several other presentations of pulmonary tuberculosis:

- acute bronchopneumonia
- pulmonary cavitation
- miliary tuberculosis
- primary complex of focal, peripheral lung disease and hilar lymphadenopathy may be noticed as an incidental finding on a chest radiograph.

Pulmonary tuberculosis is common throughout the developing world. In more developed countries, its incidence has fallen over the 20th century until recently, the reversal being caused by a combination of the acquired immunodeficiency syndrome (AIDS) and urban poverty. Primary infection follows airborne transmission from an individual with pulmonary tuberculosis. Given adequate host defences, exposure results in formation of a primary complex. The thick, lipid-containing cell wall of mycobacteria renders the organisms resistant to phagocytosis. The inhaled bacteria are, therefore, walled off by fibrosis to form a granuloma with central caseating necrosis. Immunity is mediated by the cellular immune system. Primary tuberculous pneumonia only occurs if cell-mediated immunity is inadequate to resist the initial infective challenge. Secondary pneumonia may occur following reactivation of the primary focus, often at the left or right apex.

Diagnosis

Fever, night sweats, weight loss and haemoptysis are all clinical features of pulmonary tuberculosis. The radiographic appearance supports one of the clinical presentations listed above. In addition to the routine Gram stain, sputum should also be subjected to acid-fast stain (either Ziehl–Neelsen or auramine–phenol). Three consecutive early morning specimens should be stained in this way. Sputum specimens should be treated as a potential infection hazard, with proper warning given to ward, portering and laboratory staff. The results of acid-fast stain can be provided the same day, but culture, identification and susceptibility results take several weeks because of the slow growth rate of mycobacteria. Patients who produce little or no sputum and children require either bronchoscopy or gastric aspiration to obtain diagnostic specimens. Nucleic acid amplification (polymerase chain reaction) tests can provide a much more rapid confirmation of *M. tuberculosis* infection in sputum smear-positive disease. Rapid, automated analysers have shortened the time to culture-based confirmation and generation of susceptibility testing. However, it may still require several weeks to demonstrate the presence of multidrug-resistant *M. tuberculosis*. Bacterial gene sequencing at the 16S ribosomal locus is widely used to confirm the identity of presumed *M. tuberculosis* isolates.

Treatment

Current treatment regimens employ several antimycobacterial agents to guarantee sufficient antibacterial activity in different cellular and extracellular locations: inside phagocytic cells, in granulomata and in collections of respiratory secretions. Many different regimens have been evaluated. The most effective regimens currently in use employ up to four agents in an intensive induction period of 2–4 weeks, followed by a maintenance period of 5–9 months with fewer agents. Patients are a potential source of secondary infection if acid-fast bacilli are found in sputum at the time of diagnosis. Current treatment regimens should render them noninfectious within days. Poor compliance with recommended maintenance therapy can be the cause of relapse. Commonly used antituberculous agents are rifampicin, isoniazid, ethambutol, pyrazinamide and streptomycin.

Prevention

Prevention is by intradermal inoculation of a live attenuated strain of mycobacterium (BCG) after non-reactivity has been demonstrated by tuberculin skin test. Since the main reservoir of disease in developed countries is adults with untreated pulmonary tuberculosis, secondary spread can be prevented by contact tracing and treatment. In some countries, cattle are a significant additional reservoir. Pasteurisation of milk, meat inspection and establishment of a national tuberculosis-free cattle stock are all important approaches to prevention of zoonotic tuberculosis.

Empyema

Empyema is the accumulation of purulent fluid in the pleural space. It is caused by direct extension from underlying pneumonia, infection resulting from penetrating thoracic trauma or haematogenous spread from a distant focus. Infection may be caused by a variety of bacteria including *S. aureus*, the Enterobacteriaceae, streptococci and obligate anaerobes.

Diagnosis

Pleural effusion and a gas–fluid interface may be evident on chest radiograph (a lateral view is a more sensitive means of detection), and there will also be dullness to percussion over the affected area.

The collection of purulent fluid requires drainage for diagnostic and therapeutic purposes. Anaerobic culture should be requested, preferably by communication with the laboratory prior to undertaking the drainage procedure. A thoracic surgical opinion should be sought early.

Treatment

Presumptive antibiotic therapy depends on the results of Gram stain but should include an agent active against obligate anaerobes, e.g. metronidazole.

7.5 Organisms

A checklist of the organisms discussed in this chapter is given in Box 2. Further information is given on the pages indicated.

Box 2 Organisms that infect the respiratory tract

Bacteria	see page	Fungi	see page
Streptococcus pneumoniae	245	*Aspergillus niger*	269
Staphylococcus aureus	243		
Corynebacterium diphtheriae	246–7	**Viruses**	
Klebsiella pneumoniae	248	Rhinoviruses	260
Pseudomonas aeruginosa	249–50	Coronaviruses	258
Haemophilus influenzae	251	Coxsackieviruses	260
Legionella pneumophila	252	Adenoviruses	257
Mycoplasma pneumoniae	254	Influenza virus	259
Chlamydia spp.	255	Parainfluenza viruses	259
Streptococcus pyogenes	244	Respiratory syncytial virus	259
Mycobacterium tuberculosis	253–4	Epstein–Barr virus	257
Mycobacterium spp.	253–4		
Arcanobacterium haemolyticum	73		

Self-assessment: questions

Multiple choice questions

1. Match the organism with the most appropriate means of subverting host defences:
   a. *Haemophilus influenzae*
   b. Influenza virus
   c. *Mycobacterium tuberculosis*
   d. *Streptococcus pneumoniae*

   i. IgA protease
   ii. Phagocytosis-resistant cell wall
   iii. Adhesion to epithelial receptors

2. Cigarette smoking results in:
   a. Increased mucus viscosity
   b. Impaired cilial action
   c. Reduced particle clearance from airways
   d. Increased risk of Legionella infection
   e. Susceptibility to mycoplasma infection

3. Pharyngitis:
   a. Is usually caused by a virus
   b. Always benefits from antibiotic treatment
   c. Can be caused by bacteria other than *Streptococcus pyogenes*
   d. Of bacterial origin can be distinguished from viral pharyngitis on clinical signs alone
   e. Can lead to glomerulonephritis

4. Non-infective sequelae of streptococcal pharyngitis include:
   a. Scarlet fever
   b. Rheumatic heart disease
   c. Sydenham's chorea
   d. Glomerulonephritis
   e. Quinsy

5. The common cold can be caused by:
   a. Coronavirus
   b. Epstein–Barr virus
   c. *Mycoplasma* sp.
   d. Respiratory syncytial virus
   e. Rhinovirus

6. The following respiratory pathogens are likely to be isolated from sputum specimens without special request:
   a. *Streptococcus pneumoniae*
   b. *Staphylococcus aureus*
   c. *Legionella pneumophila*
   d. *Mycobacterium tuberculosis*
   e. *Klebsiella pneumoniae*

7. Failure of pneumonia to respond to antimicrobial therapy may be because of:
   a. Incorrect diagnosis
   b. Inappropriate choice of antibiotic
   c. Wrong route of administration
   d. Reliance on radiological changes
   e. Host factors

8. Common bacterial causes of nosocomial pneumonia include:
   a. *Staphylococcus aureus*
   b. *Streptococcus pneumoniae*
   c. *Pseudomonas aeruginosa*
   d. *Mycobacterium tuberculosis*
   e. *Klebsiella pneumoniae*

9. Pulmonary tuberculosis may present as:
   a. Bronchopneumonia
   b. Pulmonary cavitation
   c. Chronic pneumonia
   d. Acute lobar pneumonia
   e. Miliary disease

10. The key diagnostic features of chronic pneumonia are:
    a. Cough
    b. Fever
    c. Purulent sputum
    d. Breathlessness
    e. Radiographic changes

Case history questions

History 1

A 3-year-old boy attended the clinic because he was irritable, off his food and had a sore left ear. His GP noticed that he had a moderately inflamed throat and a red, immobile left eardrum. The GP prescribed an oral medication that was not an antibiotic and gave the mother a bacteriology swab to take away. The mother remarked that her 1-year-old daughter also had a sore throat.

1. What condition does the boy have?
2. What did the GP prescribe?
3. What do you think the swab was for?
4. Does the little girl have the same condition?

History 2

A 16-year-old student was admitted to an intensive care unit following a severe head injury in a road traffic accident. Four days after admission, he was still in need of mechanical ventilation and had developed a fever and raised leucocyte count. One of the nurses had noticed that the patient had purulent and slightly bloodstained tracheal secretions and had sent them to the diagnostic laboratory. The Gram stain report said: 'Gram-positive cocci: further identification and sensitivities to follow'. Intravenous flucloxacillin was commenced, and fucidic acid added 2 days later when further results reached the intensive care unit. The patient had a further serious infection with *Pseudomonas aeruginosa* 2 weeks later but survived and eventually left hospital after almost a year.

1. What was the first infection?
2. Why was flucloxacillin chosen?
3. How reliable is tracheal suction as a specimen collection technique?

Data interpretation

Table 11 is the report relating to a 57-year-old male smoker with fever, confusion, diarrhoea and non-productive cough.

1. Given the clinical features in this case, what possible bacterial cause of this infection has not been mentioned on this report?

Table 11 Report for data interpretation

Test	Results		
Bronchoalveolar lavage fluid			
Microscopy	Leucocytes	+++	
	Epithelial cells	+	
	Monocytes	+	
	Gram stain	mixed bacteria	
	Acid-fast stain: no acid-fast bacilli seen		
	Mycobacteria: culture results will be issued on a separate report		
Culture	Mixed bacteria including *Moraxella catarrhalis*, *Pseudomonas aeruginosa* and viridans group streptococci		
Antibiotic susceptibilities of *M. catarrhalis* and *P. aeruginosa*			
Amoxicillin	R		
Augmentin	S		
Doxycycline	S		
Co-trimoxazole	R	S	
Gentamicin	S	S	
Ciprofloxacin	S	S	
Timentin	S	S	

R, resistant; S, sensitive.

2. Does a negative report rule out the possibility of the species mentioned in your answer to 1?
3. What is the explanation for the presence of each of the bacteria mentioned in this report?
4. What other microbiological investigations might help you to establish an aetiological diagnosis in this case?

Objective structured clinical examination (OSCE)

A 48-year-old man with fever and a productive cough was admitted after he became increasingly short of breath. He had a temperature of 38.5°C, a pulse of 120 beats/min and a respiratory rate of 22 breaths/min. Chest examination revealed reduced expansion on the right, dullness to percussion, quiet breath sounds and dullness to percussion in the right midzone and green-coloured sputum. Chest X-ray showed a clearly demarcated opacity occupying the right middle lobe. Blood gases on arterial blood collected while the patient was breathing room air confirmed a hypoxia and respiratory acidosis.

You are asked the following:

1. Does this patient have a lobar pneumonia?
2. Is his pneumonia most likely to be caused by *Streptococcus pneumoniae* infection?
3. Do other bacteria such as *Legionella pneumophila* cause lobar pneumonia?
4. Will bacteriological investigations assist the immediate management of this infection?
5. Should ceftriaxone be used as a first choice of antibiotic in resistant *Streptococcus pneumoniae* infection?

Short notes questions

Write short notes on the following:

1. Why the lungs are usually free from bacterial contamination in healthy individuals
2. Methods you know for obtaining diagnostic microbiology specimens from the lower respiratory tract; describe how to prevent contamination with the oral flora
3. Influenza and its complications
4. The clinical presentation of acute bronchitis and its treatment

Viva questions

1. Are viral upper respiratory tract infections important?
2. What microbiological tests would you use to diagnose an acute, community-acquired

pneumonia? How would the results influence your choice of antibiotic treatment?

3. In acute, community-acquired pneumonia, a specific aetiological diagnosis is now thought to be less important as a guide to immediate clinical management. What key features will determine your immediate course of action?

Self-assessment: answers

Multiple choice answers

1. a. and i.
   b. and iii.
   c. and ii.
   d. and i.

2. a. **True**.
   b. **True**.
   c. **True**.
   d. **True**.
   e. **False**. Mycoplasma infection typically affects young adults.

3. a. **True**. It is usually self-limiting. Suspected Epstein–Barr virus (infectious mononucleosis) should be investigated.
   b. **False**. Antibiotics are ineffective against viral pharyngitis and do not always benefit patients with bacterial pharyngitis.
   c. **True**. *Neisseria gonorrhoeae, Mycoplasma pneumoniae* and *Corynebacterium diphtheriae* are rarer causes.
   d. **False**. Bacterial and viral pharyngitis cannot be reliably distinguished on clinical grounds.
   e. **True**. A potential risk with streptococcal infection.

4. a. **False**. Scarlet fever is a manifestation of infection caused by an erythrogenic strain of *Streptococcus pyogenes*.
   b. **True**. Probably caused by bacterial antigens.
   c. **True**. It is closely linked with rheumatic fever.
   d. **True**. Related to bacterial antigens.
   e. **False**. Quinsy is a paratonsillar abscess.

5. a. **True**.
   b. **False**. Epstein–Barr virus causes infectious mononucleosis (glandular fever) in which pharyngitis may be a feature.
   c. **False**. *Mycoplasma* infection causes pharyngitis, bronchitis and interstitial pneumonia but does not cause the common cold.
   d. **True**.
   e. **True**.

6. a. **True**.
   b. **True**.
   c. **False**. *Legionella pneumophila* requires special culture media, direct immunofluorescence or serological tests.

   d. **False**. *Mycobacterium tuberculosis* usually requires a special request for acid-fast stain and special media.
   e. **True**.

7. a. **True**. Signs and symptoms of pneumonia can be variable and open to interpretation.
   b. **True**. Presumptive therapy is required and as response may not be immediate it is difficult to assess the choice of antibiotic.
   c. **True**. Route should be chosen to give maximum effect; this usually means intravenous.
   d. **True**. Radiological improvement is slow.
   e. **True**. Concomitant illness and a history of smoking or chest infections affect response.

8. a. **True**. Particularly associated with traumatic head injury.
   b. **False**. More typically associated with community-acquired disease.
   c. **True**. A common cause.
   d. **False**. More typically associated with community-acquired disease. Nevertheless, there are growing concerns that multidrug-resistant *M. tuberculosis* can spread within hospitals to affect other patients and staff.
   e. **True**.
   Secondary spread of less-common pathogens does occasionally occur through airborne transmission in hospitals where infection control practice is inadequate.

9. a. **True**.
   b. **True**. Seen on chest radiograph.
   c. **True**. Pulmonary tuberculosis is the most common cause of chronic pneumonia.
   d. **False**. Acute lobar pneumonia is usually caused by *Streptococcus pneumoniae* and bacterial species (not including mycobacteria).
   e. **True**. Lesions resemble millet seeds.

10. a. **False**. Cough may occur but is not diagnostic.
    b. **False**. When present, fever may be accompanied by night sweats and rigors.
    c. **False**. If a cough occurs, it may produce a purulent sputum, occasionally bloodstained.
    d. **False**.
    e. **True**. Chronic pneumonia has no consistent presentation or collection of symptoms Diagnosis is usually based on radiographic appearance.

Case history answers

History 1

1. This patient has acute otitis media.
2. It was initially treated with an oral decongestant.
3. The swab was provided so that the mother could send in a specimen of pus from the affected ear if rupture of the tympanic membrane occurred.
4. The sister probably had the same upper respiratory tract infection that predisposed the boy to secondary otitis media. The mother was advised that her daughter did not require 'prophylactic' antibiotics.

History 2

1. The first infection was a hospital-acquired (nosocomial) pneumonia, and since he was mechanically ventilated, it could also be referred to as a ventilator-associated pneumonia.
2. Flucloxacillin was given because *Staphylococcus aureus* infection was suspected; an organism more common in patients with head injury. (The fusidic acid was added 2 days later when the presence of *S. aureus* was confirmed.)
3. Tracheal aspirates from mechanically ventilated patients are prone to contamination with bacteria from the upper trachea and are, therefore, not representative of the smaller airways. Specialised bronchoscopic techniques are preferred as a means of specimen collection in ventilated patients in intensive care, but these techniques are only available in some centres.

Data interpretation answer

1. *Legionella* spp.
2. No. Neither culture-based methods nor nucleic acid amplification is the most sensitive means of diagnosing Legionnaires' disease. The urinary antigen test is currently the most sensitive means of confirming *L. pneumophila* infection.
3. The bacteria reported here could have been carried on the tip of the bronchoscope after contamination during passage through the oropharynx. *M. catarrhalis* and viridans group streptococci are oropharyngeal commensals. *P. aeruginosa* is a coloniser of the oropharynx in a proportion of hospital patients, the percentage increasing with length of hospital stay, severity of underlying disease and exposure to broad-spectrum antibiotics.
4. Legionnaires' disease can be diagnosed using a combination of serology, culture-based methods, nucleic acid amplification by the polymerase chain reaction and urinary antigen test. Serological tests for other respiratory pathogens should also be performed.

OSCE answer

1. Yes. He has a right middle lobe pneumonia.
2. Yes. This is the most common cause of community-acquired lobar pneumonia.
3. Yes. Other bacterial species including *L. pneumophila* can cause lobar pneumonia.
4. Yes. A sputum Gram stain showing neutrophils and many Gram-positive diplococci will increase the suspicion that this is a *S. pneumoniae* infection. The result should be available within minutes of receiving the sample in the laboratory.
5. No. Moderate penicillin resistance does not result in a significant increase in risk of penicillin treatment failure for *S. pneumoniae* infection unless the patient has meningitis. In this case, ceftriaxone would be a satisfactory choice of agent. But for lobar pneumonia, high-dose intravenous benzylpenicillin remains the treatment of choice.

Short notes answers

1. Review the anatomical, physiological and other defences of the respiratory tract.
2. Start with a list. A tabular answer would be acceptable.
3. Remember to mention pathogenesis, surface antigen variation, epithelial damage and subsequent staphylococcal pneumonia.
4. Three brief paragraphs on acute bronchitis (strict sense), tracheobronchitis and acute exacerbation of chronic bronchitis. If recommending antimicrobial therapy, justify in terms of pathogens and likely outcome.

Viva answers

1. Yes. They are the commonest infective reason for medical consultation and antibiotic prescription. You should mention the common cold and pharyngitis as a minimum. Mention local data on specific viral pathogens, epidemiology, public health issues and complications, if available.
2. Microscopy and culture of respiratory secretions, nucleic acid amplification tests (polymerase chain reaction (PCR)), serology, urinary antigen test for *Legionella pneumophila*. Only a clear-cut Gram or acid-fast stain result and a urinary antigen test can have immediate impact on antibiotic choice. PCR takes longer but will produce a specific result. Culture is even slower and often produces inconclusive results. Serology is rarely helpful in acute management as a rise in antibody titre may not occur until the patient has begun to recover.

3. The severity of respiratory infection is now taken as the main guide to whether the patient (i) needs hospital admission, and (ii) requires intensive respiratory care. Key features used to make these decisions are respiratory rate, blood urea, falling Pao_2 (arterial partial pressure of oxygen), falling blood pressure and involvement of both lungs or multiple lobes on chest radiograph.

8 Infections of the gastrointestinal tract and related organs

Overview

Infections of the gastrointestinal tract are amongst the commonest infective causes of death worldwide and cause a massive additional burden of morbidity, especially in developing countries. Their incidence is determined by standards of sanitation, particularly by the quality of food and water. A wide range of microorganisms can cause intestinal infection. The commoner enteric pathogens often cause a spectrum of clinical syndromes, making the laboratory confirmation of infection all the more difficult. This chapter reviews the commoner infections of the gastrointestinal tract, liver, biliary tract and pancreas.

8.1 Pathogenesis

Learning objectives

You should:

- know the principal means of transmission of infection
- understand the natural defences of the gut
- know how pathogens avoid these defences.

The principal means of transmission of gastrointestinal infections are via food, drink and by hand–mouth contact (the faecal–oral route). The initial encounter with microorganisms comes as a result of ingestion. When organisms enter the stomach they are subject to the antimicrobial effect of gastric acid. Impaired gastric acid production (e.g. gastrectomy, therapy with histamine H_2 receptor antagonists) increases the risk of enteric infection because a smaller inoculum is required for microbial survival when they reach the small intestine.

Enteric pathogens have to compete with increasing numbers of commensal organisms, particularly anaerobic bacteria. Bile and digestive enzymes in the duodenum restrict the growth of most bacterial species. Normal gut motility, peristalsis, further regulates the growth of bacteria at different levels in the intestine. The shedding of the most superficial layer of the intestinal mucosa may also limit the density of commensal species immediately adjacent to the epithelial surface. The presence of an intact indigenous microbial flora provides some resistance to infection, and interference with this commensal flora increases the risk of enteric infection. The small and large intestinal mucosa is also protected by a thin layer of mucus that acts as a lubricant and contains a variety of protective factors including IgA. Mucosal immunity is not fully understood. Humoral immunity at the mucosal surface, tissue macrophages and the gut-associated lymphoid tissue combine to prevent the entry of enteric pathogens into the host tissues and portal circulation.

Microorganisms have developed strategies to satisfy their needs and overcome these defences. Damage is caused by enterotoxin production, local invasion of the intestinal mucosa or more extensive invasion (e.g. via the gut lymphoid tissue). They may produce toxins that alter gastrointestinal physiology in favour of the infecting organism or they may invade host tissues, perhaps even surviving in macrophages. **Cholera toxin** is one of the best understood at a molecular level (Fig. 12). *Vibrio cholerae*, the cause of cholera, produces a peptide toxin that binds to ganglioside on gut mucosal cells. A change in its stereochemistry causes the active subunit (A) of the toxin to enter the cell. The active subunit then alters adenylate cyclase activity, which in turn interferes with the energy-dependent sodium pump. Sodium is not recovered from the gut lumen and water is therefore retained in the gut, hence the diarrhoea. Some other gastrointestinal pathogens also have a cholera-like toxin. However, there are other mechanisms responsible for diarrhoea such as increased peristalsis as a response to a distensive or irritant stimulus. In many cases the mechanism is not fully understood.

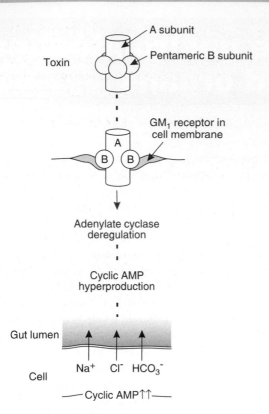

Fig. 12 The action of cholera toxin.

In viral gastrointestinal infections and hepatitis, the damage is not caused by the action of toxins but as a result of host immune response. In hepatitis, failure to mount an adequate immune response to the acute infection can result in chronic hepatitis or viral integration in the genome of host hepatocytes, eventually leading to hepatocellular carcinoma.

8.2 Diagnosis

Learning objectives

You should:

- know the signs and symptoms of gastrointestinal infections
- know the laboratory tests used
- be aware of symptoms that can have both infective and non-infective causes.

Presenting symptoms

Gastrointestinal infections may present with a large variety of signs and symptoms. Cardinal features that prompt a patient to seek medical attention include:

- diarrhoea
- vomiting

- abdominal pain
- steatorrhoea.

Diarrhoea can mean different things to different people. It is important to get the patient to specify exactly what they mean. Are the stools liquid, or just loose? How many are passed per day? Is there any blood or pus with the stool? And is there a sense of urgency to pass a stool, even if none is passed (tenesmus)? It is always helpful to examine a stool specimen personally.

Vomiting is usually more clear cut. Was there a preceding period of nausea? Its onset may be soon after ingesting an infective agent. It is therefore worth asking the patient what they had to eat and drink recently.

Steatorrhoea, or the passing of pale, bulky stools, signifies fat malabsorption, which in some cases may be the result of an enteric infection.

Abdominal pain is a feature of many different intra-abdominal (and some extra-abdominal) conditions, of which only a fraction are infective. Non-infective aetiologies should always be considered in the differential diagnosis. A full history should be sought, as with pain experienced anywhere, including position, nature, variation, radiation, time of onset, modifying factors and simultaneous symptoms. The pain associated with diarrhoea may be colicky and is caused by excessive peristaltic activity. Pain associated with hepatic, biliary and pancreatic infection can be very severe and is often located in the centre of the abdomen. Right upper quadrant pain often signifies disease in the liver or biliary tract.

Jaundice is a feature of hepatitis and biliary tract infection. In hepatitis, it is hepatocellular, while in biliary tract infection it is usually obstructive. The patient may not be visibly yellow or even have yellow sclerae when the serum bilirubin is only moderately raised. Hepatic function tests are required to confirm the nature of the jaundice. Remember that detection of conjugated and unconjugated bilirubin in the urine and the colour of the patient's stools can also be used to determine the nature of the jaundice.

Laboratory tests

Laboratory examination of stools is an essential part of the evaluation of a patient with enteric infection. Microscopy can be used to detect *Campylobacter* spp. during acute infection, a variety of enteric parasites and leucocytes. Electron microscopy is sometimes used to confirm viral enteric infection. Culture is used extensively: to detect the presence of salmonellas, shigellas, campylobacters, vibrios and other bacterial causes of enteric infection. The large number of bacteria and bacterial species present in stool specimens necessitates the use of highly selective agar media to suppress the growth of commensal organisms. *Salmonella* and *Shigella* spp. are almost always non-lactose fermenting, a feature that is employed in many types of selective system. Most laboratories use a combination of several media, e.g. xylose lysine decarboxylase (XLD) agar, desoxycholate citrate agar (DCA), an enrichment broth to increase the recovery of salmonellas (e.g. selenite broth) and a special campylobacter medium. *Campylobacter jejuni* will grow at 43°C and can be isolated on antibiotic-containing selective media grown at this temperature. Additional selective media are required if vibrios or *Escherichia coli* (enterotoxigenic, enteropathogenic or enterohaemorrhagic) are suspected. *V. cholerae* can be isolated following incubation in alkaline peptone water. *E. coli* requires the use of MacConkey agar and enterohaemorrhagic *E. coli* requires sorbitol MacConkey agar. It is, therefore, essential that the clinician communicates any relevant information to the laboratory, as this will enable the laboratory staff to select the correct media.

Preliminary identification of possible enteric pathogens usually requires confirmation by a combination of biochemical (e.g. substrate utilization) and seroagglutination test. These tests take time, so it is often 48–72 hours after specimen reception before the laboratory can confidently confirm the presence of a specific bacterial pathogen. Antibiotic-susceptibility testing is not often performed on these isolates, since antibiotic treatment is rarely indicated. In the event of a suspected outbreak of enteric infection, a number of typing methods can be used to distinguish coincidental sporadic isolates from epidemic spread of a single strain. Serotyping, bacteriophage (phage) typing and molecular typing methods all have their place in this work. Rapid methods are beginning find a place in the laboratory diagnosis of enteric infection; antigen detection ELISA (enzyme-linked immunosorbent assay) is available for confirmation of rotavirus infection; gene probes and nucleic acid amplification tests for bacterial pathogens are coming into use. The main problem in applying new molecular technologies is analogous to the problems involved in identifying bacterial pathogens from among the majority of commensal flora; in vivo molecular techniques require an extraction/purification stage, which can reduce the sensitivity of the test. Another problem is the complexity of the more common pathogenic bacterial genera. *Salmonella* spp., for example, has over 2000 serotypes, but very few type species. It is therefore likely that molecular techniques will increase the sensitivity of initial detection but traditional culture-based methods will be required for epidemiological studies in suspected outbreaks for some time to come.

In hepatitis, the common viral causes of disease can all be detected by serological methods, many of which have been developed as automated ELISAs or radio-immunoassays.

The investigation of possible enteric infection may also require endoscopy, radiological and other imaging techniques and histological studies. The complications of infection of the gastrointestinal tract and related organs include nutritionally mediated effects on the other organ systems. Nutritional, metabolic and haematological evaluation may, therefore, be required.

8.3 Management

Learning objectives

You should:

- know when antimicrobial therapy is required

- understand the value of oral rehydration

- know the public health measures that prevent enteric infections.

Chemotherapy

The more common enteric infections are fortunately self-limiting and in previously well patients do not require antimicrobial treatment. In fact, antibiotic treatment of bacterial enteric infection may have a variety of effects including increased severity of disease.

The mortality from diarrhoeal disease worldwide is mainly the result of acute dehydration, followed by malnutrition. The risk of death from acute diarrhoeal disease can be substantially reduced by rehydration and electrolyte replacement. When dehydration is severe, the initial resuscitation stage requires intravenous fluid administration. However, many patients can be managed with oral rehydration therapy using a carefully balanced mixture of salt, glucose and clean water. Early commencement of oral rehydration therapy can prevent further deterioration in many cases, and the need for more expensive fluids. This approach has been successful because the glucose content of oral rehydration salts drives an energy-dependent sodium pump in the cell membrane of intestinal mucosal cells. This system is independent of the sodium pump that is disabled in enterotoxin-caused diarrhoeas such as cholera. Oral rehydration salts are available in a pre-packed, fixed ratio mixture recommended by the World Heath Organization. A double-ended spoon for measuring salt and sugar in the correct ratio can be used to make up oral rehydration fluids in the field. Antibiotic treatment has a place in the management of a few specific enteric infections, as described below. Follow-up specimens may be needed to confirm eradication of the pathogen, especially if there is any risk of secondary infection (e.g. catering workers).

Bacterial and parasitic infections of the liver, biliary tract and pancreas require appropriate antimicrobial treatment based on knowledge of the likely pathogen. Sufficient activity of the agent at the site of infection is essential to eradicate the infective agent.

Prevention

The most important means of preventing enteric infections is the provision of pathogen-free potable drinking water. Other important public health measures include food hygiene and waste disposal. The main principles underlying safe drinking water are the separation of drinking water sources from sewage disposal routes and purification of drinking water by filtration and chlorination, or an equivalent alternative. These measures have gone a long way to prevent enteric infections such as typhoid and cholera in developed countries. The need for safe drinking water in developing countries is growing faster than the ability to provide it. The provision of pathogen-free drinking water remains a high priority public health measure worldwide. Human waste disposal is frequently linked to safe water provision because natural watercourses are often used as a convenient means of sewage disposal. A breakdown in the separation of potable water supply and sewage disposal substantially increases the risk of enteric infection. In countries where geographical and climatic factors limit the quantity of water available to the human population, alternative sewage disposal strategies can be used that require a reduced volume of water. However, availability of materials, maintenance and cultural aspect of personal hygiene all determine the effectiveness of low-technology sanitary facilities, e.g. a well-designed pit latrine is better than a flush lavatory with flies and no water.

Food hygiene is another important means of preventing enteric infection. Enteric pathogens can contaminate foodstuffs at any point between production and consumption. In general, meats and related products (e.g. dairy foods) can be vehicles for infection by microorganisms that either infect or colonise the animal source (i.e. zoonotic infection). Fruit and vegetables are prone to contamination by organisms present in the soil or in fertilising substances such as manure (especially if composted human waste, or 'nightsoil', is used). All foods are prone to contamination during storage, throughout preparation and after cooking, unless they are preserved by low pH (vinegar), high salt or high sugar concentration. A chilled environment does not prevent contamination but may limit further growth of infective organisms. The storage of uncooked and cooked meat together is a well-recognised means of contaminating food with bacterial pathogens.

Pre-exposure immunization is available for a few infections acquired via the enteric route, including typhoid fever and hepatitis A. The blood-borne hepatitis B can also be prevented by pre-exposure vaccination, or by postexposure administration of human immunoglobulin.

8.4 Diseases and syndromes

Learning objectives

You should:

- know the major infections of the gastrointestinal tract and related structures
- understand the factors contributing to their occurrence
- know the basis of their clinical management.

The main infective disease of the gastrointestinal tract and its related organs are listed in Table 12.

Although enteric fever is acquired via the gastrointestinal tract, it is considered in Chapter 18, since its principal presenting feature is fever, often in international travellers.

Food poisoning

Food poisoning may be caused by an infection of the gastrointestinal tract following consumption of heavily contaminated food, but it may also be the result of the action of preformed toxins (not necessarily microbial) in food.

Chemical toxins that cause food poisoning include **scombrotoxin** (fish from the mackerel family), **fungal toxins** (poisonous mushrooms, other fungi) and **tetrodotoxin** (from fugu, or puffer fish).

Microbial food poisoning takes several forms, with distinctive clinical presentations. If vomiting occurs only an hour or so after food consumption, it may caused by either *Staphylococcus aureus* or *Bacillus cereus* toxins. These enterotoxins are absorbed in the stomach and act via the central vomiting centre. Diarrhoea is not a typical feature of this kind of food poisoning. Attempts to isolate the causal organism from specimens of vomitus are usually unsuccessful. A food history followed by sampling of possible food sources in more likely to confirm the diagnosis.

S. aureus food poisoning is often caused by contamination of salted meat products, seafood (such as prawns) and dairy products (such as cream). *B. cereus* is a Gram-positive, spore-forming bacillus that has been associated with fried rice, especially rice that has been pre-boiled long before frying. The light heating the bacillus

Table 12 Infective disease of the gastrointestinal tract and related organs

Infection	Features
Gastrointestinal tract	
Food poisoning	Acute enteric infection caused by bacteria or toxins present in food at consumption
Infective diarrhoea	Loose and/or watery stools caused by the action of microorganisms or their toxins on the intestine
Enteric fever	See Ch. 19
Infective colitis	Inflammation of the large intestine caused by infection
Infective malabsorption	Varied, including pale, bulky, offensive stools, flatulence, diarrhoea, weight loss, anaemia
Proctitis	Inflammation of the rectum with rectal pain and a discharge
Liver	
Hepatitis	Hepatocellular damage; jaundice, pain, nausea, anorexia
Liver abscess	Focal collection of pus; fever, pain
Gall bladder and biliary tract	
Cholecystitis	Inflammation of gall bladder; fever, rigors, pain
Cholangitis	Obstruction of biliary tract; fever, jaundice, chills
Pancreas	
Pancreatitis	Inflammation of pancreas; bacterial sepsis can occur secondarily; severe, sudden-onset abdominal pain, shock

receives before the food is served stimulates germination of spores that have survived the earlier boiling process.

If the vomiting is less pronounced but there are colicky abdominal pains 12–24 hours after contaminated food consumption, the cause is more likely to be *Clostridium perfringens*. The A serotype of this Gram-positive, spore-forming bacillus produces an enterotoxin that acts on the small intestine. Diarrhoea may also be a feature. Foods most commonly implicated are precooked cold meats that have been reheated. The reheating is enough to stimulate germination of spores that survived the initial cooking stage. Culture of stool specimens for the anaerobic *C. perfringens* may be worthwhile, but only if a semiquantitative method is used and facilities for serotyping the isolate are available, since this species is a common member of the commensal colonic flora.

High-level contamination with *Salmonella* or *Campylobacter* spp. may result in a food poisoning-like syndrome; however, these species are more typically associated with an enteritis caused by bacterial invasion of the intestinal mucosa (see below). The fact that the vehicle for infection may be contaminated food means that this may be regarded as a food-borne infection for public health and legal purposes although it is not 'food poisoning' in the strictest sense.

The above syndromes do not require antimicrobial chemotherapy because they are usually self-limiting conditions. They should still be investigated using appropriate laboratory tests and food histories in order to prevent further infection from the same source. Food poisoning is a notifiable disease in many countries.

Regional and national statistics on the common causes of food poisoning are often available from public health and other official organisations.

Infective diarrhoea

Infective diarrhoea is often referred to as 'gastroenteritis'. This term is inappropriate because the stomach is not a site of invasive disease. When vomiting is a feature of enteric infection, it is thought to be initiated via a central action, rather than invasion of the gastric mucosa. The pathological process is often an enteritis, but in some specific conditions diarrhoea is caused by the action of a toxin without invasion of the intestinal mucosa (e.g. in cholera). The onset is usually between 12 and 48 hours after ingestion of the causal organism. At its worst, a secretory diarrhoea may result in torrential outpouring of fluid into the intestine, causing severe fluid loss with a risk of subsequent hypovolaemic shock and renal failure. This happens in the more severe cases of cholera.

Vibrio species

Cholera is caused by the Gram-negative, comma-shaped organism *V. cholerae*. Many patients with cholera, particularly those infected with the El Tor strain, have a less extreme diarrhoea. The main reservoir for cholera is infected individuals and it is spread most easily in conditions of poor sanitation and overcrowding, e.g. in refugee camps and poor peri-urban districts. Other *Vibrio* spp. cause diarrhoeal disease, and some vibrios may also cause a more invasive enteric infection. Some of these species are present in shellfish grown in sewage-contaminated water. Whether the diarrhoeal disease is caused by *V. cholerae* or other bacteria carrying a cholera-like toxin, basic management is the same: rehydration and prevention of spread. When laboratory facilities are available, stool specimens should be cultured for enteric pathogens, using selective agar including TCBS (thiosulphate, citrate, bile salt, sucrose) to detect growth of *V. cholerae*. Administration of tetracycline reduces excretion of bacteria and shortens the duration of symptoms. Enterotoxic *E. coli* cause a secretory diarrhoea that may mimic milder cases of cholera, especially in international travellers.

Rotavirus

In preschool infants, diarrhoea is most often caused by rotavirus infection. The infection is spread easily and is often associated with vomiting. A similar condition is caused by other viral species, collectively known as 'small round structured viruses'. There is some immunity conferred by these infections, which are rare in younger adults, but infections do occur in older adults probably because of waning immunity. These organisms have been known to cause outbreaks of diarrhoea and vomiting in hospitals, homes for the elderly and other institutions. Rotavirus can be diagnosed by ELISA performed on stool specimens, but the variety of small round structured viruses means that they are best demonstrated by electron microscopy.

Giardia lamblia (syn *G. intestinalis*)

Giardia lamblia is an anaerobic flagellate parasite of the small intestine that causes diarrhoea when large numbers of the trophozoites adhere to duodenal mucosal cells. Infection is caused by ingestion of the infective cyst stage, usually in contaminated water (the parasite is resistant to chlorination). There is a spectrum of clinical disease from severe secretory diarrhoea to asymptomatic carriage. A small percentage of those infected develop malabsorption. The cysts and, very rarely, the trophozoites can be detected in stool specimens by light microscopy or direct coproantigen test. If the diagnosis is suspected yet repeated stool microscopy is negative, duodenal aspirate or biopsy can be used to detect the trophozoite stage. Treatment is with metronidazole for at least 5 days.

Cryptosporidium species

The *Cryptosporidium* spp. are sporozoan parasites transmitted by ingestion of drinking water contaminated by the faeces of farm animals, particularly calves and lambs. Infection is limited to the intestinal epithelium and causes a secretory diarrhoea, which may last for several weeks before subsiding (in immunocompromised patients it may cause a cholera-like syndrome). There is no effective treatment. Diagnosis is confirmed by stool microscopy for the characteristic cysts, stained by a modified acid-fast method.

Salmonella and *Campylobacter* species

Infective diarrhoea can also be caused by organisms that invade the intestinal mucosa. In these infections, diarrhoea may have the features of a toxogenic, secretory infection, but the abdominal pain may be more severe and not necessarily colicky in nature. Intestinal invasion may result in bloody stools, though small amounts of blood released into the small intestine are not necessarily visible to the naked eye.

Enteric fever

Salmonella typhi and *paratyphi* are an exception from the general salmonella diarrhoea infection in that they cause a systemic illness called 'enteric fever' in which diarrhoea is uncommon in the early stages. In Europe and North America, *Yersinia enterocolitica* can also cause an invasive infection. Yersinia infection is predominantly diarrhoeal in younger children, but in older children and adults presents more as a mesenteric adenitis.

Systemic complications

Despite invasion of the intestinal mucosa, bacteria that cause infective diarrhoea rarely reach the systemic circulation. It is only in the immunocompromised and at both extremes of age that invasive bacterial intestinal pathogens tend to cause systemic infection. These infections are otherwise usually self-limiting and do not require antibiotic treatment, which may actually exacerbate some features of the infection. These infections should still be actively investigated to determine the cause of infection and to exclude the possibility of a preventable common source. In recent times, salmonellas have been associated with undercooked poultry (in some countries the majority of chicken carcasses are contaminated with salmonellas), eggs and dairy products. Campylobacters have been associated with poultry, milk and related products.

Antibiotic treatment

Diarrhoea may also be caused by antibiotic treatment. Some antibiotics suppress the normal bacterial flora of the intestine and allow the overgrowth of other species that cause diarrhoea. Clindamycin has a particularly strong association with the condition, but practically any β-lactam antibiotic can have this effect. There are a few antibiotics (e.g. erythromycin) that have a direct effect on gut motility and produce diarrhoea and colicky abdominal pain without necessarily altering the gut flora. At its most severe, antibiotic-associated diarrhoea may be accompanied by bloody stools and the formation of an inflammatory exudate on the colonic mucosa. This condition is called **pseudomembranous colitis**. It is diagnosed by demonstrating the presence of an anaerobic bacillus *Clostridium difficile* and its toxin in stool specimens. Rectal biopsy should also be performed to show pseudomembrane formation because *C. difficile* is a part of the commensal enteric flora in a high proportion of elderly people. Treatment is with either oral vancomycin or metronidazole.

Infective colitis

The major infective causes of colitis are bacillary and amoebic dysentery. The term 'dysentery' is used because the condition often causes pain originating in the inflamed colon. Diarrhoea is present as a result of either impaired fluid absorption in the proximal colon or excessive mucus production in the distal colon. Passing stools is painful, especially if the inflammation extends as far as the rectum, and there may be tenesmus. The colonic inflammation may also cause the presence of blood or pus in the stools.

Bacillary dysentery
Bacillary dysentery is caused by *Shigella* spp. The condition varies between a mild diarrhoea and severe diarrhoea with blood and pus in the stool. The former is caused by more common *Shigella sonnei*, while the most severe forms of the latter are often caused by *Shigella dysenteriae*, one of the three other species in the genus *Shigella*. Despite invasion of the colonic mucosa, bacillary dysentery does not often result in septicaemia.

Diagnosis is confirmed by stool culture for the non-lactose-fermenting Gram-negative bacillus, followed by biochemical and agglutination test.

Treatment with antibiotics known to be effective against local shigella isolates may be required in all but *S. sonnei* infection.

Amoebic dysentery
Amoebic dysentery is caused by the invasive amoebic species *Entamoeba histolytica*, following ingestion of amoebic cysts. There is invasion of the colonic mucosa by amoebae and some blood in the stool, but little pus formation. Perforation of the colon may occur in more severe infections and amoebae may reach the liver via the portal circulation, where amoebic liver abscess can develop.

Diagnosis is by stool microscopy. The presence of amoebic cysts in the stool is not diagnostic. These may be cysts of the related commensal *Entamoeba coli* or from asymptomatic carriage of *E. histolytica*. The definitive diagnosis is made either by recognising amoebic forms engulfing red blood cells or by seeing invasive amoebae in a rectal biopsy specimen. Live *E. histolytica* trophozoites are best seen in freshly passed stool preparations on a warmed microscope stage.

Treatment is with metronidazole.

The differential diagnosis includes the non-infective conditions of Crohn's colitis and ulcerative colitis.

Antibiotic-caused pseudomembranous colitis may also be an important differential diagnosis when there is a recent history of antibiotic use. Infective colitis may be part of a more extensive enteritis reaching as far as the small intestine. There is therefore considerable overlap between infective colitis and infective diarrhoea. (Haemorrhagic colitis and haemolytic uraemic syndrome, caused by verotoxin-producing strains of *E. coli* (enterohaemorrhagic), are considered in Ch. 16.)

Infective malabsorption

There are both infective and non-infective causes of intestinal malabsorption. Its features depend on the category of digestive malfunction and include pale, bulky, offensive stools, flatulence, frank diarrhoea, weight loss and ritamin B_{12}-deficient anaemia. The infections that can cause a malabsorptive syndrome include:

- bacterial overgrowth syndrome, blind loop syndrome
- tropical sprue
- *Diphyllobothrium latum* infection
- *G. lamblia* infection (see infective diarrhoea above).

Bacterial overgrowth syndrome
Bacterial overgrowth syndrome is caused by the overgrowth of commensal intestinal bacterial species in unusually high numbers, often following gastrointestinal surgery. The bacterial flora of the lower small intestinal and large intestine extends upwards into the jejunum and even the duodenum. This causes an alteration in the digestive function of the small intestine, resulting in steatorrhoea, diarrhoea and malabsorption of fat-soluble vitamins.

Radioactive carbon breath tests have been used to demonstrate intestinal bacterial overgrowth.

Treatment with metronidazole may help some patients, but in cases where bacterial overgrowth is caused by a blind loop of gut, surgical removal may be required.

Tropical sprue
Tropical sprue is a malabsorptive condition affecting adults who have resided in tropical countries. Its precise cause is unknown, but it often responds to treatment with tetracycline. Some cases resolve spontaneously.

Diphyllobothrium latum
Diphyllobothrium latum is a fish tapeworm found in populations that live around large freshwater lakes. The cysts are ingested and the tapeworm becomes established in the small intestine, where it may cause vitamin B_{12} deficiency and consequent macrocytic anaemia.

Diagnosis is by stool microscopy for the distinctive cysts. Treatment is with mebendazole.

Proctitis

Proctitis is inflammation of the rectum and like other inflammatory conditions of the lower gastrointestinal tract, may be caused by both infective and non-infective aetiologies. Infective causes are less common but include the bacteria and parasites that cause colitis (i.e. *Shigella* and *Entamoeba* spp.) as well as sexually transmitted infections (e.g. gonorrhoea) following penetrative anal intercourse. The clinical features are rectal pain and a rectal discharge; the discharge can be sampled with a swab during proctoscopy.

Investigation for *Neisseria gonorrhoeae* and *Chlamydia trachomatis* should be requested. Stool specimens should also be sent to the laboratory for microscopy and culture, whether or not there is any diarrhoea. Microscopy for *E. histolytica* and other parasite species will have to be specifically requested.

It is impossible to cover all the possible pathogens with a single antimicrobial agent. It is therefore better to wait for the result of laboratory investigations before commencing treatment.

Hepatitis

Hepatitis is a condition in which inflammatory damage occurs to hepatocytes without fibrosis or regeneration. The major metabolic functions performed by the liver include detoxification of substances carried to the liver from the small intestine via the portal circulation and from the rest of the body.

Hepatocellular damage is caused both by pathogenic microorganisms, particularly viruses, and by toxins such as therapeutic drugs and other chemicals. The microorganisms that cause hepatitis include hepatitis viruses A–E (Table 13), cytomegalovirus, various arboviruses and the spiral bacteria *Leptospira* spp. In most cases, the features of disease are directly attributable to hepatocellular damage. The jaundice this causes results in raised unconjugated bilirubin in blood and urine (the urine is not darker than usual) and raised liver enzymes. There may be discomfort or pain in the right upper abdominal quadrant and there is often nausea, anorexia and distaste for alcohol.

Hepatitis A

Hepatitis A infection ('infectious' hepatitis) is spread by the faecal–oral route and is common in children living where sewage disposal is inadequate. Hepatitis A is rare in patients over 40 years of age. In developed communities the peak incidence is in older children and young adults. The hepatitis A virus is an enterovirus with a short incubation period (2–6 weeks). Several days after the end of the incubation period, dark urine and pale stools provide evidence of cholestatic jaundice. By the time jaundice is clinically evident, the other symptoms may already have begun to subside. The patient remains infectious for around 1–2 weeks. A high proportion of infections are subclinical. Immunity is lifelong.

Diagnosis is by detection of a rising antibody titre (ELISA) or demonstration of anti-hepatitis A IgM in the serum.

There is no specific treatment, but patients should avoid alcohol for 1 year. Fulminant hepatitis is very rare and always fatal. A vaccine is available for non-immune adults. Human gammaglobulin provides short-lived protection.

Hepatitis B

Hepatitis B infection ('serum' hepatitis) is a very different disease. The infection is spread in blood, blood products and in human body secretions, e.g. during sexual intercourse. The hepatitis B virus causes a spectrum of disease ranging from fulminant hepatitis to subclinical infection. The incubation period is 6 weeks to 6 months. Hepatitis B infection may also result in late sequelae, including a carrier state, liver failure caused by chronic active hepatitis and hepatocellular carcinoma caused by malignant transformation of hepatocytes following integration of the virus into the host cell genome. The populations most at risk include male homosexuals, intravenous drug abusers, infants of mothers who are carriers, renal dialysis patients, recipients of multiple blood transfusions or multiple donor blood products and the populations of many African and Asian countries where the carrier state is more common.

Diagnosis The diagnosis is confirmed by serological studies, and a variety of methods are used for antigen and antibody detection (e.g. ELISA, radioimmunoassay). Hepatitis B surface antigen (HBsAG) is a marker for

Table 13 Viral hepatitides

Virus	Incubation (weeks)	Disease	Transmission
Hepatitis A	2–7	Infectious hepatitis	Faecal–oral
Hepatitis B	6–26	Serum hepatitis	Blood, body fluids
Hepatitis C	2–26	Most non-A, non-B hepatitis	Blood, body fluids
Delta agent	4–6	Severe hepatitis	Blood, body fluids
Hepatitis E	?	Infectious hepatitis	Faecal–oral

disease but does not distinguish active hepatitis after about 6 weeks from the time of infection, before the onset of jaundice, and usually becomes undetectable after about 3 months. The small percentage of patients that remain HBsAG positive after 6 months are carriers. Hepatitis B e antigen is an accurate marker for high-level infectivity. Antibodies to the surface antigen are protective against further infection and do not appear in significant titre in patients with chronic active disease. They may also be caused by vaccination. In the early stages of hepatitis B infection, when surface antigen is no longer detectable, the first antibody reaction to appear is to hepatitis B core antigen. Anti-core antibodies are used to confirm recent hepatitis B infection when all other tests are negative. There is little benefit to be had from specific treatment in the later stages of disease, but treatment in its early stages with interferon may reduce progression of the infection. The antiviral agent lamivudine can also be used for patients who are e antigen positive.

Control The main emphasis in hepatitis B infection is on prevention by immunoprophylaxis of high-risk groups. A genetically engineered surface antigen subunit vaccine is given into the deltoid muscle on at least two occasions. A booster dose is given if the resulting antibody response is poor. High-priority health-care workers are staff of accident and emergency units, diagnostic laboratories, blood transfusion units and renal dialysis units, and staff such as surgeons who regularly practise exposure-prone invasive procedures. In many parts of east Asia, the whole population is vaccinated during childhood because of the high incidence of hepatocellular carcinoma.

Postexposure vaccination is also practised, particularly when health-care workers have blood or other human tissues inoculated into them. They and the 'donor' both require venesection for hepatitis B serology. If the 'donor' is positive and the staff member negative, the recipient can be given purified hepatitis hyperimmunoglobulin immediately and started on a course of hepatitis B vaccination. The most common kind of injury causing potential hepatitis exposure is accidental puncture by a hypodermic syringe needle or similar device (so-called 'needle-stick' injury). The most common site of needle-stick injury is the forefinger and thumb of the non-dominant hand, during resheathing of a needle. All health-care staff should avoid resheathing used hypodermic needles and must ensure that they are disposed of safely in the proper rigid disposal container. All patients should be regarded as a potential hepatitis risk. Standard infection control precautions are designed to minimise this risk. Clinical waste and diagnostic specimens should be clearly labelled as a potential biohazard and transported with care in the recommended safe container.

Hepatitis C

Hepatitis C infection used to be called non-A, non-B hepatitis because its epidemiology suggested an infective agent distinct to hepatitis A or B viruses. The incubation period is approximately 1–3 months. Transmission is via blood and blood products. There is a higher rate of chronic hepatitis following hepatitis C infection than there is with hepatitis B. It is also the most common cause of hepatitis following blood transfusion.

Despite the fact that the virus cannot be grown in cell culture, parts of its genome have been identified and diagnostic tests developed. These are now available for laboratory confirmation of hepatitis C infection and for screening of donated blood units.

Delta agent

The delta agent is a virus associated with severe, fulminant hepatitis, but it does not cause hepatitis on its own. Instead it acts together with the hepatitis B virus to cause either severe co-infection or a superinfection in patients with chronic hepatitis. The virus is a defective RNA virus that is incapable of replicating in the absence of hepatitis B virus. Most delta agent infections have been in intravenous drug abusers. Laboratory confirmation is with ELISA or radioimmunoassay techniques.

Hepatitis E

Hepatitis E virus is an unusual cause of hepatitis in Europe and North America. It does, however, cause sporadic outbreaks of a hepatitis spread via the faecal–oral route in East Asia.

Other infectious agents

A variety of arboviruses, including yellow fever virus and hantavirus, also cause jaundice. Leptospirosis can cause a hepatitis-like clinical picture. This infection is caused by a spirochaete bacteria belonging to the genus *Leptospira*. There may be petechiae and renal failure, in addition to jaundice. The condition is considered in more detail in Chapter 20.

Liver abscess

Liver abscess is a focal collection of pus and is caused either by bacteria or by the parasite *E. histolytica*. The infection may arise following ascending pyogenic infection, particularly via the biliary tract, or following subclinical gastrointestinal infection. The patient is often febrile and usually has focal upper right quadrant pain.

Liver enlargement may be detected by manual examination, but only if the abscess is large. Diagnostic ultrasound is helpful and shows a focal, fluid-filled lesion. It can also be used to guide attempts at percutaneous drainage if the abscess is easily accessible, but complete drainage may require laparotomy. Drainage assists resolution of the abscess, and aspirated pus can be sent for bacterial culture and microscopy for amoebae. The bacterial species isolated from pyogenic liver abscesses include anaerobic bacteria, Enterobacteriaceae or *Streptococcus anginosus-constellatus*. An immunofluorescent serological test is available for invasive amoebic disease.

Initial presumptive treatment is with ampicillin, gentamicin and metronidazole. This regimen can be modified when the results of culture are known. Amoebic liver abscess can be treated with metronidazole alone.

Cholecystitis

Acute cholecystitis is an inflammation of the gall bladder that occurs most often, but not exclusively, in obese women over 50 years of age. The clinical features are fever, rigors, abdominal pain and subcostal tenderness on the right-hand side. The majority of patients have gallstones and bacteria in the gall bladder. These bacteria are of gastrointestinal origin and include Enterobacteriaceae, enterococci and anaerobic species. A severe variant, emphysematous cholecystitis, occurs in diabetics in which there is gas present in the tissues around the gall bladder. The diagnosis is confirmed by ultrasound.

Treatment is with analgesics, bed rest and antibiotics active against gastrointestinal bacteria. There is disagreement over whether to proceed to immediate cholecystectomy or wait until the acute attack has settled to arrange an elective procedure. In either case, antibiotic therapy has only a small role.

Cholangitis

Obstruction of the biliary tract can be caused by infection of the biliary tract. In some cases, this is secondary to obstruction of the common bile duct with a gallstone or a tumour (cholangiocarcinoma, pancreatic carcinoma). The clinical features are fever, jaundice and chills. In most cases, infection is caused by Enterobacteriaceae, enterococci or anaerobic bacteria. A high percentage of patients have bacteraemic spread and a positive blood culture. The condition has a high mortality rate, especially once septicaemic shock has set in.

Confirmation of the diagnosis is by a combination of blood culture and diagnostic ultrasound scan.

Treatment is with a combination of antibiotics such as ampicillin, gentamicin and metronidazole. Any underlying obstruction of the biliary tract may require surgical correction.

Pancreatitis

Acute or chronic inflammation of the pancreas causes severe, sudden-onset abdominal pain, often accompanied by shock.

Chronic pancreatitis is a recurrent disease. Several precipitating factors are recognised, including obstruction of the pancreatic duct by gallstones, excessive alcohol consumption and mumps virus infection in adults. It is not primarily an infective condition, but bacterial sepsis is one of the principal causes of mortality in acute pancreatitis. Sepsis arises either because of local or haematogenous spread of bacteria from the commensal intestinal flora or from a hospital-acquired infection.

Diagnosis is confirmed by blood culture and specimens from potential foci of infection.

Presumptive treatment is usually with intravenous antibacterial agents. Patients with the most severe disease are prone to colonisation and eventual infection with antibiotic-resistant bacteria and yeasts, which make choosing the type and duration of antimicrobial chemotherapy particularly difficult.

8.5 Organisms

A checklist of the organisms discussed in this chapter is given in Box 3. Further information is give on the pages indicated.

Box 3 Organisms that infect the gastrointestinal tract

Bacteria	**see page**	**Viruses**	**see page**
Salmonella spp.	248–9	Rotavirus	260
Shigella spp.	249	Small round structured viruses	–
Campylobacter spp.	251	Enterovirus family	–
Escherichia coli	248	Mumps family	259
Vibrio cholerae	250	Hepatitis A, B, C, and E viruses	257
Clostridium difficile	248	Delta agent	–
Yersinia enterocolitica	249		
Clostridium perfringens	247	**Parasites**	
Neisseria gonorrhoeae	252–3	*Entamoeba histolytica*	264
Streptococcus anginosus-constellatus		*Giardia lamblia* (syn *G. intestinalis*)	265
(formerly *S. milleri*)	245	*Diphyllobothrium latum*	267
Leptospira spp.	256		

Self-assessment: questions

Multiple choice questions

1. Intestinal infections can be transmitted by:
   a. The faecal–oral route
   b. Needle-stick injury
   c. Ingestion
   d. Sewage contamination of the potable water supply
   e. Consumption of shellfish

2. Diarrhoea can be caused by:
   a. Toxin-mediated fluid uptake from the intestinal lumen
   b. Bacterial invasion of gut-associated lymphoid tissues
   c. The action of bacterial toxin
   d. Increased peristalsis
   e. Inflammation restricted to the rectal mucosa

3. In the laboratory diagnosis of bacterial enteric infection:
   a. Selective media are used to reduce growth of commensal species
   b. More than one selective medium is used for primary isolation in most diagnostic laboratories
   c. Confirmation of an organism's identity may require both biochemical and agglutination tests
   d. Microscopic examination of stool specimens has no diagnostic value
   e. Antimicrobial susceptibility testing is not routinely performed

4. The following precautions are used in hospitals to prevent patient-to-patient spread of enteric infections:
   a. Avoid resheathing hypodermic syringe needles
   b. Dispose of stools, urine and body secretions as hazardous waste
   c. Postexposure vaccination
   d. Use of gloves, aprons and handwash for those in physical contact with the patient
   e. Chlorination of drinking water supply

5. Which of the following methods are used to prevent food-borne infection:
   a. Cooking
   b. Separation of raw and cooked meat in storage
   c. Freezing
   d. Storage in brine (salt solution)
   e. Storage in vinegar

6. Food poisoning:
   a. Is caused by bacteria or toxins present at the time of consumption
   b. Is always caused by microorganisms or their products
   c. Should be diagnosed by culture of vomit
   d. May be caused by *Staphylococcus aureus*
   e. Can result in symptoms as late as 48 hours after ingestion

7. The predominant clinical feature of enteric infection with the following organisms is watery diarrhoea:
   a. *Clostridium perfringens*
   b. *Salmonella typhi*
   c. *Shigella dysenteriae*
   d. *Shigella sonnei*
   e. Enterotoxigenic *Escherichia coli*

8. *Vibrio cholerae*:
   a. Is a comma-shaped Gram-negative bacterium
   b. Grows optimally at slightly acid pH
   c. Can cause a torrential watery diarrhoea
   d. Infection can cause hypovolaemic shock
   e. Infection does not respond to antibiotic therapy

9. Rotavirus infection:
   a. Occurs most often in preschool children
   b. Only rarely causes vomiting
   c. Can cause institutional outbreaks
   d. Can be confirmed by stool antigen detection
   e. Does not confer protective immunity

10. Bloody stools are a frequent finding in infections caused by:
    a. Small round structured viruses
    b. *Entamoeba histolytica*
    c. Rotavirus
    d. *Shigella dysenteriae*
    e. Enterohaemorrhagic *Escherichia coli*

11. Entamoebal infection:
    a. Is most often caused by *Entamoeba coli*
    b. Is restricted to the colonic epithelium
    c. May result in liver abscess
    d. Can be confused with ulcerative colitis
    e. Is confirmed by finding amoebic cysts in the stool

12. Concerning the serological diagnosis of hepatitis B infection:
    a. HBsAG (hepatitis B surface antigen) is a marker of infectivity
    b. A positive e antigen test indicates low infectivity

c. HBsAG remains detectable in chronic hepatitis

d. Antibodies to HBsAG do not always indicate past infection

e. Anti-hepatitis B core antigen is the first detectable antibody after infection

13. Liver abscess:
    a. Rarely causes local pain or tenderness
    b. Is always caused by bacteria
    c. Should be diagnosed by culture of aspirated contents
    d. Can be diagnosed by immunofluorescent antibody test
    e. May be caused by *Streptococcus anginosus-constellatus*

14. In cholangitis:
    a. There is both obstructive and infective biliary tract disease
    b. The classical presentation is chills, fever and jaundice
    c. Antibiotic therapy is only an adjunct to surgery
    d. There is a negligible risk of septicaemia
    e. Infection is usually caused by intestinal pathogens

Case history questions

History 1

> Three medical students celebrate their examination results by going out for a meal at a nearby Chinese restaurant. They choose a selection of dishes, including crispy duck, spare ribs, chicken chow mein and fried rice, with which they have some bean sprouts and bamboo shoots. On the way home, one of them is violently sick, and by 11 p.m., one of the others is vomiting, while the other has an unsettled stomach. None of them has diarrhoea.

1. Were the students' symptoms caused by an invasive infection or a toxin?
2. What organisms would you associate with these symptoms?
3. Would you request any bacteriological tests in this case?
4. What investigation would be useful?

History 2

> A 30-year-old man attended the clinic with a history of intermittent, mild diarrhoea lasting over 3 months.

> He had had a bout of more severe diarrhoea, nausea, loss of appetite and 'indigestion' at first, but all the symptoms apart from the diarrhoea had subsided. He had not been overseas recently. Three consecutive stool specimens were obtained for exclusion of bacterial and viral enteric pathogens, but no pathogen was detected.

1. What organism might be responsible for this patient's symptoms?
2. If the patient has not travelled abroad, how did he acquire this infection?
3. If stool microscopy is negative, what other diagnostic microbiology test might help?
4. What treatment might you use?

Data interpretation

A faecal specimen is taken from a woman who had diarrhoea on the way home from an Australian restaurant where she ate a plate of New Zealand green mussels.

Salmonella enteritidis was isolated but no other intestinal bacterial pathogens.

1. Can this patient blame the salmonella infection on the restaurant?
2. What would be needed to prove the mussels were the cause of her infection?
3. Does this laboratory result have an alternative explanation?
4. What antibiotic treatment would you choose?

Objective structured clinical examination (OSCE)

An 8-year-old boy developed loose, watery stools which persisted over 2 weeks before his mother sought medical advice. On examination, he was pale and listless but did not have clinical signs of gross dehydration. He had an otherwise unremarkable medical history and had previously been fit and healthy. A sample of diarrhoea stool was sent for laboratory examination. No bacterial intestinal pathogens were isolated. Cryptosporidium cysts were noted on microscopy.

You are asked the following:

1. Is dehydration possible in the absence of clinical signs?
2. Does this child need rehydration therapy?
3. Can cryptosporidial infection be life-threatening?
4. Should antibiotic treatment be considered in this case?
5. Are other members of the family at risk from the same infection?

Short notes questions

Write short notes on the following:

1. How the normal gastrointestinal tract is protected against infection
2. How the laboratory would confirm a diagnosis of enteric infection caused by a common bacterial pathogen
3. The role of antibiotic therapy in the management of enteric infection
4. What is pseudomembranous colitis (PMC)
5. The relationship between infection and the malabsorption syndrome
6. Approaches used to prevent hepatitis B infection

Viva questions

1. Why are some intestinal pathogens so difficult to demonstrate in clinical samples?
2. What type of hepatitis do you fear most? Give your reasons.

Self-assessment: answers

Multiple choice answers

1. a. **True**. One of the most important routes.
   b. **False**. Needle-stick injuries are associated with blood-borne infection.
   c. **True**. Food and drink are major sources.
   d. **True**. A particular problem in developing countries.
   e. **True**. Can accumulate microorganisms such as vibrios from contaminated water.

2. a. **False**. In toxigenic diarrhoea, fluid uptake from the lumen is reduced.
   b. **False**. Bacterial invasion of Peyer's patches may result in ulceration but is not a direct cause of diarrhoea.
   c. **True**. For example cholera toxin.
   d. **True**. This causes a colicky pain.
   e. **False**. Inflammation restricted to the rectum is proctitis and does not necessarily cause loose or liquid stools.

3. a. **True**. Stool specimens contain high numbers of commensal species.
   b. **True**. Any relevant clinical information should be sent with the specimen to assist in the choice of media.
   c. **True**.
   d. **False**. Stool microscopy can be used for recognition of enteric parasites, preliminary diagnosis in campylobacter infection and to detect leucocytes.
   e. **True**. Because antibiotic treatment is rarely required.

4. a. **False**. This is a precaution against blood-borne infection.
   b. **True**. These are potent sources of infection.
   c. **False**. This is a precaution against blood-borne infection.
   d. **True**.
   e. **False**. Chlorination of drinking water is unlikely to have any impact on the spread of enteric infection within the hospital.

5. a. **True**. Cooking will kill most species.
   b. **True**. Cross-contamination in storage is a common source of infection.
   c. **True**. This prevents growth of any infective organisms.
   d. **True**. High salt concentration preserves, as do low pH and high sugar concentration.
   e. **True**. Provides a low pH environment.

6. a. **True**.
   b. **False**. Non-microbial causes of food poisoning include scombrotoxin, mushroom and puffer fish poisoning.
   c. **False**. Culture of vomit is rarely contributory.
   d. **True**. *S. aureus* usually causes vomiting within one or two hours through production of an enterotoxin in the stomach.
   e. **True**. This is more likely if poisoning is with *Clostridium perfringens*, which produces an enterotoxin in the small intestine.

7. a. **False**. *C. perfringens* type A can cause food poisoning in which there is colicky abdominal pain and, less commonly, vomiting and diarrhoea up to 48 hours after consumption.
   b. **False**. *S. typhi* is an important cause of enteric fever, in which diarrhoea is unusual in the early stages. Initial constipation is more common.
   c. **False**. *S. dysenteriae* causes bacillary dysentery, which is often very severe. There is a colitis, with blood and pus in the stool.
   d. **True**. Other *Shigella* spp. can cause a severe dysentery.
   e. **True**. May mimic mild cholera and is often seen in international travellers.

8. a. **True**.
   b. **False**. Optimal growth of *V. cholerae* is at an alkaline pH.
   c. **True**. In severe cholera.
   d. **True**. Owing to the severe fluid loss.
   e. **False**. Treatment of cholera with tetracycline will both shorten the duration of diarrhoea and reduce excretion of vibrios.

9. a. **True**. A similar infection is with 'small round structured viruses'.
   b. **False**. In rotavirus infections, vomiting commonly accompanies diarrhoea.
   c. **True**. Infection spreads easily.
   d. **True**. Using ELISA (enzyme-linked immunosorbent assay).
   e. **False**. The reduced incidence of rotavirus infection in adults is explained by protective immunity following childhood infection.

10. a. **False**. Small round structured viruses cause watery diarrhoea.
    b. **True**. There is amoebic invasion of the colonic mucosa.

c. **False**. Causes watery diarrhoea and vomiting.
d. **True**. Severe infections result in blood and pus in the stools.
e. **True**. These strains produce a verotoxin that binds to gut mucosa causing damage and haemorrhage.

11. a. **False**. *Entamoeba coli* is a non-pathogenic commensal; cysts of *E. coli* must be distinguished from those of *Entamoeba histolytica* in stool specimens.
   b. **False**. Amoebic dysentery can either be locally invasive or result in dissemination to the liver.
   c. **True**. Abscesses can also occur in the lungs and brain.
   d. **True**. This also is an inflammation of the large intestine.
   e. **False**. The diagnosis is confirmed by finding amoebic trophozoites (amoebae) ingesting red blood cells in the stool.

12. a. **True**. It does not, however, distinguish active, convalescent and carrier states.
   b. **False**. The e antigen is associated with high level infectivity.
   c. **True**. If it is still positive after 6 months, this indicates a carrier state.
   d. **True**. They may be caused by vaccination.
   e. **True**. It is used to confirm recent infection.

13. a. **False**. Usually presents with focal upper right quadrant pain.
   b. **False**. Some liver abscesses are caused by the protozoan parasite *Entamoeba histolytica*.
   c. **False**. Aspiration of liver abscess contents is often difficult and in amoebic disease may not contain a detectable parasite, so aspiration is performed more for therapeutic purposes.
   d. **True**. This detects amoebic disease.
   e. **True**.

14. a. **True**. Infection can occur secondary to an obstruction such as gallstone.
   b. **True**. This is sometimes known as Charcot's triad.
   c. **False**. Antibiotic treatment is essential. It is in acute cholecystitis that antibiotics are only an adjunct to surgery.
   d. **False**. There is a high risk of septicaemia, septic shock and, therefore, death.
   e. **False**. The bacteria causing this infection are usually intestinal commensals; intestinal pathogens such as *Salmonella* and *Shigella* spp. are rarely implicated.

Case history answers

History 1

1. Only a toxin could have acted so quickly.
2. *Bacillus cereus* and *Staphylococcus aureus*, of which *B. cereus* is the more likely in this setting.
3. No, culture of vomit specimens is rarely helpful.
4. Food history of the students and any other diners at the restaurant that evening. If there has been a large outbreak of food poisoning, case-control studies may be done, but in this case the likely vehicle for toxin was the fried rice. Kitchen practice at the restaurant might need improving to prevent further problems of this kind.

History 2

1. The protozoan parasite *Giardia lamblia*, which would not have been searched for unless a request was made for enteric parasites. Other parasites might also cause this clinical picture (e.g. *Cryptosporidium* sp.) though the upper gastrointestinal symptoms make this unlikely.
2. Indigenous cases of giardiasis occur through consumption of contaminated drinking water. *G. lamblia* cysts are relatively resistant to chlorine and may survive despite attempts to eradicate them.
3. Endoscopy for duodenal aspirate or biopsy can be used to confirm giardiasis. Failing that, the gelatin capsule string test can be used to obtain duodenal trophozoites.
4. Metronidazole for 5 days for *G. lamblia* infection.

Data interpretation answer

1. No. The onset of diarrhoea was too soon after eating at the restaurant to implicate any food consumed there.
2. An indistinguishable isolate of *Salmonella enteritidis* from the mussels. This rarely occurs.
3. It is most probable that the salmonella infection was obtained at some time prior to visiting the restaurant. In Australia, *Salmonella enteritidis* is much less common than *Salmonella typhimurium* and the former is often associated with recent travel in southeast Asia.
4. None. Uncomplicated salmonellosis in an otherwise healthy adult does not normally require antibiotic therapy.

OSCE answer

1. Yes. Listlessness is a sign of dehydration.
2. Rehydration may be necessary with oral rehydration salt solution after 2 weeks of continuous diarrhoea.
3. Yes, because it causes dehydration. This is a potential hazard in small children and in the setting

of human immunodeficiency virus infection and the acquired immunodeficiency syndrome.

4. No antibiotic has been found to be effective in cryptosporidial infection.

5. Yes. Either from a common environmental source or from an infected family member.

Short notes answers

1. Defences of the gastrointestinal tract could be listed in anatomical sequence. Give examples of pathogens excluded by specific defence mechanisms and how impaired defences contribute to disease.

2. Follow the sequence of microscopy, culture, confirmatory tests. *Salmonella*, *Shigella* and *Campylobacter* spp. are the best examples to choose. Remember the importance of selective media.

3. Remember that most bacterial enteric infections do not require antimicrobial chemotherapy. List the exceptions: cholera, campylobacter, at extremes of age, parasitic infection, enteric fever. Explain the contribution antimicrobial therapy makes.

4. A brief account of PMC should cover its epidemiology, pathogenesis, diagnosis, treatment and prevention. Cannot be answered without reference to *Clostridium difficile*.

5. Needs to include bacterial overgrowth syndrome, tropical sprue, fish tapeworm (*Diphyllobothrium latum*) and giardiasis.

6. Cover aspects including pre- and postexposure vaccination, avoiding contact with body secretions, urine and stools of infected person, careful disposal of clinical waste, syringe needles, etc.

Viva answers

1. There is a problem of looking for needles in haystacks. You have to find bacteria that may only be a small portion of the total range and number of bacteria normally present in faeces. That requires several types of selective agar. Some (e.g. campylobacter) only grow under special atmospheric conditions. Others are closely related to commensal bacteria (e.g. *Escherichia coli* O157:H7). Some parasites may be present at very low count or present intermittently (e.g. *Giardia lamblia*).

2. Hepatitis A and B can be prevented by vaccination, and hepatitis B exposure can be managed by postexposure hyperimmune globulin. Hepatitis C, however, has a higher rate of conversion to chronic active hepatitis and cannot be prevented by vaccination. It may be transmitted by needle-stick or similar sharps injury and can dictate a need to withdraw from exposure-prone procedures.

9 Urinary tract infections

Overview

Urinary tract infection (UTI) is seen commonly in both general and hospital practice. The more severe types of urinary tract infection are encountered less frequently but often require hospital admission for inpatient management. A specific aetiological diagnosis and antibiotic susceptibility testing is required in UTI to avoid treatment failure caused by antibiotic resistance. Careful collection of diagnostic specimens will help to avoid the problem of assessing the medical significance of bacterial isolates and the unnecessary treatment that may result.

9.1 Pathogenesis

Learning objectives

You should:

- understand the relationship of structural features and coexisting conditions with susceptibility to urinary tract infections
- understand how infecting microorganisms contribute to pathogenesis.

Only the lower part of the urethra has a resident bacterial flora. The rest of the urinary tract is normally sterile and is kept free of bacteria by the flushing effect of urine flow. Local phagocyte activity may also play a small role in non-specific defences. Mucosal IgA and secretions from prostatic and urethral glands may have a minor antibacterial effect. Entry of microorganisms into the urinary tract is usually along the urethra by the 'ascending' route, following colonisation of the periurethral area by enteric organisms. More rarely, organisms reach the urinary tract by haematogenous spread.

Structural features of the urinary tract are important contributors to infection: the relative shortness of the female urethra is thought to be the main reason why females are more susceptible to urinary tract infections (UTIs) than males throughout life. It is likely that sexual intercourse assists access of bacteria into the bladder, since celibate women experience fewer episodes of infection than sexually active women. The use of a contraceptive diaphragm increases the risk of UTI. Interference with urine flow also increases the risk of UTI. Causes include prostatic hypertrophy, neurogenic bladder, anatomically abnormal kidney and bladder or kidney stones. Microorganisms may gain access to the urinary tract during urinary catheterisation or surgical instrumentation. Indwelling catheters provide a permanent portal of entry for microbial pathogens and act as a nidus of infection.

The infecting organisms play an active part in the pathogenesis of UTI, though the importance of this is less well understood. Probably the most important microbial factor is the ability to adhere to urinary epithelial cells. Some strains of *Escherichia coli*—the most common cause of community-acquired UTI—possess pili with protein components that preferentially interact with galactose-containing receptor sites on epithelial cell surfaces. These are more commonly found in patients with UTI. *Proteus* sp. possess urease, which produces ammonia in the urine. This raises the pH and causes precipitation of phosphate crystals, leading to stone formation. Renal stones increase the risk of further infection, as does any foreign body in the urinary tract, since they provide a site where antibiotics are less effective.

9.2 Diagnosis

Presenting symptoms

The common features of urinary tract infection are an urgent desire to urinate (urgency), frequent urination (frequency) and painful urination (dysuria). The urine may have an offensive odour. In lower urinary tract infection, there may also be a feeling of fullness in the lower abdomen, or pain above the symphysis pubis. In infection of the upper urinary tract, pain when present is in the loin and tenderness may be present over the affected kidney. Fever and other features of systemic infection are also common. In children, UTI may present as bedwetting.

Laboratory tests

Laboratory confirmation of the diagnosis is by microscopy and culture of a urine specimen, which should be collected without contamination by urethral, perineal or enteric flora. Usually this can be achieved by collection of a midstream specimen of urine (MSU) from the patient (Fig. 13).

Urine specimens deteriorate rapidly at room temperature. Several approaches have been adopted to overcome this problem. Rapid transport to the laboratory and immediate processing is the ideal. If not possible, samples can be refrigerated to prevent deterioration, but cellular contents will continue to lyse even at lower temperatures. Borate crystals are used by many laboratories as a preservative for urine specimens submitted from general practice.

In the laboratory, microscopic examination of the specimen is used to count the number of neutrophils and erythrocytes and to record the presence of casts and epithelial cells. Significant pyuria is said to be present when they are greater than 10^8 cells/ml urine. This is usually indicative of UTI. UTI can occur in the absence of pyuria. Epithelial cells in specimens from female patients usually indicate vaginal contamination. Casts are best sought for in a deposit from centrifuged urine. White cell casts may be the result of infection in upper urinary tract.

The significance of the bacteria isolated from urine culture is judged by the number of colony-forming units (cfu) of bacteria per millilitre and the number of bacterial species present. If the patient is asymptomatic and a Gram-negative species has been isolated, a threshold of $> 10^5$ cfu/ml is generally used. When symptoms of UTI are present, the number may be much lower than that and yet still significant. Lower numbers may also be significant in Gram-positive infections. Accurate determination of numbers is therefore important and is usually achieved by culture of a known volume of urine, followed by colony count. Contamination of the specimen is indicated by very low counts of organisms, mixed species or the presence of epithelial cells.

Pyuria may be recorded in the absence of bacterial growth. The reasons include antibiotic treatment prior to specimen collection and infection with organisms that do not grow on routine media for urine culture, e.g. mycobacteria, mycoplasma, nutritionally variant bacteria and anaerobic bacteria. Antibiotic use and the presence of these other microbial species can be detected by additional laboratory tests.

9.3 Management

Chemotherapy

No single agent can be recommended for treatment of UTI on account of the range of potential pathogens and the prevalence of antibiotic resistance amongst them. The choice of agent should be based on knowledge of local susceptibility data and can be changed if the causal organism turns out to be resistant. There are several agents used only for treatment of uncomplicated lower UTI, which are therefore less likely to promote antibiotic resistance. These include

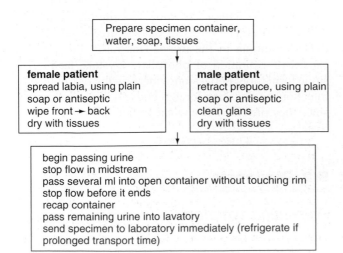

Fig. 13 Collection of a midstream specimen of urine (MSU).

nitrofurantoin, nalidixic acid and trimethoprim. None of these is suitable in early pregnancy, when a β-lactam such as ampicillin or a cephalosporin should be used instead. Resistance to ampicillin and related antibiotics is common. Patients with an indwelling urinary catheter or a physically abnormal urinary tract are unlikely to eradicate organisms causing UTI, despite antibiotic treatment.

Prevention

Some women find that emptying the urinary bladder immediately after sexual intercourse helps to prevent UTI. Urinary catheterisation or instrumentation of the urinary tract should be avoided if at all possible. It should not be performed to diagnose lower UTI and, where essential, should be performed as a strictly aseptic procedure.

9.4 Diseases and syndromes

Learning objectives

You should:

- know the major infections of the urinary tract
- understand the factors contributing to their occurrence
- know the basis of their clinical management.

The main infective diseases are listed in Table 14.

Cystitis

Cystitis is an infection of the urinary bladder, usually limited to the bladder epithelium. It is more common in females than males throughout life and is most common in young adult women. The causal species are members of the perineal skin and enteric flora. *E. coli* is the single commonest species. Other common causes of cystitis include *Staphylococcus saprophyticus*, other Entero-

bacteriaceae and, less commonly, *Staphylococcus aureus* and *Candida albicans* (the last often associated with diabetes mellitus). The principal pathogenicity feature of species associated with cystitis is the ability to adhere to bladder epithelial cells.

Dysuria and urinary frequency are the main clinical features of cystitis. These and urgency are the result of irritation of the bladder mucosa by inflammation. Vaginitis caused by *Trichomonas* sp., *Mycoplasma* sp. or anaerobic bacteria may cause similar symptoms.

Laboratory diagnosis is by microscopy and culture of an MSU. The peak of bacteriuria precedes the peak urinary leucocyte count. The criteria used to judge the significance of urinary isolates are reviewed in Clinical diagnosis. The methods used are only semiquantitative and therefore have a margin of error. If there is any doubt about the relevance of laboratory isolates, it is often worthwhile repeating the urine culture, with further advice to the patient about specimen collection.

Management

Treatment is usually commenced before laboratory results are available, the choice being based on local susceptibility data. The results of susceptibility tests should be available by 48 hours from the time the specimen arrives in the laboratory. Some laboratories report the results of urine culture after 24 hours if MSU specimens with significant pyuria are subjected to immediate antibiotic testing. It is wise to enquire whether adult women might be pregnant, as this will affect antibiotic choice. For uncomplicated cystitis, a 1- or 3-day course of antibiotic treatment is recommended. The results of treatment for longer periods are no better. Adult women presenting with their first episode of dysuria and frequency can be treated successfully with a single dose of an appropriate urinary antibiotic. If there is any doubt about the presence of complicating factors, or extension of infection to the upper urinary tract, a longer course of treatment should be started. The distinction between lower and upper UTI is particularly difficult to make in children, who should be given a longer course of treatment and investigated for underlying causes (see Ch. 16). Patients with cystitis should be advised to take one of their doses of antibiotics at bedtime to ensure high

Table 14 Infective diseases of the urinary tract

Infection	Occurrence	Features
Urethral syndrome	Common	Symptoms of cystitis but no positive bacterial culture
Asymptomatic bacteriuria	Common	Should be treated in pregnant women and before urological procedures
Cystitis	Uncommon	Infection of bladder, usually epithelium; dysuria, urinary frequence
Pyelonephritis	Uncommon	Infection of kidney, often of parenchyma; flank pain, renal tenderness, fever
Perinephric abscess	Uncommon	Pus under the renal capsule but above the medulla; fever, loin pain
Prostatitis	Uncommon	Inflammation of prostate gland; similar symptoms to pyelonephritis
Genitourinary tuberculosis	Uncommon	Usually a postprimary spread; sterile pyuria or asymptomatic

levels in residual bladder urine overnight. They should also be advised to empty the bladder just before going to bed. A high fluid intake should be recommended during the day to increase the flushing effect of urine flow.

Cystitis may relapse or recur. Relapse usually occurs shortly after the end of treatment, is caused by the same species or strain and results from antibiotic resistance, poor compliance, extension of infection to the upper urinary tract, bladder stones, diverticulae or similar factors. Recurrence may occur any time after completion of treatment and is usually caused by different organisms. Precipitating factors amenable to medical intervention are much less common.

Pyelonephritis

Pyelonephritis is an infection of the kidney, often involving the renal parenchyma. Infection of the upper urinary tract usually follows extension from the bladder via the ureters. More rarely it is caused by haematogenous spread. The species commonly isolated in pyelonephritis are *E. coli*, other Enterobacteriaceae and *S. aureus*. Host factors that contribute to the pathogenesis of pyelonephritis include indwelling urinary catheter, neurological diseases, renal stones, ureteric reflux and pregnancy. Bacterial factors implicated in pathogenesis include P-pili.

Diagnosis
Patients may have dysuria and frequency and no other features of UTI despite bacterial invasion of the renal parenchyma ('subclinical' pyelonephritis). Renal involvement is usually evident as flank pain, renal tenderness and fever. There is a high incidence of bacteraemia in these patients.

Laboratory diagnosis is by urine microscopy and culture. The laboratory should be informed that pyelonephritis or upper UTI is suspected, so that low bacterial counts are not dismissed as insignificant. White cell casts should be searched for in a centrifuged urine deposit. Peripheral blood should be collected for culture. Localisation studies are sometimes performed to help to distinguish between lower and upper UTI. In practice, many clinicians rely on the response to initial treatment. The most reliable method is cystoscopy with selective sampling from the bladder and from each ureter. Imaging techniques such as ultrasound scan and intravenous urogram may help here.

Management
Treatment for 2 weeks with a bactericidal antibiotic should be sufficient for uncomplicated pyelonephritis, providing that the initial management is in hospital. Complicated infection (e.g. with renal stones or other underlying host factors) requires a longer course of antibiotics. The underlying urinary tract pathology will also require correction.

Perinephric abscess

A perinephric abscess is a collection of pus located underneath the renal capsule, but external to the renal medulla. Infection is caused most often by *S. aureus*, but other bacteria (e.g. the Enterobacteriaceae) and yeasts such as *C. albicans* may be implicated.

Diagnosis
The clinical picture is similar to that of acute pyelonephritis, with fever and loin pain. Urine cultures are usually negative but should still be performed to help to exclude pyelonephritis. Blood culture should be performed as a matter of course. Ideally pus should be obtained from the abscess by needle aspiration, but this may not always be possible. Drainage of the collection of pus helps to accelerate resolution of the infection.

Management
Presumptive treatment is with antistaphylococcal antibiotics such as flucloxacillin. Modification to the treatment regimen may be required when the results of culture and susceptibility tests become available.

Prostatitis

Prostatitis is an inflammation of the prostate gland, either acute (usually infective) or chronic (usually non-infective). A variety of bacterial species can cause prostatitis, often without obvious predisposing factors. These are the same range of organisms that cause lower UTI: *E. coli*, *Enterococcus faecalis*, *S. aureus*, and possibly *Corynebacterium* spp., etc. The symptoms of acute prostatitis overlap with those of pyelonephritis, but some patients also have perineal pain after sitting.

Establishing a specific bacteriological diagnosis can be difficult. Laboratory-based localisation tests (e.g. coating bacteria with anti-human fluorescent antibody) are insufficiently specific. The best method of collecting a specimen for bacterial culture is to obtain the first few millilitres of urine passed, an MSU and, finally, urine passed after prostatic massage. This procedure is rarely performed.

The penetration of many antibiotics into prostatic tissue is poor. Oral agents that appear to achieve satisfactory levels in the prostate include trimethoprim and ciprofloxacin.

Genitourinary tuberculosis

Extrapulmonary tuberculosis may cause damage to structures in the genitourinary tract, particularly the kidney, but spread to other structures in the genitourinary tract may follow. Infection is usually post-primary disease caused by *Mycobacterium tuberculosis* and is often insidious in onset. It is more common in Asian populations.

Diagnosis

Renal tuberculosis often presents as sterile pyuria but may, if chronic, be discovered incidentally by abdominal X-ray. To obtain laboratory confirmation of renal tuberculosis, three consecutive early morning urine collections should be made. These can be processed in the diagnostic laboratory to suppress faster growing commensal bacteria and then cultured for mycobacteria on Lowenstein–Jensen medium or similar medium. Acid-fast stain is of limited value because commensal mycobacteria are often present in the distal urethra and on the perineum. Tuberculosis of other sites in the genito-urinary tract is often diagnosed histologically in biopsy material. A thorough search should be initiated for tuberculous foci elsewhere in the body, particularly in the lungs.

Management

Treatment is with a combination of antituberculous agents under expert supervision for a prolonged period, according to local protocols. Prevention is with BCG (bacille Calmette–Guérin) vaccination in childhood and by tracing and treating the contacts of new cases.

Urethral syndrome (abacterial cystitis)

Urethral syndrome affects adult women; there are symptoms of cystitis but no positive bacterial culture. The microbial cause is usually not known, even after detailed investigation. Some cases are caused by chlamydias, trichomonas or mycoplasmas arising from genital infection.

Antibiotic treatment usually has no beneficial effect, but some authorities recommend a short trial of anti-microbial chemotherapy.

Asymptomatic bacteriuria

By definition, asymptomatic bacteriuria is detected only incidentally in most cases and has no accompanying pyuria. It is common in the elderly. It may represent the early stages of UTI in some cases, but studies have shown that it is unlikely to be the cause of chronic renal damage and usually does not require antibiotic treatment.

However, during pregnancy, asymptomatic bacteriuria may progress to pyelonephritis and can cause intrauterine growth retardation or even precipitate premature labour. Treatment is, therefore, recommended in pregnant women. The possible risk of introducing infection further up the urinary tract or of causing bacteraemia means that treatment of asymptomatic bacteriuria prior to urological instrumentation is prudent.

9.5 Organisms

A checklist of the organisms discussed in this chapter is given in Box 4. Further information is given on the pages indicated.

Box 4 Organisms that infect the urinary tract

Bacteria	see page	Fungi	see page
Corynebacterium spp.	246–7	*Candida* spp.	269
Escherichia coli	248		
Klebsiella spp.	248	**Parasites**	
Proteus spp.	249	*Trichomonas* sp.	265
Pseudomonas aeruginosa	249–50		
Enterococcus faecalis	245		
Staphylococcus saprophyticus	243		
Staphylococcus aureus	243		
Mycoplasma sp.	254–5		
Chlamydia sp.	255		

Self-assessment: questions

Multiple choice questions

1. The major defences of the urinary tract against infection include:
   a. Urethral gland secretions
   b. Local phagocytic cells
   c. Urine flow
   d. Colonisation resistance
   e. The vesicourethral sphincter

2. Entry of microbial pathogens into the urinary tract:
   a. Is most often via the bloodstream
   b. Is often from around the urethral meatus
   c. In females, is assisted by sexual intercourse
   d. Is more likely when a urinary catheter is present
   e. Is more common in males

3. The following factors increase the risk of infection by interfering with urine flow:
   a. Anomalous ureter
   b. Neurogenic bladder
   c. Prostatic hypertrophy
   d. Indwelling catheter
   e. Contraceptive diaphragm

4. In community-acquired UTI, *Escherichia coli*:
   a. Causes stone formation through urease activity
   b. Is the most common cause of infection
   c. Is usually sensitive to orally active antibiotics
   d. Is often ampicillin resistant
   e. Does not cause pyelonephritis

5. When collecting a urine specimen for culture:
   a. The patient should avoid contact between the perineum and the container
   b. A urinary catheter is a good collection method
   c. The first few drops of urine must be collected
   d. The area around the urethral meatus should first be cleaned
   e. The preferred specimen is a midstream urine sample

6. The following methods are used to prevent deterioration of urine specimens during transport to the laboratory:
   a. Borate crystals
   b. Refrigeration
   c. Early morning specimen collection
   d. Immediate processing
   e. Incubation in transit

7. The number of bacteria per mililitre of urine in a midstream specimen (MSU) is:
   a. Raised prior to significant pyuria in UTI
   b. Used as an indicator of UTI
   c. Usually $>10^3$/ml in cystitis
   d. The only factor used to assess the significance of culture results
   e. Often $<10^5$/ml in staphylococcal UTI

8. Pyelonephritis is:
   a. Easily distinguished from cystitis
   b. An infection that carries significant risk of septicaemia
   c. Always associated with a urine bacterial count of $>10^5$/ml
   d. A recognised complication of cystitis
   e. Best treated with an antibiotic such as nitrofurantoin

9. Acute prostatitis:
   a. Is usually caused by bacteria
   b. Typically causes pain on standing up
   c. Can be diagnosed easily using standard laboratory methods
   d. Is usually caused by the same species that cause other UTIs
   e. Is best treated with a β-lactam antibiotic

10. Tuberculosis of the urogenital tract:
    a. Usually presents shortly after onset of the disease
    b. Most commonly affects the kidney
    c. May spread to any structure in the urogenital tract
    d. Is very uncommon in Asian people
    e. May be accidentally diagnosed on abdominal X-ray

Case history questions

History 1

A 29-year-old woman visited her GP complaining of a burning sensation when passing urine, which was more frequent than usual. The GP chose to wait for the results of urine culture before prescribing any antibiotics. When the culture showed no bacterial growth, the GP called the woman back and gave her a short course of trimethoprim, after arranging for further tests.

1. What is the woman's condition called?
2. Why did the GP prescribe an antibiotic?
3. What other tests were arranged on the second visit?

History 2

A 21-year-old female medical student was admitted to hospital with a fever and loin pain. After obtaining diagnostic cultures, the house officer prescribed empirical antibiotics and ordered her to drink 3 litres of water in the next 24 hours. Shortly after this, the student experienced severe pain radiating into the groin. An X-ray was hurriedly arranged. After seeing the student on his ward round the next morning, the consultant remarked on the length of antibiotic treatment required.

1. What is the infection?
2. What is the most likely causal pathogen?
3. Can you explain the sudden onset of pain?
4. What do you think the radiograph showed?
5. How long did the consultant want treatment to continue?

Data interpretation

A midstream urine specimen from a 79-year-old woman with urinary frequency gave the following interim results.

Microscopy:
—leucocytes >10–$20/\mu L$ ($< 100/\mu L$)
—epithelial cells   ++
—Gram stain   Gram-positive cocci, Gram-negative bacilli

Culture: mixed bacteria including *Enterococcus faecalis*, coagulase-negative staphylococci and *Escherichia coli*.

Antibiotic susceptibilities were to follow.

1. What is the most likely explanation for this result?
2. What action would you take?
3. In what circumstances might this culture result require further investigation?

Objective structured clinical examination (OSCE)

A 64-year-old man became febrile while on the urology day case ward. He had a feeling of wanting to pass urine but was unable to manage even a drop. He complained of pain in his lower abdomen, and a tender central mass was found rising out of the pelvis behind the symphysis pubis. Rectal examination suggested an enlarged prostate. A urinary catheter was passed using standard aseptic technique and a specimen of the urine sent for analysis. A blood culture was then collected.

You are asked the following questions.

1. Which was more likely: (a) systemic infection led to urinary retention or (b) urinary tract infection led to fever?
2. Are these events most likely to have been triggered by a prostatic abscess?
3. Will the results of laboratory urine analysis influence your choice of antibiotic?
4. Are the results of blood culture likely to influence your choice of antibiotic?
5. Does this patient requires urgent urological instrumentation?

Short notes questions

Write short notes on the following:

1. The factors that contribute to the pathogenesis of urinary tract infection
2. The reason for the development of signs and symptoms in urinary tract infection
3. The management of cystitis
4. Relapsing and recurrent urinary tract infection

Viva questions

1. What is meant by 'pre-analytical problems' with laboratory investigation of UTI?
2. It has been said that little can be done to prevent UTI. Do you share this view?

Self-assessment: answers

Multiple choice answers

1. a. **False**. Urethral secretions only play a small role.
   b. **False**. Local phagocytes only play a small role.
   c. **True**. This helps to flush organisms out of the system.
   d. **False**. Above the distal urethra there is no significant resident flora to provide 'colonisation resistance'.
   e. **False**. The sphincter regulates bladder emptying but does not prevent infection.

2. a. **False**. The most common route of entry is the 'ascending' route.
   b. **True**. Often with enteric organisms.
   c. **True**. Celibate women experience fewer episodes of infection.
   d. **True**. Indwelling catheters provide a permanent portal of entry and act as a nidus for infection.
   e. **False**. Since UTI is less common in males of all ages, it can be inferred that microbial entry is also less common.

3. a. **True**.
   b. **True**.
   c. **True**.
   d. **False**. Urinary catheters allow constant bladder drainage. They increase the risk of infection by providing a route for microbial access and by acting as a nidus of infection within the bladder.
   e. **True**.

4. a. **False**. It is *Proteus* sp. that produce a urease and assist stone formation.
   b. **True**. Some strains have pili that allow the organisms to adhere to the urinary epithelial cells.
   c. **True**.
   d. **True**. This is relatively common.
   e. **False**. *E. coli* is a common cause of pyelonephritis.

5. a. **True**. To prevent contamination.
   b. **False**. Catheterisation purely for specimen collection should be avoided since it will increase the risk of UTI.
   c. **False**. The first few drops of specimen should be discarded to avoid contamination with the urethral flora.
   d. **True**. The meatus is a source of organisms.
   e. **True**. This is referred to as an MSU.

6. a. **True**. Often used in samples from general practice.
   b. **True**. Although some cell lysis occurs even at lower temperatures.
   c. **False**. Early morning specimens are for diagnosis of genitourinary tuberculosis.
   d. **True**. Rapid transit and immediate processing are best practice.
   e. **False**. Incubation in transit would accelerate the deterioration of cellular contents of urine specimens.

7. a. **True**. However, pyuria can be recorded in the absence of bacterial growth.
   b. **True**.
   c. **False**. Counts are usually $>10^5$/ml in cystitis, but counts as low as 10^3/ml may be considered significant if there are symptoms.
   d. **False**. Other factors taken into consideration include the results of previous culture, presence of epithelial cells, pyuria and the number of bacterial species present.
   e. **True**. When symptoms of a UTI are present.

8. a. **False**. Localisation tests may be needed to distinguish these; it is often difficult.
   b. **True**. There is flank pain and renal tenderness.
   c. **False**. The bacterial count in pyelonephritis may be less than 10^5/ml, so the laboratory will need informing.
   d. **True**. It usually follows spread from the bladder.
   e. **False**. Nitrofurantoin is a urinary antiseptic and is unsuitable for infections involving the kidney.

9. a. **True**. It is chronic prostatitis that is usually non-infective.
   b. **True**. There may also be perineal pain after sitting.
   c. **False**. Prostatitis may be difficult to diagnose and cultures may be helpful.
   d. **True**. *Escherichia coli, Enterococcus faecalis, Staphylococcus aureus*, etc.
   e. **False**. The antibiotic chosen needs to penetrate the prostate gland, e.g. trimethoprim or a quinolone.

10. a. **False**. Genitourinary tuberculosis usually has a chronic presentation.
    b. **True**. The kidney is usually the initial site in the urogenital tract to be infected.
    c. **True**.

d. **False**. It is more common in Asian peoples than in many other population groups.
e. **True**.

Case history answers

History 1

1. A bacterial cystitis, or 'urethral syndrome'.
2. Antibiotics are usually ineffective, but some authorities recommend a trial of a short course.
3. Culture for mycoplasma, chlamydia and trichomonas and other difficult-to-cultivate causes of cystitis.

History 2

1. Pyelonephritis.
2. *Escherichia coli*.
3. Ureteric colic caused by dislodgement of a renal stone.
4. Small stone at one of the pelviureteric junctions, ureteric entry into the pelvis or the urethral valve.
5. Since this is a complicated UTI, the consultant wanted to ensure removal of the stone and more than 2 weeks of antibiotic treatment would be needed, followed by careful repeat cultures. Pyelonephritis with ureteric obstruction carries a high risk of septicaemia.

Data interpretation answer

1. The low leucocyte count, presence of epithelial cells and mixed bacterial growth all point to contamination by perineal flora during specimen collection.
2. If the patient has not commenced antibiotic therapy and symptoms persist, a repeat specimen should be collected. The patient should be given clear, unambiguous instructions on how to collect a good quality midstream urine specimen.
3. If there was a higher leucocyte count and the epithelial cells were absent, mixed enteric bacteria such as *E. coli* and *E. faecalis* may point to a vesico-colic fistula. More detailed urological investigations would be indicated.

OSCE answer

1. (a) This sounds like urosepsis.

2. No. They are more likely to have started with benign prostatic hypertrophy, then continued as lower UTI, retention and finally systemic sepsis.
3. Yes. Gram stain of a spun urine deposit may distinguish between a Gram-negative bacillus such as *Escherichia coli* and Gram-positive cocci such as *Enterococcus faecalis* or *Staphylococcus aureus*.
4. Yes, but not until the preliminary results are available, which will be at least 5 hours but more often 24–48 hours later. You should not wait for the results before commencing therapy.
5. No. Not until the acute sepsis has been brought under control. Uncontrolled local or systemic infection significantly increase the risk of complications for urological surgery.

Short notes answers

1. Cover both host and bacterial factors. Remember to state the relative importance of each.
2. Deal with cystitis (including the 'urethral' syndrome) and pyelonephritis. Overlap between symptom complexes is worth mentioning, since it prevents easy distinction between syndromes.
3. Discuss the use of urinary antiseptics, agents for use in pregnancy, duration of treatment, non-therapeutic measures and follow-up specimens. Points of discussion include short versus longer-course treatment and the timing of follow-up specimens.
4. Could be answered in tabular format.

Viva answers

1. Collection and transport of urine specimens have a major impact on the quality of the results reported by the laboratory. Outline the issues and how they can be overcome.
2. No. Catheter-associated UTI can be prevented or delayed by use of closed urine drainage systems and aseptic technique. Postcoital UTI in women can be helped by urination immediately after intercourse. Recurrent UTI can sometimes be prevented and often suppressed by long-term, low-dose antibiotic therapy. Correction of underlying urinary tract pathology such as kidney stones, prostatic hypertrophy or bladder diverticulae will reduce the risk of secondary UTI.

10 Infections of the genital tract

Overview

Infection arises in the genital tract either as a result of sexual activity or through infection with members of the indigenous flora. These infections can be caused by different species, as either single or multiple infections. Any one sexually transmitted infection is a marker for risky behaviour that could lead to any other similarly transmitted infection. The practical difficulties of achieving an aetiological diagnosis and delivering antimicrobial chemotherapy, combined with the social context of sexually transmitted disease, make it necessary to treat most genital tract infections empirically. Infections of the female pelvis are particularly difficult to diagnose early and may lead to infertility or tubal pregnancy. Screening, contact tracing and education are all employed to reduce the risk of further spread of disease.

10.1 Pathogenesis

Learning objectives

You should:

- know the characteristics of the likely pathogens
- know the factors that make an individual susceptible to genital infections.

Numerically, most of the infections of the genital tract in both males and females are transmitted as a result of sexual intercourse, when organisms are exchanged during intimate contact. Many of these species are fastidious organisms that survive for only short periods, if at all, away from human body. Some are obligate intracellular parasites, while bacterial species such as *Neisseria gonorrhoeae* cannot survive prolonged periods away from a body surface. Infections transmitted in this way are thought to be maintained in the human population by a core group of sexually promiscuous individuals who share their diseases with less promiscuous individuals in the wider population. The risk of contracting sexually transmitted disease is therefore proportional to the number of sex partners and the amount of sexual activity, i.e. the total sexual contact previously experienced by both members of a pair. Early age of first sexual encounter is also a recognised risk factor for infection. There is thought to be an additional risk of disease if there is a pre-existing infection, which in some cases may act as a cofactor for the pathogenesis of another infection. Pathogenic bacteria may gain access to the upper female genital tract via the tail or filament of an intrauterine contraceptive device (IUD). Other contraceptive practices can alter the risk of sexually transmitted infection, either by providing a barrier to the spread of infection between partners or by altering hormonal status, which may affect susceptibility to ascending infection in women by altering the composition of cervical mucus. Women are most susceptible to gonococcal infection in the latter part of the menstrual cycle, particularly during menstruation. Some infective agents have a means of establishing themselves on epithelial surfaces: *N. gonorrhoeae* has adhesive pili that attach to receptor sites on the urethral epithelium. *Chlamydia trachomatis* initial bodies have a preference for columnar epithelium. The penetration of superficial epithelial layers by most agents of sexually transmitted disease is significantly assisted by the microtrauma caused by sexual intercourse.

Infection in the organs of the female pelvis may also arise following miscarriage, abortion, childbirth or other gynaecological procedures. In these cases, infection is usually caused by organisms present in the indigenous flora of the lower genital tract. The presence of necrotic material (e.g. products of conception), haematoma or foreign body (e.g. intrauterine device) within the uterus provides a nidus for infection, particularly with anaerobic bacteria.

10.2 Diagnosis

Learning objectives

You should:

- know the likely presenting symptoms

- know how to conduct a clinical examination

- understand what samples should be taken and what tests to request.

Clinical features

Infections of the genital tract in both sexes produce symptoms referable to the structures involved. Conditions affecting the external genitalia are the most easily detected, yet they may become extensive if the patient is reluctant to seek medical advice. The most common features of external genital infection are ulcerative or vesicular lesions. Infections of the lower genital tract may present with a discharge. Discharge is more common in males than in females, who have a much higher percentage of subclinical disease. The nature of the discharge may help in a clinical diagnosis. Inguinal lymphadenopathy may be present in a variety of conditions, and the appearance of the skin overlying the inguinal nodes may be an important clinical sign. Other symptoms that need to be asked about include the nature of any pain relating to the genital tract. This can be local, referred or more generalised. It may be brought on by sexual intercourse in females (dyspareunia). Women patients should be asked about menstrual flow and any intermenstrual bleeding, as well as the possibility of pregnancy (which may affect antibiotic choice). The intimate nature of the questions asked by the attending physician may prevent the patient providing all the relevant information, particularly during the initial stages of clinic visit. A comprehensive sexual, contraceptive and travel history should all be taken, sensitively. The patient should be encouraged to volunteer anything else that they think relevant before the end of the visit.

The clinical examination should be done under optimal conditions, with an assistant present and all the materials required for specimen collection to hand. A systematic examination of the external genitalia, the lower and upper genital tract should be performed, since any one sexually transmitted infection is an indicator of risky behaviour that could have led to a second or coinfection. If sexually transmitted infection is possible, all other body sites involved in sexual contact should also be sampled, e.g. oropharynx and rectum. Bimanual examination of the pelvic organs should be performed routinely in women with suspected pelvic infection.

Laboratory tests

Genital ulcers or vesiculating lesions that might be caused by bacterial infection should be microscopically examined for causal pathogens by Gram stain and dark ground microscopy. Viral infections of the external genitalia can often be diagnosed by their macroscopic appearance, but sometimes diagnostic specimens are required to confirm the aetiological diagnosis. Purulent genital discharge should be cultured and, from male patients, Gram stained. Samples of a genital discharge can be examined under the microscope in the clinic. In male patients with no significance discharge, specimens may have to be obtained with a fine Dacron swab inserted into the distal urethra. In female patients, the swab should be inserted into the uterine cervix only after a vaginal speculum has been passed and vaginal secretions cleaned from the external os with large cotton swabs. Swab specimens taken for culture of *N. gonorrhoeae* should either be used to inoculate agar plates in the clinic or be put into a suitable transport medium (e.g. Stuart's) and sent to the laboratory immediately. Swabs for *C. trachomatis* should be placed directly into chlamydia transport medium, if cell culture is to be attempted. Direct fluorescent antigen detection is also available.

Laparoscopy is the best means of obtaining microbiological specimens from women with pelvic inflammatory disease. Other methods are less satisfactory and prone to contamination with organisms from the lower genital tract. Patients with pelvic inflammatory disease and fever should have blood cultures taken.

10.3 Management

Learning objectives

You should:

- understand the significance of resistance and coinfection in response to therapy

- be aware of the potential for patients to fail to follow therapy

- understand primary and secondary preventive measures.

Chemotherapy

The antibiotic treatment of genital infections used to be much simpler: there were fewer diseases, fewer pathogens, antibiotic resistance was not a significant issue and the importance of compliance was little appreciated. All of these factors have now conspired to make the treatment of genital infection much more complex. It is true that treatment regimens can still be worked out for some of the more clearcut clinical syndromes, but the recognition of the potential for more than one pathogen to cause the same clinical picture, and for more than one infection to coexist in the same patients, means that it is often impossible to rely on a single antimicrobial agent. Antibiotic resistance has become a significant factor in some of the more common genital infections. *N. gonorrhoeae*, for instance, became resistant to the sulphonamides not long after their introduction. It took the same species longer to develop resistance to penicillin, first by a stepwise increase in minimum inhibitory concentration and then by the acquisition of transferrable (plasmid-carried) penicillinase-mediated resistance. This species has now acquired resistance to a more recently introduced group of antibiotics, the quinolones. Not all instances of treatment failure in genital infection result from antibiotic resistance. Some are caused by coinfection with another infective agent, e.g. *C. trachomatis*, which necessitates use of a second antibiotic. But perhaps the greatest challenge in treating genital infections is the wide variation from the therapy recommended and prescribed by the physician. A high proportion of patients cease taking their medication as soon as symptoms subside, and then may even sell the remaining medicines to sexual contacts who were more reluctant to seek proper treatment. Some abscond and are lost to the formal follow-up that is so important to ensure the success of therapy. In parts of the developing world where sexually transmitted infections are very common, there may be no formal health-care involvement in the provision of antimicrobial chemotherapy.

Prevention

Genital infection caused by sexually transmitted pathogens can be most effectively prevented by sexual abstinence, or by monogamous relationships. It is precisely because adolescents and young adults are less likely to form this type of relationship that they are at much greater risk of sexually transmitted infection, yet prove resistant to traditional approaches to disease control. Barrier methods of contraception therefore need emphasis as a fall-back preventive strategy. Condoms can be effective when employed properly, which entails ease of access and familiarity with the method of application. The above are examples of primary prevention. Prevention of secondary infection relies on screening of high-risk populations and contact tracing, followed by properly supervised treatment and patient education. The populations consistently shown to exhibit the most risky behaviour are the older teenage/younger adult group, homosexual/bisexual men, prostitutes and, in developing countries, adult males. Health education resources have been targeted at these populations with variable effect. Heterosexual individuals have shown little inclination to reduce their level of risk, while male homosexuals have substantially modified their sexual behaviour, though there is some concern that safe sex practices may be on the wane.

Non-sexually transmitted genital infections in women can be prevented in some cases by high standards of hospital hygiene. Ensuring that products of conception or haematomas are not left in utero after delivery and gynaecological procedures will also help to reduce the risk of uterine infection.

10.4 Diseases and syndromes

Learning objectives

You should:

- know the major infections of the genital tract
- know the factors contributing to their occurrence
- know the basis of their clinical management.

The main infective diseases are listed in Table 15. Although the acquired immunodeficiency syndrome (AIDS) and other sequelae of infection with the human immunodeficiency virus (HIV) are transmitted sexually in many, the presenting features of these conditions are usually found in other organ systems. For this reason, AIDS is considered in Chapter 17, Infections in immunocompromised patients.

Genital herpes

Genital herpes is a painful, vesiculating infection of the external genitalia and lower genital tract caused by herpes simplex virus types I and II, for which humans are the only reservoir. Transmission is via intimate contact, with transfer of virus in secretions either into sites of microscopic trauma or where the epithelium is altered by disease. Herpes simplex virus infects squamous epithelial cells and forms an intranuclear inclusion body. This is followed by formation of giant cells and cytolysis. Oedema gathers locally to cause vesiculation. On dry surfaces, these will eventually crust over, but on moist surfaces, vesicles become macerated, lose their tops and become painful, inflamed ulcers. During a first attack, lesions may last between 2 and 4 weeks, with new lesions formed during this time. There may be systemic symptoms, including fever and myalgia, and a high proportion also have a painful urethritis. The lesions may spread from the external genitalia to nearby structures including the thigh, perianally and into the

Table 15 Diseases of the genital tract

Infection	Occurrence	Features
Genital herpes	Common	Painful vesiculating infection of the external genitalia and lower genital tract
Genital warts	Common	Papillomata on external genitalia or perianal area
Urethral discharge in males	Common	Purulent discharge
Vaginal discharge	Common; infective and non-infective causes	Type of discharge is indicative of cause
Cervicitis	Diagnosis often delayed	Inflammation of the uterine cervix
Pelvic inflammatory disease	Diagnosis often delayed	Acute often with fever; non-specific features
Epididymitis	Diagnosis often delayed	Tender epididymis to palpation, local pain, may be urethritis-type features
Early syphilis	Sexually transmitted	Initial painless papule followed by painless ulcer/chancre; secondary syphilis involves symmetrical, erythematous, maculopapular rash and erosive lesions spreading over body; late manifestations are gummas or neurosyphilis
Chancroid	Sexually transmitted; rare in Europe, USA	Ulceration of external genitalia
Lymphogranuloma venereum	Sexually transmitted	Lymphadenopathy
Granuloma inguinale	Sexually transmitted in Asia, Caribbean	Painless papule that enlarges; pseudobuboes and inguinal lymphadenopathy can occur
Intrauterine infection	Uncommon; postpartum or postabortion	Offensive lochia, fever
Scabies	Intimate contact	Infestation of mite in burrows causes irritation
Pubic lice	Sexual contact	Irritating infestation of lice on pubic hairs

vagina. Female patients usually have a more severe form of the condition. Women may also shed the virus from the cervix for several weeks after symptoms subside.

The virus is able to persist in latent form in sacral sensory nerve ganglia, from where it may cause recurrent infections whenever restricting factors are removed, e.g. during severe illness, immune compromise, pregnancy or emotional stress. Recurrent attacks last 1 to 2 weeks and are often less severe, but viral shedding and infection of the partner still occur. The majority of primary infections will be followed by at least one recurrence in the ensuing year.

Diagnosis

The diagnosis is usually suspected on clinical grounds. The diagnosis can be confirmed by viral culture, or nucleic acid amplification (polymerase chain reaction). Alternatively, material from vesicles can be stained using the Giemsa method and examined microscopically for giant cells with intranuclear inclusion bodies (the Tzanck smear).

Control

No therapy prevents the development of viral latency, and available treatments are of little benefit to most people with recurrent infection. When treatment is required, the agent used is aciclovir. Topical creams have a limited effect during a primary attack and must be applied carefully to avoid autoinoculation and secondary infection. Given orally, the drug can reduce the duration of an acute attack and does reduce viral shed-

ding, but it must be given continually to prevent recurrent attacks. Intravenous aciclovir is effective at reducing viral shedding and shortening acute primary attacks, but this treatment requires hospital admission. Currently, severe first attacks are best treated by hospital admission for intravenous treatment. Recurrent attacks can be managed by continuous oral therapy if particularly troublesome, but withdrawal of treatment may result in severe recurrence. Antiviral resistance is increasingly recognised, particularly in immunocompromised patients. No vaccine is currently available.

Genital warts

External genital or perianal papillomata are caused by the human papillomavirus (HPV). HPV can be transmitted during sexual intercourse but presumably also requires inoculation into squamous epithelium in association with minor trauma. Genital warts are noticed by most patients because of their nuisance value. They may produce exuberant papillomatous growth (the exophytic variety) or take on a more flattened appearance. Sometimes there is also pruritus and a local burning sensation. The differential diagnosis includes condyloma latum, molluscum contagiosum and skin tags. In recent years, genital warts have received much attention as a precursor to squamous carcinoma, particularly of the uterine cervix.

Viral DNA from HPV types 16 and 18 has been demonstrated in cancerous cervical tissue. It is thought that malignant transformation is caused by deregulation of epithelial cell DNA, following viral integration. Not all 57 types of HPV are associated with cervical dysplasia, intraepithelial carcinoma or overt malignancy. Not all infections with higher-risk HPV types lead to carcinoma. However, the cofactors involved in the progress from initial HPV infection to cervical cancer (which may take up to 20 years) have not been fully identified. Other genital infections may increase the probability of malignant transformation. Genital warts should not be dismissed as a trivial condition in either male or female patients.

Diagnosis

The diagnosis is mainly by recognition of their macroscopic appearance, if present on the external genitalia. Cervical warts are more difficult to detect but can be seen more easily if acetic acid solution is painted over the cervical surface. Warts will become white with this treatment; the 'acetowhite' reaction.

Control

The traditional treatment has been to paint podophyllin on the lesions once a week for 5 weeks as a local cytotoxic agent. This is less effective than trichloroacetic acid solution. Some warts are very refractory to treatment and require ablation with cryotherapy, electrocautery or laser treatment. Patients with genital warts should be encouraged to abstain from intercourse and ask their partner to seek treatment. No vaccine is available yet.

Syphilis

Syphilis is caused by *Treponema pallidum*. It can occur up to 1 year after infection and has primary, secondary and latent stages (Table 16).

Infection is spread by sexual or other mucosal contact (congenital syphilis, see Ch. 14). The bacterium enters the tissues via microscopic trauma and reaches other parts of the body via the bloodstream. A painless papule appears at the site of primary inoculation after 2 to 3 weeks. This rapidly breaks down to form a painless ulcer or chancre, which has a slightly indurated margin. The spirochaete *T. pallidum* can be found in exudate from the chancre during this time. Chancres may be small and can go unrecognised especially by homosexual men and by women patients. The main alternative diagnosis is chancroid, which tends to be painful and often has a more prominent margin. The chancre heals spontaneously and at about the same time lesions of secondary syphilis appear. These include a symmetrical, erythematous, maculopapular rash that starts centrally and spreads to palms and soles; superficial erosions appear on apposed external body surfaces (perianal, vulvar, axillary, etc.); grey erosions appear on mucosal surfaces (called condyloma latum) and a folliculitis occurs that can result in hair loss. The erosive lesions and rash contain spirochaetes and are infectious. Non-specific systemic symptoms are common during secondary syphilis. After secondary syphilis, the disease becomes latent until years to decades later, when late manifestations (e.g. gummas or neurosyphilis), referred to as tertiary syphilis, occur in around 25% of untreated patients (see Ch. 19).

Diagnosis

Clinical diagnosis may be difficult, particularly during the secondary stage of the disease. If a primary chancre is noticed, diagnosis can be confirmed by darkground microscopy for spirochaetes. *T. pallidum* cannot be grown in the laboratory and, in the early stages of primary syphilis, serological tests may be negative. During secondary syphilis, both the group-specific tests (e.g. VDRL (Venereal Disease Research Laboratory)) and specific treponemal tests (e.g. FTA (fluorescent treponemal antibody)) will be positive in all cases. Exudate from erosive lesions should also be examined by darkground microscopy for detection of spirochaetes.

Control

Treatment is with a single intramuscular dose of a benzathine penicillin (alternative treatment is tetracycline or erythromycin), and follow-up serology (VDRL) should be performed at 1, 3, 6 and 12 months. A positive syphilis serological test should prompt the physician to consider HIV serology. Syphilis is a notifiable disease in many countries, and all contacts should be traced for screening and for treatment if required.

Table 16 Syphilis

Stage	Lesion	Laboratory diagnosis
Primary	Chancre	Darkground microscopy of exudate
Secondary	Maculopapular rash	Serological tests: TPHA usually positive; VDRL raised
Tertiary	Aortic aneurysm, neurosyphilis, gummas	Serological tests: FTA-Abs positive; TPHA, VDRL may be negative

TPHA, *Treponema pallidum* haemagglutination; VDRL, Venereal Disease Research Laboratory test; FTA, Fluorescent treponemal antibody, absorbed test.

Chancroid

Chancroid is an ulcerative condition of the external genitalia caused by *Haemophilus ducreyi* infection. This sexually transmitted disease is rare in Europe and North America but is common in tropical countries. The causal organism, *H. ducreyi*, has an uncertain relationship to other organisms in the genus. The initial lesion is a papule, which breaks down to form a painful ulcer with a heaped-up, inflamed edge. Far more males develop chancroid than females. The most common sites are on the penis—the coronal sulcus, the glans and the shaft—but lesions also occur on the thighs adjacent to penile lesions. There may also be painful inguinal lymphadenopathy.

Diagnosis
Gram stain and culture of exudate from the ulcer base forms the basis of diagnosis. The typical appearance of *H. ducreyi* is chains of Gram-negative bacilli ('streptobacilli'), which have been described as 'schools of fish'. No single agar medium is ideal for culture, but incubation in 5% carbon dioxide at 33–34°C is recommended.

Treatment
Erythromycin, trimethoprim, ciprofloxacin and single-dose ceftriaxone have all been successfully used to treat chancroid. Secondary prevention can be achieved by screening and treatment, particularly of commercial sex workers.

Lymphogranuloma venereum

Lymphogranuloma venerum is a genital infection in which lymphadenopathy is the predominant feature. It is caused by *C. trachomatis*. The *C. trachomatis* strains responsible for this sexually transmitted infection are L1, L2, and L3; these are distinct from the serotypes that typically cause other urogenital or ocular infections. The inguinal lymph nodes enlarge, and the overlying skin becomes discoloured and wrinkled. Eventually, the skin may break down to form sinuses.

Diagnosis
The diagnosis can be confirmed by serology. Although the antigen used in the complement fixation test (CFT) is only group specific, a high titre is specific for lymphogranuloma venereum. Biopsy material or lymph node exudate can be cultured for chlamydias, when available.

Control
Treatment is with erythromycin or a sulphonamide. No vaccine is available.

Granuloma inguinale

Granuloma inguinale is a sexually transmitted infection caused by an uncultivatable Gram-negative bacterium, *Calymmatobacterium granulomatis*. This condition is prevalent in parts of Asia and the Caribbean and causes a painless papule that enlarges slowly. Inguinal lymphadenopathy is rare, but local extension can produce pseudobuboes. The diagnosis can be confirmed by Giemsa stain of a tissue smear, which reveals the black, intracellular Donovan bodies. The condition has been treated successfully with erythromycin, tetracycline, chloramphenicol and co-trimoxazole.

Urethral discharge in males

Discharge from the male urethra has many causes, but when an adult male seeks medical assistance, the cause is often urethritis caused by a sexually transmitted infection. Purulent discharge from the urethra may be caused by either *N. gonorrhoeae* or *C. trachomatis* (serotypes A–K). Although *N. gonorrhoeae* typically causes a more obviously purulent discharge, there is overlap in the clinical presentation and a high proportion of dual infection. Non-gonococcal urethritis is often referred to as 'non-specific urethritis', even though it usually has a specific cause. The patient may have dysuria, but some patients have urethritis without a clinically evident discharge.

Diagnosis
Diagnosis is by microscopy, culture and antigen detection. A Gram stain performed on a smear of purulent urethral discharge is a good means of detecting *N. gonorrhoeae*, which appear as intracellular Gram-negative diplococci. Even if bacteria are not seen, the presence of segmented neutrophils should be sought, because these provide evidence of a urethritis. A wire-mounted thin alginate swab should be inserted into the distal urethra and turned 180° to obtain epithelial cells for detection of *C. trachomatis*, which is an intracellular pathogen. These should be smeared carefully for direct fluorescent antigen testing. The swab can then be placed in chlamydia transport medium for subsequent chlamydia cell culture. PCR-based tests are now available in many centres.

Treatment and control
Patients require presumptive antimicrobial therapy while they are still in the clinic. Gonococcal urethritis can be treated with a single large dose of ampicillin combined with probenicid, if penicillinase-producing strains are uncommon. If they are prevalent locally, or if an alternative is required on account of a penicillin allergy, ceftriaxone may be considered. Otherwise, a 10-day course of erythromycin will be required. Patients with urethritis should be given simultaneous treatment for possible chlamydial infection. This requires a 7–10-day course of tetracycline. Follow-up cultures are advisable, and failure to cure urethritis fully may be the result of an

unrecognised chlamydial infection. Attempts have been made to produce a vaccine directed against gonococcal pili and thus prevent bacterial adhesion to the urethral epithelium, but these have been unsuccessful. There are no effective vaccines against the two main microbial causes of urethritis.

Vaginal discharge

A number of infective conditions may cause a vaginal discharge, but there are many non-infective causes as well. The leading infective causes include:

- candidiasis
- trichomoniasis
- bacterial vaginosis.

Cervicitis can also result in vaginal discharge. The nature of the discharge can help towards a specific aetiological diagnosis, but there is considerable overlap between clinical entities; consequently, laboratory confirmation is usually sought.

Candidiasis Vaginitis caused by the yeast *Candida albicans* is typically associated with a thick, creamy discharge and a white, curd-like inflammatory exudate. The condition is not necessarily transmitted sexually and is often associated with tight underwear, ecological disturbance resulting from antibiotic use or variation in hormonal background during particular phases of the menstrual cycle.

Trichomoniasis Vaginitis caused by the flagellated protozoan *Trichomonas vaginalis* is sexually transmitted, and the male partner is usually asymptomatic. The discharge is described as frothy, thin and offensive.

Bacterial vaginosis In bacterial vaginosis, there is a thin discharge with a distinctive odour, which the patient may well notice. The condition is caused by a disturbance in vaginal flora that results in an overgrowth of commensal anaerobic bacteria; the metabolic products of these include volatile amines, hence the smell. Species including *Gardnerella vaginalis* and *Mobiluncus* sp. have been implicated as possible causes of the condition, but isolation of these organisms does not help in the clinical management of individual patients.

Diagnosis

A sample of the discharge can be examined under the light microscope for yeasts, motile trichomonad trophozoites and the so-called 'clue-cells' (epithelial cells with adherent bacteria) that occur in bacterial vaginosis. Addition of potassium hydroxide to the specimen results in pungent odour in patients with bacterial vaginosis: called the 'whiff' test. The specimen should also be cultured for yeasts, *T. vaginalis* and *N. gonorrhoeae*.

Control

Treatment is according to laboratory findings. Candidiasis can be treated with either nystatin or an imidazole intravaginally. Failure of treatment should lead to a trial of oral therapy. Both bacterial vaginosis and trichomonad vaginitis can be treated with metronidazole. Vaginal discharge caused by gonococcal infection should be treated as cervicitis. Little can be done to prevent infective vaginitis, other than avoiding the excessive use of antibiotics and advising women prone to candidiasis to wear looser underwear.

Cervicitis

Inflammation of the uterine cervix is usually caused by sexually transmitted infection with either *N. gonorrhoeae* or *C. trachomatis*. Cervicitis is the female counterpart of urethritis in adult males. Unfortunately, it is not so easily noticed and a large proportion of cases go undiagnosed. The consequence of undiagnosed cervicitis is ascending infection of the female genital tract: endometritis, salpingitis, tubo-ovarian abscess or disseminated gonococcal infection (DGI). The most important non-infective sequelae include infertility or, if the fallopian tubes remain patent, an increased risk of tubal pregnancy.

Diagnosis

The clinical features of cervicitis include vaginal discharge in some cases, pain during sexual intercourse (dyspareunia), intermenstrual bleeding and other less specific features. Asymptomatic patients may present at the clinic because a partner has been found to have a sexually transmitted infection. Bimanual pelvic examination should be performed to help to detect ascending infection.

A vaginal speculum should be used to provide adequate access to the cervix. The mucus covering the vaginal surface of the cervix should be cleaned away with a fresh cotton swab. A sterile swab can then be used to obtain a sample for laboratory confirmation of the diagnosis, by insertion into the endocervix. A second swab should be inserted and turned to pick up epithelial cells for detection of *C. trachomatis*. There is evidence that *Mycoplasma hominis* and *Ureaplasma urealyticum* may also contribute to cervical infection. Some centres may be prepared to accept specimens for confirmation of their presence by antigen detection. Microscopy of Gram-stained cervical discharge can produce misleading results and is therefore not performed in most clinics. Coinfection with the two leading pathogens may occur at this site.

Treatment

Treatment is with ciprofloxacin or ceftriaxone, and doxycycline or azithromycin (tetracyclines should not be used if the patient might be pregnant). The patient will require advice, follow-up and screening of sexual contacts.

Pelvic inflammatory disease

Pelvic inflammatory disease (PID) is a term used to refer to infections of the female pelvic organs; it is usually sexually transmitted. Infection of the fallopian tubes, the adjacent structures and abscesses in the pouch of Douglas usually occur as a result of ascending sexually transmitted infection from the lower genital tract. *N. gonorrhoeae* and *C. trachomatis* are prominent causes of PID. However, many cases are polymicrobial and feature other species such as anaerobic bacteria, streptococci, *Mycoplasma* and *Ureaplasma* spp.

Diagnosis

The clinical features may be non-specific and the diagnosis can be missed or confused with non-infective conditions. In acute PID, the patient often has a fever and requires hospital admission. The differential diagnosis includes appendicitis, inflammatory bowel disease, tubal pregnancy and ruptured ovarian cyst. A more chronic presentation may go undiagnosed for a long time. Features that may indicate PID include lower abdominal pain, dyspareunia, irregularities of menstrual flow, tenderness to pelvic examination and palpable adnexal mass.

Focal collections should be sampled for microscopy and culture in view of the polymicrobial nature of PID, but these may be difficult to access. Any method involving an approach via the vagina is prone to contamination with regional bacterial flora. Passage of a needle via the vagina for aspiration from the pouch of Douglas (culdocentesis) is painful and similarly prone to specimen contamination. The preferred method is to obtain bacteriological specimens at laparoscopy, after which they should be transferred to the diagnostic laboratory immediately.

Treatment and control

Presumptive therapy is directed towards *N. gonorrhoeae*, *C. trachomatis*, anaerobic bacteria and streptococci. Various combinations of antibiotics are recommended such as ceftriaxone, metronidazole and doxycycline. The choice of antibiotics may have to be altered in the light of culture results. When optimal antimicrobial chemotherapy is commenced early, infection may resolve without surgical drainage. PID can theoretically be prevented by early diagnosis and treatment of cervicitis.

Intrauterine infection

Infections of the uterus are uncommon and arise in several specific settings.

Endometritis Endometritis may occur as a consequence of ascending infection with *N. gonorrhoeae* or *C. trachomatis* but is rarely diagnosed as a distinct entity. Infection may arise postpartum or postabortion, when bacteria from the vaginal flora gain access and establish an acute endometritis. This process is assisted by the presence of retained products of conception, e.g. placental remnants. Postpartum, the patient will have offensive lochia and a fever. Historically, this was often caused by *Streptococcus pyogenes*, but anaerobic and other bacteria may also be implicated. Extension of infection into the myometrium and spread via the bloodstream may develop rapidly. Blood cultures and a specimen of vaginal discharge should be collected before commencing treatment. A third-generation cephalosporin combined with metronidazole would be satisfactory empirical therapy. Many such cases turn out to be hospital-acquired infection. Postabortion infections commonly involve anaerobic bacteria, and *Clostridium perfringens* in this setting can be rapidly fatal.

Pelvic actinomycosis A more insidious intrauterine infection is pelvic actinomycosis, caused by the bacterium *Actinomyces israelii*. Infection occurs more commonly in women with IUDs and in only a small percentages of cases results in clinically evident disease. These patients may have any of the features of cervical or uterine infection. The majority of patients who come to medical attention have had actinomyces-like organisms noted on a routine cervical smear. In most cases, these are commensal organisms and do not signify active infection. Most cases of IUD-associated actinomycosis can be managed by removal of the IUD, but penicillin treatment is advised if the patient has symptoms attributable to infection.

Epididymitis

Epididymitis is an infection of the epididymis caused by a variety of bacterial species. In men under the age of 35 years, most cases of epididymitis are caused by ascending sexually transmitted infection, usually with *N. gonorrhoeae* or *C. trachomatis*. But in older men, infection is more often caused by Enterobacteriaceae, staphylococci or *Corynebacteria* spp. The epididymis is tender to palpation and there may be local pain. If the infection has arisen from ascending, sexually transmitted infection there may be clinical features of urethritis. The condition may be difficult to distinguish from testicular torsion, in which case a surgical opinion is required.

Specimens for diagnostic microbiology are difficult to obtain but may be possible by careful needle aspiration. The specimen should be taken to the laboratory immediately for microscopy and culture. Treatment is with a long-acting penicillin, or with a cephalosporin (e.g. ceftriaxone) and a tetracycline.

Scabies

Scabies is an irritating infestation of the skin with the mite *Sarcoptes scabei*. It can involve any skin surface below the neck but is usually found in the skin folds around the fingers or wrist, and the perineum, where transmission is result of intimate contact. The female mite burrows into the stratum corneum to lay her eggs, and her faeces provoke an allergic reactions, causing the irritation, which may be severe enough to cause excoriation by the patient's fingernails.

Diagnosis is made by examining the burrows with a hand lens. Sometimes the female mite can be removed for microscopic confirmation by probing with a sterile syringe needle. Treatment, which should include any contacts, is with topical application of the insecticide lin-

dane or malathion. The insecticide should be applied from the neck to the toes.

Pubic lice

The louse *Pthiris pubis* can cause an irritating infestation of the perineum. It is spread by sexual contact. Close examination may reveal adult lice or the immature stage, nits, adhering to the shaft of pubic hairs. On microscopy, the adult stage looks like a miniature crab, hence the colloquial term for the condition, 'crabs'. Treatment is with malathion or an alternative insecticide.

10.5 Organisms

A checklist of the organisms discussed in this chapter is given in Box 5. Further information is given on the pages indicated.

Box 5 Organisms that infect the genital tract

Bacteria	see page	Viruses	see page
Chlamydia trachomatis	255	Herpes simplex virus	257
Corynebacteria	246–7	Human papillomavirus	258
Neisseria gonorrhoeae	252–3	Human immunodeficiency virus	260
Mycoplasma hominis	254–5		
Ureaplasma urealyticum	254–5	**Parasites**	
Treponema pallidum	255	*Trichomonas vaginalis*	265
Haemophilus ducreyi	251		
Gardnerella vaginalis	–	**Arthropods**	
Mobiluncus spp.	–	*Sarcoptes scabei*	272
Anaerobic bacteria	247–8, 252	*Pthiris pubis*	272
Streptococcus pyogenes	244		
Streptococcus spp.	244–5		
Actinomyces israelii	247		
Fungi			
Candida albicans	269		

Self-assessment: questions

Multiple choice questions

1. The following statements describe the pathogenesis of genital tract infections:
   a. Not all genital tract infections are sexually transmitted
   b. Risk of sexually transmitted infection increases with a new sex partner
   c. Contraceptive use can increase the risk of infection
   d. Some contraceptive methods can reduce the risk of infection
   e. Increased age of first sexual encounter leads to increased risk of infection

2. The following statements describe clinical features of genital tract infection:
   a. Urethritis always causes a purulent discharge
   b. Male patients with dyspareunia probably have urethritis
   c. Only a very small proportion of patients with genital tract infections have no local symptoms
   d. Ulceration or vesiculation are common features of external genital tract infections
   e. Patients may not divulge key features of genital tract infections unless asked

3. Pair the appropriate specimen collection technique with the clinical problem:
   a. Urethritis   i. Vaginal swab
   b. Cervicitis   ii. Laparoscopic aspirate
   c. Vaginal discharge iii. Fine-tipped alginate swab
   d. Pelvic abscess   iv. Endocervical swab

4. The following methods are 100% reliable in the prevention of sexually transmitted infections:
   a. Barrier contraception
   b. Monogamous sexual relationship (by both partners)
   c. Health education
   d. Contact tracing and treatment
   e. Celibacy

5. Genital herpes is:
   a. A vesiculating infection
   b. Usually less severe in female patients
   c. Always caused by herpes simplex virus type II
   d. Typically recurrent after the first infection
   e. A condition that persists in latent form

6. Genital warts are:
   a. Caused by herpes simplex virus type II
   b. Best treated with topical podophyllin for 5 weeks
   c. Either exophytic or flat
   d. Associated with subsequent cervical dysplasia
   e. Sexually transmitted

7. The term 'early syphilis' can refer to:
   a. Latent, postsecondary disease
   b. The macular rash stage of syphilis
   c. The chancral stage
   d. The gummatous stage
   e. Neurosyphilis

8. In chancroid:
   a. The causative agent is *Haemophilus ducreyi*
   b. The initial lesion is a painful ulcer
   c. Women are more prone to the condition than men
   d. A characteristic Gram-stain appearance may help in diagnosis
   e. Erythromycin can be used for treatment

9. In lymphogranuloma venereum (LGV):
   a. The causative agent is *Chlamydia trachomatis* types A–K
   b. Infection is sexually transmitted
   c. There is pseudoinguinal lymphadenopathy
   d. Diagnosis can be confirmed by CFT (complement fixation test)
   e. Overlying skin may break down to form sinuses

10. The principal infective causes of urethral discharge in an adult male are:
    a. Herpes simplex virus type II
    b. *Trichomonas vaginalis*
    c. *Ureaplasma urealyticum*
    d. *Chlamydia trachomatis* types A–K
    e. *Neisseria gonorrhoeae*

11. Infective causes of vaginal discharge in an adult female include:
    a. *Neisseria gonorrhoeae*
    b. *Trichomonas vaginalis*
    c. *Gardnerella vaginalis*
    d. *Candida albicans*
    e. *Lactobacillus* sp.

12. Infection of the uterine cervix:
    a. Causes vaginal discharge in some cases
    b. May lead to salpingitis, and tubo-ovarian abscess
    c. Causes infertility only rarely
    d. Causes asymptomatic disease in a high proportion of cases

e. Women to be a major reservoir of gonococcal disease

13. The following species are commonly isolated from women with pelvic inflammatory disease (PID):
   a. *Neisseria gonorrhoeae*
   b. Obligate anaerobic bacteria
   c. *Chlamydia trachomatis*
   d. Streptococci
   e. *Streptococcus pyogenes*

14. Postpartum endometritis:
   a. Can be caused by *Streptococcus pyogenes*
   b. Is more often caused by *Neisseria gonorrhoeae*
   c. Rarely causes a fever in the first 48 hours after delivery
   d. Can be hospital acquired
   e. May extend into the myometrium

15. The following statements about epididymitis are correct:
   a. It is usually a sexually transmitted disease in young adults
   b. It may be caused by Enterobacteriaceae
   c. The affected epididymis is tender
   d. It may be confused with testicular torsion
   e. Tetracyclines have no place in the treatment of epididymitis

16. In scabies:
   a. The clinical features are caused by the louse *Pthiris pubis*
   b. Local irritation can be severe
   c. Male and female lice can be found in burrows in the skin
   d. Other potential sites of infestation include skin around the wrist and fingers
   e. Insecticide application in the affected area is sufficient to eradicate infestation

Case history questions

History 1

An 18-year-old student said that he had been treated for gonorrhoea by his GP 2 weeks ago but complained of dysuria and a urethral discharge in spite of finishing the course of tablets his GP had given him. On examination, a small amount of almost clear fluid was expressed from the patient's urethra.

1. What explanations can you give for the persistent symptoms?
2. What investigations would you arrange in the clinic?
3. What would your choice of antibiotic be?
4. What advice would you give the patient?

History 2

A 25-year-old hairdresser complained of lower abdominal pain on and off for the last month, a feeling of heaviness in the pelvis and pain during sexual intercourse. When asked she said she could not remember any of her recent partners saying anything about genital infections. A tender mass was felt to the left side during pelvic examination.

1. If the patient has a genital infection, what is it likely to be?
2. What would be the best approach to obtaining a microbiological specimen?
3. What would be your choice of presumptive treatment?
4. What non-infective complications of infection might you expect in this patient?

Short notes questions

Write short notes on the following:

1. The relationship between sexual activity and infection of the genital tract
2. The principal reasons for treatment failure in gonococcal infection
3. The connection between genital infection and cervical carcinoma
4. The clinical course of early syphilis
5. Bacterial vaginosis

Self-assessment: answers

Multiple choice answers

1. a. **True**. In women, infections can follow birth, abortion or gynaecological procedures.
   b. **True**. Risk is proportional to the number of sex partners.
   c. **True**. Oral contraceptives may alter hormonal status and, thus, the composition of the cervical mucus.
   d. **True**. Methods such as condom use can provide a physical barrier.
   e. **False**. Younger age of first sexual encounter increases risk.

2. a. **False**. Urethritis may not cause a noticeable discharge.
   b. **False**. Dyspareunia (painful or difficult coitus) occurs only in female patients.
   c. **False**. A high proportion of patients, especially females with cervicitis, are asymptomatic.
   d. **True**. These are the most common features.
   e. **True**. Patients are often embarrassed by both the condition and the examination.

3. a. and iii.
   b. and iv.
   c. and i.
   d. and ii.

4. a. **False**. Barrier methods of contraception do not give 100% protection against genital infection even when used properly since they only limit the degree of genital contact. Microscopic trauma may even be increased by the friction barrier methods generate.
   b. **True**. Thus avoiding a risky sexual contact.
   c. **False**. This increases awareness of risks but may not alter risk-taking behaviour.
   d. **False**. This is an important aspect of control of sexually transmitted diseases but is no way near 100% effective.
   e. **True**. Although other methods of infection of the genital tract (e.g. gynaecological procedures) do exist.

5. a. **True**. It is also painful.
   b. **False**. Herpes is often more severe in females.
   c. **False**. Genital infection is more commonly caused by HSV II, but an increasing proportion of cases are now caused by HSV I because of changing patterns of sexual behaviour.

   d. **True**. The attacks are often less severe.
   e. **True**. In sacral sensory nerve ganglia.

6. a. **False**. Genital warts are caused by human papillomavirus.
   b. **False**. Although podophyllin is often used as described, better cure rates are obtained with trichloroacetic acid or other methods.
   c. **True**. There may also be accompanying pruritus and a burning sensation at the lesions.
   d. **True**. They are a potential precursor for squamous carcinoma.
   e. **True**. Access to epithelial cells is also required, probably through minor trauma.

7. a. **True**. Infection can be latent for up to a year.
   b. **True**. The macular rash follows healing of the initial chancre.
   c. **True**. This early union develops from the initial painless papule.
   d. **False**. Gummas are a features of late tertiary syphilis.
   e. **False**. Neurosyphilis is a feature of late, or tertiary, syphilis.

8. a. **True**. The organism is common in tropical countries.
   b. **False**. In chancroid the initial lesion is a painful papule.
   c. **False**. Men are about eight times more likely than women to develop chancroid.
   d. **True**. *H. ducreyi* forms chains of bacilli (streptobacilli) that look a little like schools of fish.
   e. **True**. Trimethoprim, ciprofloxacin and single-dose ceftriaxone can also be used.

9. a. **False**. The causative agent of LGV is *C. trachomatis* types L1–L3.
   b. **True**.
   c. **False**. Pseudolymphadenopathy (pseudobuboes) is a feature of granuloma inguinale. In LGV, there is genuine inguinal adenopathy.
   d. **True**. A high titre is specific for LGV.
   e. **True**. Initially the skin becomes discoloured and wrinkled before sinus formation.

10. a. **False**. HSV II may cause urethritis during acute herpetic infection but this is usually not associated with purulent discharge.

b. **False**. Trichomonad infection of the male urethra is usually asymptomatic.

c. **False**. The role of ureaplasma in non-gonococcal urethritis is controversial and it is not currently considered a major cause of purulent urethral discharge.

d. **True**.

e. **True**.

11. a. **True**. A purulent discharge.
    b. **True**. A frothy, thin, offensive discharge.
    c. **False**. *G. vaginalis* is associated with bacterial vaginosis, an alteration of the vaginal flora that results in a non-infective vaginal discharge.
    d. **True**. It causes a thick creamy discharge.
    e. **False**. *Lactobacillus* sp. is part of the indigenous vaginal flora and not known to play a causal role in vaginal discharge.

12. a. **True**.
    b. **True**. It can be asymptomatic and so forms a source of ascending infection.
    c. **False**. Damage to the fallopian tubes following sexually transmitted cervical infection is an important cause of reduced fertility.
    d. **True**. This can lead to serious sequelae.
    e. **True**. The woman may only be diagnosed when a partner seeks treatment.

13. a. **True**. A prominent cause of PID.
    b. **True**. Hence an antibiotic to cover these organisms is often included in treatment.
    c. **True**. A prominent cause.
    d. **True**. PID is often polymicrobial, including streptococci.
    e. **False**. *S. pyogenes* is a rare isolate in PID. It is, however, associated with nosocomial postpartum endometritis.

14. a. **True**. The classic cause.
    b. **False**. *N. gonorrhoeae* is a rare cause of postpartum endometritis.
    c. **False**. Fever usually occurs within the first 2 days after delivery; a fact that is widely used in the definition of puerperal fever.
    d. **True**. Many cases are nosocomial.
    e. **True**. Spread via the bloodstream can also occur.

15. a. **True**. Usually with *Neisseria gonorrhoeae* or *Chlamydia trachomatis*.
    b. **True**. In men over 35 years of age.
    c. **True**. There may be local pain.
    d. **True**. Hence a surgical opinion should be sought if there is any doubt.

e. **False**. Tetracyclines are widely used to treat the possible chlamydia component of infection in epididymitis.

16. a. **False**. Scabies is caused by the itch mite *Sarcoptes scabei*.
    b. **True**. Patients can present with excoriation.
    c. **False**. Only the females can be found in skin burrows.
    d. **True**.
    e. **False**. Insecticide needs to be applied from the neck down.

Case history answers

History 1

1. This could result from antibiotic resistance, inappropriate choice of treatment, chlamydial coinfection, reinfection by an untreated partner or he might be lying about compliance with the prescribed treatment.

2. Gram stain and direct chlamydia fluorescent antigen of a smear preparation of urethral discharge. Culture of discharge for *Neisseria gonorrhoeae* and *Chlamydia trachomatis*.

3. In view of the possible treatment failure, single-dose intramuscular cefoxitin and a 1-week course of tetracycline would be suitable, but in areas where penicillin-resistant gonococci are rare, high-dose ampicillin with probenicid would be an acceptable alternative to cefoxitin.

4. Avoid intercourse until completion of treatment and encourage sexual partner(s) to attend for screening and any treatment that might be necessary.

History 2

1. This is probably pelvic inflammatory disease and could be a tubo-ovarian abscess.

2. Aspiration of any focal collection at laparoscopy.

3. Treatment should cover *Neisseria gonorrhoeae*, *Chlamydia trachomatis*, anaerobes and streptococci. Cefoxitin and doxycycline are recommended as a presumptive choice.

4. Infertility and tubal pregnancy are both more likely following pelvic inflammatory disease.

Short notes answers

1. This question can be tackled in terms of acquisition, penetration and damage, from a host and pathogen point of view. Use examples.

2. Reasons to be covered: antibiotic resistance (sulphonamides, penicillin, tetracycline,

quinolones), second pathogen
(*Chlamydia trachomatis*) and failure of
compliance.

3. Outline the pathogenesis of cervical carcinoma
starting with human papillomavirus infection.

Remember the role of second genital infections as
cofactors.

4. A chronological sequence should be followed.
5. Cover the microbiology, clinical presentation and
diagnosis.

11 Infections of the central nervous system

Overview

Fortunately, infection of the central nervous system is an uncommon event. When infection does occur, it carries a high risk of mortality. Even when adequately treated, it often leads to neurological impairment. Prompt recognition and early treatment help to reduce the risk of mortality and serious morbidity. Preventive strategies are now available against some of the bacterial pathogens of the nervous system.

11.1 Pathogenesis

Learning objectives

You should:

- understand how infection of the CNS can occur
- know the events that follow infection
- know which microorganisms are likely to be involved and why.

The central nervous system (CNS) is well protected against invasion by pathogenic microorganisms. Not only is it surrounded by the rigid, bony skeleton, but it is also supplied by a capillary circulation that has an unusually non-leaky vessel wall with tight endothelial intercellular junctions and a low rate of pinocytosis. Access to the CNS is normally denied to microorganisms (and, incidentally, many antibiotics unless there is local acute inflammation). The cerebrospinal fluid (CSF), produced by the choroid plexus and circulated in the subarachnoid space over the surface of the brain, is kept sterile, and the phagocytic capacity of adjacent tissues is very limited.

The first stage in the process that leads to infection is usually mucosal colonisation. This is followed by spread via the bloodstream, penetration of the blood–brain barrier and spread in the CSF. Vascular permeability in meningitis is roughly proportional to bacterial number and leucocyte number. High numbers of microorganisms cause local energy metabolism to switch to anaerobic glycolysis, with a consequent rise in lactate concentrations and fall in CSF glucose (relative to serum glucose). Inflammation causes local irritation, which may trigger abnormal neuronal activity. Pus collection, and subsequent fibrosis, particularly around the brainstem can lead to interference with cranial nerve function. When the inflammation is spread over the surface of the cerebral cortex, features of raised intracranial pressure are not predominant. However, focal pus collection (i.e. brain abscess) is likely to increase intracranial pressure.

Certain microorganisms are more capable of causing CNS infection than others. In the case of some bacterial species (*Escherichia coli*, *Neisseria meningitidis*, group B streptococci), the common factors appear to be expression of adhesins, IgA protease and polysaccharide capsule; these assist initial mucosal colonisation and subsequent resistance to phagocytosis. Some viral pathogens of the nervous system have a specific tropism for nervous tissue (e.g. poliovirus and rabies virus, see Chs 22 and 18). Different organisms are more likely to cause CNS infection in patients with compromised defences (e.g. *Listeria monocytogenes* and *Cryptococcus neoformans*). There is an increased risk of recurrent meningeal infection in patients with penetrating cranial trauma and in those with compromised immune defences, particularly complement deficiency and following splenectomy.

11.2 Diagnosis

Learning objectives

You should:

- know the clinical features of infection
- know which laboratory tests are useful.

Clinical features

The clinical features of CNS infection can be considered in four groups:

- general features of infection
- meningeal irritation
- localising features
- raised intracranial pressure.

The general features of infection are those encountered in any acute infection: fever, malaise, loss of appetite, nausea and prostration. Meningeal irritation causes headache, neck stiffness and possibly two eponymous signs: Kernig's sign (resistance to straightening of the knee when the leg is flexed to 90° at knee and thigh) and Brudjinski's sign (resistance to passive flexion of the neck). In severe cases, epileptic seizures may occur. Localising features are those clinical neurological signs that point to a focal lesion in the CNS. The signs of raised intracranial pressure include headache (increases on lying down and diminishes shortly after getting up in the morning), a reduced conscious level and the presence of papilloedema.

Laboratory tests

The principal laboratory contribution to the diagnosis of CNS is the examination of CSF obtained by lumbar puncture. Lumbar puncture, correctly performed, carries little risk in a patient with meningitis, but it should be avoided in patient with suspected brain abscess or evidence of raised intracranial pressure, because it may precipitate uncal herniation. Normal CSF is crystal clear. Contamination of the specimen with visible blood sometimes occurs when the lumbar puncture ruptures small venules. This 'traumatic tap' can be distinguished from pathological causes of bloodstained CSF by collecting into a series of three numbered containers and asking for erythrocyte counts on all three (the red cell count should fall significantly in a traumatic tap). Lumbar puncture is thought to be safe during septicaemia as long as a traumatic tap is avoided. A sample of 5–10 ml CSF should be collected into sterile plastic universal containers for microscopy and culture. Some CSF should also be collected into the appropriate container for protein and glucose estimation. Simultaneous blood samples should be obtained for culture and for serum glucose estimation.

Newer imaging techniques such as computed tomography (CT) and magnetic resonance imaging (MRI) have become an essential part of the acute evaluation of patients with CNS infection. If there is any doubt about the presence of a space-occupying lesion and resulting raised intracranial pressure, a CT or MRI scan should be performed prior to lumbar puncture.

The laboratory should be able to process CSF specimens rapidly and produce results that indicate the presence or absence of a treatable infection in a short time frame. Microscopy of a Gram-stained centrifuged CSF deposit will confirm the presence of bacteria in the majority of bacterial meningitides. A corrected sedimentation rate (CSR) and total and differential leucocyte count help to distinguish viral and bacterial meningitis. In some cases where no bacteria can be seen on Gram stain, the presence of bacterial infection can still be confirmed by nucleic acid amplification (polymerase chain reaction (PCR)). CSF protein and glucose estimation are another set of parameters used to diagnose CNS infection. The glucose level must be compared against the serum glucose performed at the same time (CSF glucose should be no less than 40% of serum level). Changes are less pronounced, if present at all, in CSF from patients with brain abscess.

CSF is cultured in the laboratory using enriched, non-selective media to grow fastidious bacterial species. Viral infections are confirmed by collection of throat and rectal swabs for viral cultivation, and possibly by detection of antiviral IgM in the serum. In patients with encephalitis, specific diagnosis requires the collection of a brain biopsy.

11.3 Management

Learning objectives

You should:

- be aware of the need for prompt treatment and how to choose the most suitable agent(s)

- understand which agents will penetrate to the brain

- know what preventive measures can be used for CNS infection.

Chemotherapy

The serious complications and potential fatal outcome of CNS infection necessitate prompt, appropriate antimicrobial chemotherapy. It is therefore necessary to commence chemotherapy long before the results of antimicrobial susceptibility tests become available. Sometimes the results of rapid tests such as CSF Gram stain and antigen detection can guide the choice of treatment. But more often the choice of agent has to be based on knowledge of the most likely infective agent(s). Protocols for the presumptive treatment of the common CNS infections are revised periodically in order to reflect changes in antimicrobial susceptibility patterns and other epidemiological changes.

Penetration of many antimicrobial agents into the CNS is poor, even when the meninges are inflamed. The best penetration is achieved by agents that have small, lipid-soluble molecules. Chloramphenicol, active against most strains of *Streptococcus pneumoniae* and *N. meningitidis*, is widely used for treating CNS infection caused by these organisms. There may also be some theoretical benefit over newer antibacterial agents that are more bactericidal, since these may cause increased liberation of cell wall components that increase inflammatory damage temporarily. The β-lactam agents, however, are less able to penetrate the blood–brain barrier, sometimes achieving only 2–5% serum concentration. If used, they should therefore be administered intravenously in high doses. The third-generation cephalosporins (e.g. cefotaxime) have gained a place in the treatment of bacterial CNS infections because of their activity against the more common pathogens and their improved availability in the CSF. Gentamicin, vancomycin and erythromycin do not pass through the non-inflamed blood–brain barrier in useful concentrations.

There are very few antiviral agents that can be used to treat viral CNS infection, but it is likely that a number of new agents will become available in the near future. Those currently available include aciclovir and ganciclovir.

Fluconazole has some use in the treatment of fungal CNS infection. Amphotericin is also used but can cause toxicity problems.

Other types of chemotherapy (e.g. corticosteroids) may have their place in the management of certain CNS infections.

When CNS infection results in a focal lesion (i.e. a brain abscess), neurosurgical intervention may be more important than antimicrobial chemotherapy.

Prevention

Most infections of the CNS are of a sporadic, non-epidemic nature and are therefore difficult to prevent. Epidemic spread of certain strains of meningococci can be prevented by vaccination of high-risk populations, e.g. military recruits and Hajj pilgrims. If a high-risk population can be identified for other common bacterial pathogens, a vaccine may help to prevent disease, e.g.

Haemophilus influenzae capsular type B conjugate vaccines. *L. monocytogenes* infection is best prevented by food hygiene practices. Public health laboratories can run periodic checks to ensure that microbiological food standards are adhered to.

Secondary prevention of bacterial meningitis refers to the administration of prophylactic antibiotics to immediate, intimate contacts of cases of meningococcal meningitis.

11.4 Diseases and syndromes

Learning objectives

You should:

- know the major infections of the central nervous system
- know the factors contributing to their occurrence
- know the basis of their clinical management.

The diseases of the CNS are listed in Table 17.

Acute meningitis

Acute meningitis is a microbiological emergency. It involves acute inflammation of the leptomeninges (pia and arachnoid mater). Appropriate presumptive chemotherapy given promptly can halt or reverse the progress of a disease that, if untreated, carries a high mortality rate. Initial transmission of the infective agent is often by droplet infection, i.e. the respiratory route. Colonisation of the nasopharynx then occurs, which is followed in some cases by dissemination via the cerebral circulation.

Viral meningitis In viral meningitis, the infecting organism first causes a systemic infection with primary viraemia, before progressing to viral meningitis. The more common agents of viral meningitis are mumps virus, echovirus, coxsackievirus and other members of

Table 17 Diseases of the central nervous system

Infection	Features
Meningitis	
Acute	Acute inflammation of the leptomeninges (pia and arachnoid mater)
Chronic	Cranial nerve palsies, neurological complications
Recurrent	Episodes separated by disease-free periods; usually associated with a CSF leak or a compromised immune system
Encephalitis	Inflammation of the cerebral cortex
Brain abscess	A focal pyogenic lesion in the cerebrum
Slow viral infections	
Common viruses	Rare degenerative panencephalitis; can occur in AIDS
Prions	Degenerative fatal brain condition

the enterovirus group. Herpes simplex virus (particularly HSV type II), lymphocytic choriomeningitis virus, poliovirus and a variety of other agents may cause meningitis less commonly. Transmission is by either the faecal–oral or the respiratory route. Viral meningitis is usually milder than bacterial infection and is self-limiting, requiring only supportive care.

Bacterial meningitis Bacterial meningitis is often a much more serious disease. Though less common, bacterial meningitis contributes most of the mortality and severe morbidity attributed to all meningitis. The major issue in diagnosing meningitis is therefore distinguishing bacterial from viral infection. The clinical presentation may provide some clues, but there is sufficient overlap between severe viral and moderate bacterial meningitis to cause difficulty in individual cases.

Diagnosis

Viral infection tends to have a longer and more insidious build-up and may be associated with an upper respiratory tract infection and a non-specific rash. In bacterial meningitis caused by *N. meningitidis*, there is a characteristic purpuric rash in around half the patients, particularly over the extensor surfaces of the limbs. Progression of this rash to ecchymoses, or the development of shock, is a poor prognostic sign. Patients will have the features of a febrile illness and signs of meningeal irritation. Conscious level deteriorates relatively late in the course of infection. Signs of raised intracranial pressure are rarely seen.

The benefits of performing a diagnostic lumbar puncture outweigh the small, theoretical risks associated with the procedure. Blood culture should always be performed because around 30% of those affected have a concomitant septicaemia, and some patients have a bacterial pathogen recovered from the blood but not the CSF. If CSF is sent for biochemical estimations, peripheral blood should also be sent for a serum glucose. Although CSF microscopy, culture and susceptibility testing should all be requested, Gram stain and cell count/differential should be performed as urgent procedures.

CSF results suggesting a diagnosis of meningitis are shown in Table 18. Around 80% patients with untreated acute bacterial meningitis have bacteria visible on CSF Gram stain. This figure falls to around 60% if the patient has previously received antibiotics. There is some degree of overlap between rapidly available CSF results in bacterial and viral meningitis.

Other bacterial pathogens cause acute meningitis less often: e.g. *E. coli*, group B streptococci and *L. monocytogenes* in neonates (see Ch. 15), and *L. monocytogenes* and *C. neoformans* in the immunocompromised (see Ch. 18). The milder nature of viral meningitis means that the aetiological agent is often not sought. Surveys suggest that the common viral causes of meningitis include enteroviruses such as mumps virus, echovirus and coxsackieviruses.

In patients with no laboratory evidence of bacterial meningitis on preliminary CSF testing, the following causes should be considered:

- common
  —prior antibiotic treatment
  —viral infection
- less often
  —tuberculous meningitis
  —leptospirosis
  —neurosyphilis
  —cryptococcosis
  —neoplastic disease.

Treatment

Presumptive chemotherapy should be chosen on the basis of epidemiological factors, modified by the results of CSF Gram stain, leucocyte count and biochemistry. In unvaccinated preschool children (<5 years of age), *H. influenzae* is the most common bacterial pathogen, followed by *S. pneumoniae* and *N. meningitidis*. These patients should be given intravenous ceftriaxone or ampicillin and chloramphenicol (ampicillin should be given in sufficiently high dose to guarantee penetration into the CSF). Older children and adults can be given intravenous benzylpenicillin every 2–4 hours, since *N. meningitidis* and *S. pneumoniae* are the principal pathogens in this age group. CSF results that support a diagnosis of meningitis are shown in Table 18.

It may be necessary to modify presumptive antimicrobial chemotherapy in the light of culture and susceptibility results. In some locations, ampicillin resistance among *H. influenzae* or penicillin-resistance among *S.*

Table 18 Results of initial cerebrospinal fluid investigations

Form of meningitis	Neutrophils (per mm^3)[a]	Lymphocytes (per mm^3)[a]	Protein (g/l)	Glucose	Gram stain
Pyogenic	500–2000		1–3	Low	Bacteria may be seen
Viral		50–500	0.5–1	Normal	Nil
Tuberculous	100–600		1–6	Low	Nil

[a]$\times 10^6$/l.

pneumoniae may be common enough to make the presumptive use of these agents inadvisable. Third-generation cephalosporins (e.g. cefotaxime) may be a suitable alternative. The optimal duration of chemotherapy is subject to debate, but for the three main bacterial pathogens it should be between 7 and 14 days, depending on the species isolated.

Postinfective neurological sequelae such as neurogenic deafness, cranial nerve palsies and blindness are common, particularly after *H. influenzae* meningitis. Several studies have indicated that early treatment with glucocorticosteroids may reduce the incidence of these complications. Hydrocephalus may also occur as a result of inflammation around the arachnoid villi. Epidemic meningococcal meningitis, which is usually caused by type A or occasionally type C *N. meningitidis*, can be prevented by administration of a polysaccharide vaccine. Hajj pilgrims, military recruits and other members of closed or confined communities are worth vaccinating. Unfortunately, the most common type of *N. meningitidis* causing endemic meningococcal meningitis is type B, which is poorly immunogenic. A vaccine is not currently available. The *H. influenzae* capsular type B conjugate vaccine has had a significant effect on the incidence of invasive *H. influenzae* infection in some populations. The vaccine is given to infants under the age of 1 year.

Contacts. Family and other intimate contacts of patients with *N. meningitidis* or *H. influenzae* meningitis should be given a 48-hour prophylactic course of rifampicin.

Chronic meningitis

Chronic meningitis is a distinct clinical entity with a different epidemiology and range of causal agents from acute meningitis. In chronic meningitis, fever and features of meningeal irritation are less pronounced, while there is increased likelihood of cranial nerve palsies and other neurological complications. The most common cause is *Mycobacterium tuberculosis*. The condition can also be caused by *L. monocytogenes* and other bacteria; herpes simplex, lymphochoriomeningitis and other viruses; *C. neoformans* and other fungi; and by neoplastic disease.

Diagnosis
Lumbar puncture should be performed. The leucocyte count will be raised, but to a lower extent than in acute bacterial meningitis. In tuberculous meningitis, protein concentration may be very high. No bacteria will be visible on Gram stain, but acid-fast stain of CSF will show bacilli in around 25% patients. If 5–10 ml CSF is centrifuged, and the acid-fast-stained deposit examined for at least 30 minutes by an experienced microscopist, up to 80% of cases may be detected. Gram-positive bacilli present at microscopy or after culture should not be dis-

missed as 'contaminants' since CSF is normally sterile, and Gram-positive bacilli may actually be *L. monocytogenes*. CSF should also be examined for *C. neoformans* by microscopy of India ink preparation and a latex agglutination test. Oligonucleotide probes and nucleic acid amplification (PCR) are being employed in larger centres to obtain a rapid diagnosis of tuberculous meningitis. Other foci of tuberculosis should also be sought. The CSF should be cultured on Lowenstein–Jensen or similar medium, but slow growth of this species results in culture taking weeks to months before reports can be issued.

Treatment
Presumptive therapy may have to be commenced on the basis of suggestive clinical signs and suspicious nonspecific CSF findings. Four agents are used, of which at least two penetrate the blood–brain barrier effectively, e.g. rifampicin, isoniazid, ethambutol and pyrazinamide. There is a high rate of neurological sequelae.

Recurrent meningitis

Episodes of meningitis separated by disease-free periods can occur. The microbial causes of recurrent meningitis are numerous, but the condition is usually caused either by a CSF leak or through a compromised immune system. The causal agents differ from those causing acute bacterial meningitis in that they are upper respiratory tract commensals such as *S. pneumoniae*, other streptococci, *H. influenzae* and *N. meningitidis*. Different organisms may cause infection on each occasion. In hospital-acquired infection, Enterobacteriaceae and *Staphylococcus aureus* are more common. Detailed investigation of a source is required in patients with recurrent infection.

Encephalitis

Inflammation of the cerebral cortex is usually caused by a viral infection and may occur as an extension of meningeal infection. A large number of viruses, including herpes simplex virus, rabies virus and various arboviruses, can cause encephalitis. (Rabies and arbovirus infections are dealt with in Ch. 19 and human immunodeficiency virus (HIV) infection in Ch. 18.) Viral invasion of neural tissue occurs after initial spread via the bloodstream. Damage is in proportion to the invasion of neurones, and the severity of infection, therefore, reflects how long the disease is allowed to go unchecked by immune defences or chemotherapy.

Diagnosis
The most important decision to be made in diagnosing encephalitis is whether it is caused by herpes simplex or

another viral agent, because herpes simplex infection is potentially treatable. The clinical features (fever, depressed conscious level, seizures and possibly mood change) do not necessarily help to make this distinction. Electroencephalogram (EEG) may demonstrate a characteristic pattern and computed tomographic scans may slow localisation in one or other temporal lobes, but a definitive diagnosis of herpes simplex encephalitis can only be made by obtaining an open brain biopsy. If CT or MRI scan demonstrates a focal lesion in the temporal lobe (the commonest site), biopsy should be taken from this site. Material obtained at biopsy should be used for the following: viral culture, direct immunofluorescence, nucleic acid amplification (PCR) and histopathology.

Treatment

Confirmed herpes simplex virus encephalitis should be treated with intravenous aciclovir. There is a high rate of late neurological sequelae, and recovery is slow.

Brain abscess

Brain abscess arises as a result of spread from a primary ear infection (e.g. acute otitis media or mastoiditis), direct spread following trauma or haematogenous spread from a distant site (especially the lungs). Abscesses have a particular predilection for the boundary between grey and white matter, where the collateral circulation is least efficient. In its early stage, the lesion is a focal cerebritis, which then becomes a collection of pus with an inflamed margin.

Diagnosis

A substantial proportion of patients have no fever or signs of meningeal irritation. Signs of a space-occupying lesion may only present later in the development of the disease. When brain abscess is suspected, lumbar puncture should be avoided, at least until the possibility of raised intracranial pressure has been excluded. The diagnosis is usually made using imaging techniques. Confirmation of an infective aetiology often has to wait until the patient undergoes craniotomy. Brain abscesses are caused by a wide variety of bacteria and may be multibacterial. Causative species include streptococci, Enterobacteriaceae and anaerobic bacteria. In order to obtain the best possible diagnostic yield, pus collected at craniotomy should be transferred to the laboratory quickly to avoid death of anaerobic and microaerophilic bacteria in transit. Some laboratories have the facilities to perform gas-liquid chromatography, which demonstrates the fatty acid metabolites of anaerobic bacteria present in pus, even when those bacteria are no longer viable.

Treatment

Presumptive antimicrobial chemotherapy is with a combination of metronidazole, and an extended-spectrum cephalosporin given intravenously. Surgical intervention is the mainstay of management for brain abscess in all but its earliest stages, and it is probable that antimicrobial chemotherapy contributes little by itself to the eventual outcome.

Slow virus infection

There are a variety of chronic or degenerative brain syndromes attributed to viral infection. These fall into two main groups:

- rare degenerative complications of common viral infections
- syndromes thought to be caused by unconventional, protein infection agents known as 'prions'.

The first category includes subacute sclerosing panencephalitis (measles virus), progressive multifocal leucoencephalopathy (JC virus) and rubella panencephalitis (rubella virus). The first two conditions have been recognised for several decades as rare, inevitably fatal degenerative brain syndromes. These conditions have become increasingly common because of the influence of AIDS.

The second category has come to public notice much more recently and includes conditions such as **kuru** (a transmissible, degenerative brain condition found among hill tribes in Papua New Guinea), **Creutzfeldt–Jakob disease** (CJD), **Gerstmann–Straussler syndrome**, and related conditions in domestic animals (scrapie, bovine spongiform encephalopathy and visna). A transmissible protein-like agent is thought to be the cause of each of these conditions, but the relationship between these conditions and the exact means of transmission have yet to be worked out. Of particular note is the resistance of 'prions' to temperatures normally reached during autoclaving. In fact, these infective agents are highly resistant to most physical and chemical means of decontamination. There is no diagnostic test short of brain biopsy, and no effective chemotherapy for any of these diseases. The European outbreak of new variant CJD has been linked to the bovine spongiform encephalopathy outbreak. Operating theatre equipment used to handle neural or lymphatic material in patients with a possible diagnosis of CJD is a possible infection hazard to patients in whom it is subsequently used. The equipment has to be either destroyed, which can be very costly, or decontaminated in sodium hydroxide plus sterilised at an unusually high temperature.

11.5 Organisms

A checklist of the organisms discussed in this chapter is given in Box 6. Further information is given on the pages indicated.

Box 6 Organisms that can infect the central nervous system

Bacteria	see page	Viruses	see page
Haemophilus influenzae	251	Herpes simplex virus	257
Neisseria meningitidis	252–3	Mumps virus	259
Streptococcus pneumoniae	245	Coxsackievirus	260
Other streptococcal spp.	244–5	Echovirus	259
Escherichia coli	248	Lymphocytic choriomeningitis virus	–
Staphylococcus aureus	243	Rubellavirus	261
Listeria monocytogenes	246	Measles virus	259
Mycobacterium tuberculosis	253–4	JC virus	–
Treponema pallidum	255	Arboviruses	261
		Rabies virus	260
Fungi		Prions	11
Cryptococcus neoformans	269		

Self-assessment: questions

Multiple choice questions

1. The following contribute to the defence of the central nervous system (CNS) against infection:
   a. The cranial vault
   b. Leaky capillary circulation
   c. Low rate of pinocytosis
   d. Cerebrospinal fluid (CSF) distribution via the subarachnoid space
   e. Secretory IgA

2. Features of meningeal irritation include:
   a. Headache, increased by lying down
   b. Fever
   c. Papilloedema
   d. Neck stiffness
   e. Positive Kernig's sign

3. The following laboratory tests contribute to the immediate management of acute meningitis:
   a. Gram stain of centrifuged CSF
   b. CSF glucose concentration
   c. Latex agglutination antigen tests
   d. CSF leucocyte count
   e. CSF protein concentration

4. In viral infections of the CNS:
   a. Specific diagnosis is usually confirmed by laboratory tests
   b. Throat swab and faecal specimen may be required for a specific aetiological diagnosis
   c. Brain biopsy is required to confirm the diagnosis in some conditions
   d. CSF microscopy may contribute to the diagnosis
   e. CSF glucose level falls only slightly

5. The following infections can be prevented by vaccination:
   a. Herpes simplex type II encephalitis
   b. *Haemophilus influenzae* meningitis
   c. Recurrent meningitis
   d. *Neisseria meningitidis* meningitis
   e. Mumps meningitis

6. In a patient with meningitis, the following feature would make you consider a bacterial aetiology:
   a. Rapidly deteriorating conscious level
   b. Purpuric rash on the buttocks
   c. Sublingual temperature of 37.8°C
   d. CSF leucocyte count of 1500×10^6 cells/l $(1500/\text{mm}^3)$
   e. CSF protein level of 2 g/l

7. The following statements about lumbar puncture are correct:
   a. It should be avoided in septicaemic patients
   b. Laboratory tests on CSF obtained can guide immediate therapy
   c. CSF obtained should be collected into a traumatic tap
   d. It is safe in the majority of patients suspected of having advanced brain abscess

8. Match the organism with the most appropriate risk group:
   a. *Streptococcus pneumoniae*   i. Military recruits
   b. *Haemophilus influenzae*   ii. Immunocompromised patients
   c. *Neisseria meningitidis*   iii. The elderly
   d. *Listeria monocytogenes*   iv. Preschool children

9. Causes of 'aseptic meningitis' include:
   a. Neurosyphilis
   b. Antibiotic-treated *Haemophilus influenzae* infection
   c. *Mycobacterium tuberculosis*
   d. Fulminant *Neisseria meningitidis* infection
   e. *Cryptococcus neoformans*

10. In chronic meningitis:
    a. Cranial nerve palsies occur
    b. A non-infective aetiology is the most common cause
    c. *Cryptococcus neoformans* can be confirmed by microscopy of India ink CSF preparation
    d. A finding of Gram-positive bacilli at CSF microscopy should be regarded as contamination of the specimen
    e. Microscopy for acid-fast bacilli should be prolonged

11. In recurrent meningitis:
    a. A different bacterial pathogen may be isolated in each episode
    b. *Streptococcus pneumoniae* is a common isolate from CSF
    c. The underlying cause may be a communicating CSF leak
    d. Features of meningeal irritation are less common in second and subsequent episodes
    e. Lymphocytic choriomeningitis virus is a common cause

12. Concerning encephalitis:
    a. Severity of disease is proportional to the delay before immune defences or chemotherapy check viral invasion

b. The most common causal agent is the mumps virus

c. A specific diagnosis should be made by CSF examination

d. Herpes simplex infection is treatable with aciclovir

e. Electroencephalogram may contribute to a specific diagnosis

13. The following bacterial species are commonly associated with brain abscess:
    a. Streptococci
    b. *Staphylococcus aureus*
    c. Anaerobic spp.
    d. Enterobacteriaceae
    e. More than one of the above

14. 'Slow virus' infections of humans include:
    a. Subacute sclerosing panencephalitis
    b. Rubella panencephalitis
    c. Gerstman–Straussler syndrome
    d. Kuru
    e. Scrapie

Case history questions

History 1

An 18-month-old child was brought to his GP by his mother who said he was 'not well'. Apart from being hot and a bit listless, the GP found nothing else of note. The mother was told that it was probably one of the viruses going round and advised to use paracetamol syrup for the temperature. The mother called the GP 4 hours later. She was worried that her son was really quite drowsy and wanted to lie in the dark all the time. The GP called on a home visit shortly afterwards and examined the child again. This time he noted an axillary temperature of 38.9˚C, neck stiffness and a purpuric rash over the buttocks. He immediately gave the child an intramuscular injection of ampicillin and arranged for emergency admission to the local paediatric unit. On arrival, the child was shocked with rapidly progressing ecchymotic lesions over all four limbs and the abdomen. An urgent lumbar puncture and blood culture were performed, intravenous antibiotics commenced and resuscitation procedures instituted, but the child died shortly after.

1. What infection was most likely, and what complications had set in by the time of hospital admission?
2. What was the most probable causal agent?
3. Which antibiotics would most often be used in a child of this age with this infection?

History 2

A 24-year-old professional man was admitted to hospital with a recent history of fever, fits and changed behaviour. CT scan showed diffuse inflammatory changes, greatest in the left temporal lobe. A lumbar puncture was performed to achieve a specific aetiological diagnosis, after which treatment with intravenous aciclovir was commenced.

1. What is the diagnosis likely to be?
2. What aetiological agents need to be considered?
3. What additional diagnostic procedure should have been performed?
4. What advice might you give the relatives after the initial response to therapy?

Data interpretation

A laboratory report was issued on a specimen of CSF from a patient with headache, mild fever and a drooping right eyelid. His chest radiograph had a right apical opacity and ipsilateral hilar lymphadenopathy. These were the results:

> leucocytes: 150×10^6 cells/l (150/mm^3); 90% neutrophils
> erythrocytes: nil
> Gram stain: no bacteria seen
> acid-fast stain: no bacteria seen
> cryptococcal antigen: negative
> culture: no bacterial growth
> mycobacterial PCR (polymerase chain reaction): genus negative/*M. tuberculosis* complex negative
> mycobacterial culture: continuing. A further report will be issued if culture is positive.

1. What specific infection needs to be considered in this clinical setting?
2. Do the results of microscopy rule out this diagnosis?
3. What does the PCR result add to your assessment of the likely diagnosis?
4. How long will it be before you can expect a final culture result: at the earliest, and at the latest?

Objective structured clinical examination (OSCE)

A 52-year-old woman was admitted because of progressive worsening headache and fever. These features and some left-sided focal neurological signs prompted a CT scan, which revealed right-side enhancement with contrast but no focal space-occupying or cavitating lesion. As there was no evidence of raised intracranial pressure, lumbar puncture was performed and the CSF obtained sent for laboratory investigations. The leucocyte cell count was 20×10^6 cells/l ($20/mm^3$). These were predominantly neutrophils. No red cells or bacteria were seen. Presumptive antimicrobial therapy has been commenced. You are asked:

1. Do you think these features strongly suggest a diagnosis of cerebral abscess?
2. Is it likely that a primary source of bacterial infection is present in adjacent structures?
3. Would CSF biochemistry be unhelpful in this setting?
4. Do you think a combination of intravenous gentamicin and metronidazole would be a good choice of antibiotics for this patient?
5. Surgical drainage is almost certainly required; do you agree?

Short notes questions

Write short notes on the following:

1. How microbial invasion of the CNS can cause acute neurological damage
2. Factors that enter into the choice of antibacterial agents for the treatment of acute meningitis
3. The principal post-infective sequelae of meningitis and how might they be prevented
4. The acute management of suspected brain abscess

Viva questions

1. What are the main clinical features of an infection of the CNS? What are the limitations of using these in reaching a diagnosis?
2. Why is acute meningitis a microbiological emergency? What action would you take in the first hour after admitting a patient with suspected meningitis?

Self-assessment: answers

Multiple choice answers

1. a. **True**.
   b. **False**. Intracranial capillary endothelium is usually not leaky in the absence of inflammation.
   c. **True**. This reduces the points of exit through the vessel walls.
   d. **False**. The subarachnoid space is the principal route followed by infecting organisms after they have entered the CSF.
   e. **True**. Some pathogens act by producing an IgA protease, to avoid this defence.

2. a. **False**. Headache on lying down is a feature of raised intracranial pressure.
   b. **False**. Fever is not specific to meningitis.
   c. **False**. Papilloedema is a feature of raised intracranial pressure.
   d. **True**. This is known as Brudjinski's sign.
   e. **True**. This is resistance to straightening of the knee when the leg is flexed to 90° at knee and thigh.

3. a. **True**. This is a rapid test that confirms the presence of bacteria in around 80% of acute untreated cases of meningitis.
   b. **False**. The useful glucose indicator is not the absolute concentration. It is the CSF level in relation to serum glucose (important, for example, in diabetics, etc.).
   c. **True**. A rapid antigen method to detect bacteria.
   d. **True**. This is an indicator of infection with bacteria rather than a virus.
   e. **True**. Protein levels generally rise in acute bacterial infection.

4. a. **False**. Since the majority of viral CNS infections are self-limiting meningitides, the tests required to achieve a specific aetiological diagnosis in viral meningitis are usually not done on the grounds of making little contribution to management.
   b. **True**. The virus is usually of respiratory or faecal–oral origin.
   c. **True**. A specific aetiological diagnosis can only be made by examination of a brain biopsy.
   d. **True**. Leucocyte, glucose and protein levels are indicative of the type of pathogen.
   e. **False**. CSF glucose level may fall significantly in some cases of viral meningitis, especially those caused by lymphocytic choriomeningitis and mumps viruses.

5. a. **False**. There is no vaccine.
   b. **True**. Capsular type B conjugate vaccine, which is used for high-risk groups.
   c. **False**. This is usually a consequence of a compromised immune system or a CSF leak. Different pathogens may be involved in different episodes.
   d. **True**. Type A or C can be prevented with a polysaccharide vaccine. However, type B is poorly immunogenic.
   e. **True**. Mumps vaccine is among the group offered to all children in the UK.

6. a. **True**. Viral infections tend to have a longer development.
   b. **True**. Indicative of *Neisseria meningitidis*.
   c. **False**. A moderate pyrexia is not specific to bacterial meningitis.
   d. **True**. Less extreme levels are seen in viral and tuberculous meningitis.
   e. **True**. Protein levels generally rise in bacterial infections.

7. a. **False**. Septicaemia is not a contraindication for carefully performed lumber puncture.
   b. **True**. Gram stain, microscopy, leucocyte count and biochemistry.
   c. **False**. A plastic container should be used for CSF to avoid adhesion of leucocytes to a glass surface.
   d. **False**. Bloodstained CSF may indicate subarachnoid haemorrhage.
   e. **False**. Suspected brain abscess should always prompt computed tomographic (CT) or magnetic resonance (MR) scan prior to lumbar puncture, which should be avoided if there is any evidence of a space-occupying lesion.

8. a. and iii.
   b. and iv.
   c. and i.
   d. and ii.

   There is a degree of overlap between the major at-risk groups for all the organisms listed; however, the most appropriate associations are the ones given above.

9. a. **True**. In secondary and tertiary syphilis.
   b. **True**. An indication of partially treated infection.
   c. **True**. It is rarely acute.
   d. **False**. In fulminant meningococcal meningitis, it would be very unusual to find no sign of bacteria in one of the tests: Gram stain, direct antigen agglutination test and bacterial culture.

e. **True**. *C. neoformans* can cause aspectic meningitis particularly in the immunocompromised.

10. a. **True**. Together with other neurological complications.
    b. **False**. The most common cause of 'chronic meningitis' is *Mycobacterium tuberculosis*.
    c. **True**. The clear capsulated cryptococci show against the black background.
    d. **False**. CSF is normally a sterile fluid: the presence of Gram-positive bacilli may be evidence of *Listeria monocytogenes*.
    e. **True**. It may take 30 minutes to detect the bacilli.

11. a. **True**. Recurrent meningitis usually reflects a weakness in the brain's defences.
    b. **True**. This is a common upper respiratory tract commensal.
    c. **True**. This allows a passage for infection.
    d. **False**. Less-pronounced signs of meningeal irritation are associated with chronic meningitis, not recurrent infection.
    e. **False**. Lymphocytic choriomeningitis virus is a cause of 'aseptic' meningitis; the causes of recurrent meningitis are predominantly bacterial.

12. a. **True**. Damage is in preportion to the invasion of the neurones.
    b. **False**. Mumps virus is a less common cause of encephalitis but was among the commoner causes of viral meningitis until vaccination was introduced.
    c. **False**. The specific aetiological diagnosis requires brain biopsy for viral culture, ELISA and direct immunofluorescence.
    d. **True**. Ganciclovir is also used.
    e. **True**. There may be a typical pattern.

13. a. **True**.
    b. **True**.
    c. **True**.
    d. **True**.
    e. **True**. Brain abscesses are often polymicrobial, the bacteria listed being among the common causal agents. The fastidious nature of some of these species means that more species than the laboratory isolates may be present in any given case.

14. a. **True**. A rare degenerative condition.
    b. **True**. Vaccination is available for rubellavirus.
    c. **True**. A transmissible protein-like agent (prion) is thought to be involved.
    d. **True**. Found among hill tribes in Papua New Guinea and is related to dietary habits.

e. **False**. Scrapie is a slow virus or 'prion' disease of sheep. Some authorities believe it is the cause of bovine spongiform encephalopathy. There is at present no evidence that scrapie can be transmitted to humans.

Case history answers

History 1

1. Acute bacterial meningitis. Possible answers include septicaemic shock, disseminated intravascular coagulation (DIC) and adrenocortical haemorrhage (Waterhouse–Freidrichson syndrome, the cause of shock in meningococcal meningitis).
2. *Neisseria meningitidis*.
3. Ampicillin or third-generation cephalosporin (e.g. cefotaxime).

History 2

1. Encephalitis.
2. Herpes simplex encephalitis is likely in view of the temporal lobe involvement. However, other viral aetiologies might be considered depending on likely exposure: HIV, arbovirus or rabies.
3. Brain biopsy for histology, direct immunofluorescence, ELISA (enzyme-linked immunosorbent assay) and viral culture.
4. It might be wise to introduce tactfully the possibility of residual neurological damage.

Data interpretation answer

1. Tuberculous meningitis.
2. No. The most careful microscopic examination of CSF for acid-fast bacilli will only pick up a positive result in around a quarter of cases.
3. Very little. PCR (or nucleic acid amplification) is little more sensitive than carefully examined acid-fast stain and will only rarely produce a positive result on microscopy-negative CSF.
4. With the newer automated systems, around 12–14 days, but classically up to around 6 weeks when relying on manual culture systems.

OSCE answer

1. No. These features suggest an earlier stage of intracranial infection: cerebritis.
2. Yes. Such infections often follow local spread of infection from chronic suppurative otitis media, dental abscess or sinusitis.
3. No. A very high CSF protein and low relative CSF glucose would suggest tuberculous meningitis as an important differential diagnosis.

4. No. Gentamicin has poor CNS penetration. Even if it did reach the site of inflammation, this combination would leave important gaps in cover such as for streptococci.
5. No. Early diagnosis and treatment of cerebral abscess at the focal cerebritis stage has increased the success of a primarily medical approach to this infection.

Short notes answers

1. Mention the role of bacterial cell wall components in stimulating lymphokine production, increased vascular permeability, etc. Inflammation, oedema, vasculitis, basal collection of pus and hydrocephalus should all be covered.
2. Probably best to list presumptive agents by age of patient and likely bacterial pathogens. Then cover issues relating to antimicrobial resistance.
3. Cranial nerve palsies, neurogenic deafness, blindness and hydrocephalus. Prevent by an early start to appropriate antibacterial chemotherapy and use of adjunctive glucocorticosteroids.
4. Diagnosis: avoid lumbar puncture before CT or MRI scan. Lumbar puncture only if no focal lesion or scan

evidence of focal cerebritis. Look for evidence of ENT (ear, nose and throat) pathology, and cyanotic heart disease. Arrange for neurosurgery for diagnostic and therapeutic reasons. Presumptive therapy with penicillin, metronidazole and chloramphenicol. Refer to variations for Enterobacteriaceae and staphylococci.

Viva answers

1. You can describe these as the consequences of generalised infection, meningeal irritability, raised intracranial pressure and focal neurological signs. The reason the laboratory and imaging studies are essential is that clinical features of the main disease syndromes overlap and do not predict the specific aetiology or progression of infection with sufficient accuracy to determine clinical management.
2. Prompt commencement of appropriate antibiotic therapy and, where necessary, other supportive measures will reduce mortality and morbidity. Initial actions need to include rapid diagnosis, immediate presumptive chemotherapy, recognition of disease severity and poor prognosis indicators that will suggest a need for intensive care.

12 Infections of the eye and surrounding structures

Overview

The eye is relatively well protected against infection, and the common infections of the eye are usually eradicated without serious consequences. The wide range of potential microbial pathogens and the restricted range of antibiotics available for treatment of eye infections make treatment of conditions other than conjunctivitis particularly difficult. Moreover, infections of the cornea and posterior chamber can cause blindness or loss of visual acuity. In order to reduce the risk of such serious complications, these rarer infections need to be recognised early and referred for specialist treatment.

12.1 Pathogenesis

Learning objectives

You should:
- understand the defences of the eye against infection
- know how infection occurs.

The contents of the eye are maintained in a sterile state by anatomical and non-specific defences. The eyelids provide both a barrier against minor trauma and, in the blinking reflex, a means of spreading the tear film and clearing particulate material from the conjunctival epithelium. Lysozyme, present in tears, has some antibacterial activity and may also increase aggregation of bacteria, thereby making them easier to clear. The integrity of the conjunctiva is another barrier to microbial invasion, and minor trauma of this layer increases the risk of infection of the underlying cornea. The cornea is avascular and lacks the phagocytic defences of other tissues. Infection of the anterior chamber of the eye may be limited to this area by the lens, its supporting ligament and the iris. There is a net flow from the vitreous to the aqueous humour, further reducing the opportunity for infection to spread in the opposite direction. Haematogenous access is limited by the tight junctions of the vascular endothelium of vessels supplying the eye.

Infection becomes established in the eye by direct inoculation, which is often assisted by trauma or by spread from adjacent tissues or the bloodstream. Damage can occur through the inflammation alone, and it is inflammation that causes the earliest signs of ophthalmic infection, e.g. red eye, swollen eyelid or clouded cornea. The most serious infections of the eye may lead to blindness and sometimes even to death. Blindness or a loss of visual acuity caused by infection is multifactorial, affecting any of the structures between the cornea and the retina.

12.2 Diagnosis

Learning objectives

You should:
- be aware of the causes of red eye
- know the features of infection of different structures in the eye
- understand what tests are suitable and what are the limitations of these tests.

Clinical features

The most evident sign of eye infection is a red eye, but not all red eyes are infected, and not all eye infections cause red eye. If redness is caused by infection of blood vessels in the conjunctival epithelium, particularly in the periphery of the eye, it is likely to result from conjunctivitis, but redness in only the vessels surrounding the iris (the limbus) may be the result of keratitis, uveitis or non-infective conditions such as glaucoma.

Acute inflammation usually results in an inflammatory exudate, present as a discharge from the eye. If this is profuse and contains many neutrophils, it will stick the eyelids together when allowed to dry, e.g. overnight.

Inflammation of the conjunctival epithelium causes a thickening of this layer over the sclera where it is more mobile. Over the inner surface of the eyelids it may form papillae, projections with a vascular tuft at the centre, or follicles, which are avascular projections.

In corneal infection, the cornea may take on a hazy appearance, caused partly by the presence of inflammatory cells on its inner surface. Inflammation in the anterior chamber of the eye may cause a crescent-shaped collection of pus in the dependent part, called a 'hypopyon'.

Other features that should be searched for include fever, enlargement of lymph nodes in the neck, ocular trauma, swelling or other lesion on the eyelids, proptosis (projection of the eye from its socket) and limitation of eye movement (ophthalmoplegia). Finally, fundoscopic examination may reveal further signs of infection.

Laboratory tests

Laboratory confirmation of the microbial cause of eye infection is difficult. Even in conjunctivitis, the organisms isolated from purulent exudate are not necessarily those causing the infection. They may be indigenous flora of the facial skin, and the underlying cause may be a fastidious bacterial species or obligate intracellular organism. A full diagnostic workup therefore includes swabs for microscopy using Gram, Giemsa, periodic acid–Schiff (PAS) and silver stains; culture for aerobic and fastidious bacteria, viruses and fungi; and other more specific tests.

In practice, a smaller range of tests are usually selected on the basis of epidemiological and clinical features, taking into account the extent to which the results will affect management of the condition. So, for example, many cases of viral conjunctivitis are not confirmed by specific laboratory tests because the condition is self-limiting and does not require specific chemotherapy. However, when a specimen of anterior or posterior chamber fluid is obtained by an ophthalmic surgeon, the unrepeatable nature of the specimen makes it worthwhile requesting the fullest possible range of diagnostic tests (preferably by prior arrangement with the laboratory).

12.3 Management

Learning objectives

You should:

- be aware of which route to use when giving drugs
- understand the requirement for high-purity antibiotics
- be aware of the importance of prompt treatment
- understand the need for prophylaxis in minor eye injuries.

Chemotherapy

Infection of the conjunctiva and anterior chamber are easily accessible to topically applied antimicrobial agents. These infections can, therefore, be treated with either eye drops or ointment. Drops are preferred for adults since they are spread in the tear film over the conjunctival epithelium. In children drops may be washed out by tears, so ointments are used instead. Even severe infections can be treated with antimicrobials in this form as long as they are administered frequently, e.g. hourly for 12 hours. Specially strong formulations of eye drops may be required. Infections of the posterior chamber and uveal tract cannot be treated with topical agents; however, most agents do not reach adequate therapeutic levels in the eye when given intravenously unless there is acute inflammation. For this reason, intravenous antibiotics are usually supplemented by subconjunctival or intravitreal agents. Vitrectomy may be required for diagnostic and therapeutic purposes, in which case a first intravitreal dose can be given at this time. The range of antibiotics that can be given intravitreally is limited to those available in special high-purity formulations. Infection of the structures immediately surrounding the eye cannot be treated with topical antibiotics but may respond to the appropriate intravenous antibiotic agent(s).

It is known that serious eye infections are less likely to result in blindness or reduced visual acuity if they are treated with the appropriate agent(s) promptly. The wide range of potential pathogens means that every attempt should be made to obtain satisfactory diagnostic specimens before commencing chemotherapy. However, it is often necessary to commence treatment without a specific microbiological diagnosis and, sometimes, without any laboratory clues at all. The need for ophthalmic surgery and an individualised antimicrobial regimen, often in the absence of laboratory confirmation of the infective agent, dictates a team approach to treatment of these infections.

Prevention

The causal role of minor trauma and ophthalmic surgery in eye infection has long been recognised. Corneal abrasions dealt with in accident and emergency departments are usually examined for foreign bodies (which should be removed), treated with topical antibiotic and covered with an eye patch until the effects of local anaesthesia wear off. Ophthalmic surgery is carried out under scrupulously clean conditions, and any implanted material must of course be sterile.

12.4 Diseases and syndromes

Learning objectives

You should:

- know the major infections of the eye and its surrounds
- know the factors contributing to their occurrence
- understand the basis of their clinical management.

The main diseases of the eye are listed in Table 19.

Conjunctivitis

Conjunctivitis is the most common eye infection encountered in medical practice and is usually dealt with in general practice. It can be caused by bacteria, viruses and occasionally fungi (Table 20). The most important distinction to be made is between a self-limiting viral conjunctivitis and a bacterial infection that requires antimicrobial therapy. In conjunctivitis, the eye is usually red because of dilated epithelial blood vessels. These extend to the periphery of the eye. Viral conjunctivitis is normally accompanied by a moderate discharge, unlike the more pronounced, predominantly neutrophil discharge found in bacterial infection. Follicles on the tarsal surface are a feature of viral conjunctivitis, whereas papillae occur mainly in bacterial infection. If follicles persist for more than a few weeks, a diagnosis of inclusion conjunctivitis cased by *Chlamydia trachomatis* should be considered.

Table 20 Causes of conjunctivitis

Infective agent	Epidemiology
Viruses	Common, often self-limiting
Staphylococcus aureus	Common, purulent
Neisseria gonorrhoeae	Neonates
Chlamydia trachomatis	Neonates
	Severe, in developing countries
Haemophilus influenzae	Children
Moraxella lacunata	Unusual

Viral conjunctivitis

The most common viral agents of conjunctivitis in most developed countries are the adenoviruses, which cause a concomitant fever and sore throat in children (pharyngoconjunctival fever) or a keratoconjunctivitis with preauricular lymphadenopathy in adults. Epidemics caused by transmission by health-care workers using ophthalmological instruments have been reported. Many other viruses have been implicated as a cause of conjunctivitis.

Bacterial infection

Staphylococcus aureus is the most common bacterial cause of conjunctivitis. *Haemophilus influenzae* in children and *Neisseria gonorrhoeae* and chlamydiae in neonates also cause conjunctivitis. A variant of *H. influenzae*, *Haemophilus aegypti*, can also cause the infection. Some strains of *H. influenzae* have been implicated in a potentially fatal conjunctivitis-associated disease, Brazilian haemorrhagic fever, which affects children. *Moraxella lacunata* is a small Gram-negative coccobacillus that sometimes causes conjunctivitis associated with dermatitis at the angles of the eyelids.

Trachoma

C. trachomatis deserves to be singled out as a cause of eye infection since it is the most common infective cause of blindness worldwide. Serotypes A–C are implicated in trachoma, a severe inclusion conjunctivitis found in poorer locations throughout the world and spread by flies or inanimate objects. The organism is an obligate intracellular bacterium that causes severe chronic inflammation of the conjunctival epithelium. This distorts the eyelid, drawing the eyelashes inward, which causes conjunctival and corneal abrasion. Tear secretion and drainage are impaired by scarring,

Table 19 Infections of the eye and its surrounds

Infections	Occurrence	Features
Conjunctivitis	Common	Inflammation of the conjunctival epithelium
Keratitis	Common	Inflammation of the cornea
Endophthalmitis	Less common	Inflammation of the uveal tract or posterior chamber; usually an intraocular infective cause
Orbital cellulitis	Less common	Inflammation of the periocular tissues

leading to a dry eye surface. Secondary bacterial infection follows.

Inclusion conjunctivitis

Inclusion conjunctivitis is a much milder disease, caused by *C. trachomatis* serotypes D–K, and is spread by sexual contact. There are follicular inclusions, which can be confused with viral infection but which last more than 4 weeks. Diagnosis is made by taking conjunctival cells with an alginate swab or platinum spatula. Laboratory confirmation is by culture in cell monolayer, direct immunofluorescence or by Giemsa stain of epithelial cells (the last is the least sensitive).

Treatment

Treatment of bacterial conjunctivitis is with topical antibiotic drops. A variety of preparations are available, which include agents such as chloramphenicol, bacitracin and neomycin. If *N. gonorrhoeae* infection is suspected, the patient should also be given intramuscular procaine penicillin or oral amoxicillin plus probenicid. Chlamydial infection can be treated with an oral tetracycline, but pregnant women and children should be treated with oral erythromycin. Topical antibiotics do not improve the response to treatment. The eye should not be covered during conjunctivitis, since it is at increased risk of pressure necrosis. Patients should be instructed to take special care with personal hygiene including avoiding touching the affected eye and sharing towels.

Keratitis

Keratitis is inflammation of the cornea. Patients with corneal infections are at significant risk of losing vision in the affected eye. Infections are caused by bacteria, fungi, viruses and, very rarely, by protozoa. Bacterial keratitis is caused by *Streptococcus pneumoniae*, *Pseudomonas aeruginosa*, staphylococci and other bacteria. Bacterial enzymes reduce the thickness of the cornea and may cause corneal perforation. There is pain in the eye, increased tear formation and photophobia. The cornea loses its normal translucency, and keratic precipitates will be visible on slit lamp examination. If significant pus formation occurs, it collects in the dependent part of the anterior chamber as a hypopyon. Pseudomonas infection is associated with the use of soft contact lenses. The most common viral cause of keratitis is herpes simplex virus. In adults, corneal herpes infection results from reactivation of dormant virus from an earlier infection. This affects all layers of the cornea and often causes a branching ('dendritic') ulcer. Fungal keratitis occurs after contact with soil or vegetable matter and is more common in hot, humid climates. The more commonly isolated fungi are filamentous species such

as *Fusarium* sp., but yeasts (*Candida* spp. etc.) are occasionally found. Varicella-zoster virus can also cause a reactivation keratitis.

Treatment

Patients with keratitis require referral to a specialist for a full diagnostic workup, including microscopy, culture and possibly biopsy. Treatment of bacterial keratitis must be started promptly after the diagnosis has been made to avoid corneal perforation. Antibiotics can be given in the form of concentrated drops, as long as they are given every 15–30 minutes round the clock. Herpes keratitis can be treated with aciclovir drops.

Endophthalmitis

Endophthalmitis is inflammation of the uveal tract or posterior chamber, usually caused by an intraocular infection. It usually arises de novo and not as a result of conjunctival or orbital infection. *Bacillus cereus* is the common bacterial cause, following corneal trauma, but other bacterial species, including staphylococci, streptococci, *Pseudomonas* sp. and *H. influenzae*, have been implicated. Following cataract surgery and lens implantation, *Staphylococcus epidermidis* and the anaerobe *Propionibacterium acnes* are the common bacterial causes. Fungal endophthalmitis is becoming more common, probably as a result of blood-borne infection following intravascular cannulation or parenteral nutrition. Consequently, a high proportion of these cases have positive blood cultures.

Diagnosis

Uveal tract infections, such as chorioretinitis, are difficult to distinguish from other posterior chamber infections on clinical grounds alone. Clinical signs are less pronounced than in infections of the anterior chamber, and a wide variety of organisms can cause uveal tract infection. Two particular conditions will be highlighted: *Toxoplasma gondii* infection, which results in a chorioretinitis, following intrauterine infection (see Ch. 15) and cytomegalovirus infection. Cytomegalovirus retinitis is a particular problem in the immunocompromised, especially in human immunodeficiency virus-associated disease (Ch. 18). Collection of diagnostic specimens from the eye is best done as an operative procedure. Intravitreal antibiotics can be administered at the same time.

Treatment

The choice of agent depends on the epidemiological setting and the most likely microbial pathogen. However, presumptive therapy is often with a combination of several antimicrobial agents, which can be reviewed once the results of laboratory tests are known.

Orbital cellulitis

Orbital cellulitis is inflammation of the periocular soft tissues. It is caused by a variety of bacteria and fungi, of which the most common are *S. aureus* and *H. influenzae* (the latter is the most common in children). The condition arises most often following an infection of the periorbital sinuses but may also occur as a complication of trauma or infection at a distant site.

Orbital cellulitis goes through several distinct stages, from localised inflammation to cellulitis, subperiosteal abscess and, finally, cavernous sinus thrombosis. The eye protrudes from the socket (proptosis) and is unable to move (ophthalmoplegia), the eyelids are swollen and there is fever. The infection is a progressive one and has a high mortality rate if untreated.

Collection of diagnostic specimens is problematic and treatment is often commenced on a presumptive basis. In adults, a penicillinase-resistant β-lactam is often used, against staphylococci, and in children an agent known to be effective against *H. influenzae* (e.g. ampicillin) is used.

12.5 Organisms

A checklist of the organisms discussed in this chapter is given in Box 7. Further information is given on the pages indicated.

Box 7 Organisms that infect the eye and surrounding structures

Bacteria	see page	Fungi	see page
Staphylococcus aureus	243	*Candida* spp.	269
Staphylococcus epidermidis	244	*Fusarium* spp.	269
Streptococcus pneumoniae	245		
Pseudomonas aeruginosa	249–50	**Viruses**	
Haemophilus influenzae	251	Herpes simplex virus	257
Haemophilus aegypti	251	Varicella-zoster virus	257
Moraxella lacunata	253	Adenoviruses	257
Neisseria gonorrhoeae	252–3	Cytomegalovirus	257
Chlamydia trachomatis	255		
Propionibacterium acnes	–	**Parasites**	
Bacillus cereus	246	*Toxoplasma gondii*	263–4
		Acanthamoeba spp.	264

Self-assessment: questions

Multiple choice questions

1. The eye is protected against infection by:
   a. Eyelids
   b. Lacrimal secretions
   c. Efficient corneal phagocytosis
   d. Conjunctival epithelium
   e. The tear film

2. A unilateral red eye:
   a. Always indicates the presence of infection
   b. Extending to the lateral edge of the sclerae is a feature of conjunctivitis
   c. Can result from posterior chamber infection
   d. With purulent discharge is caused by bacterial infection
   e. Is not a feature of uveitis

3. The following organisms cause conjunctivitis:
   a. Adenovirus
   b. *Staphylococcus aureus* only rarely
   c. *Moraxella lacunata*
   d. *Haemophilus influenzae*
   e. *Chlamydia trachomatis*

4. Keratitis:
   a. Is a severe conjunctival infection
   b. May be caused by herpes simplex infection
   c. Leads to formation of a hypopyon in some cases
   d. Results in corneal perforation only as a late complication
   e. Can be caused by wearing contact lenses

5. Endophthalmitis:
   a. Following lens implants is often caused by propionibacteria
   b. After corneal trauma is most often caused by staphylococci
   c. Is best diagnosed by aspirating anterior chamber contents
   d. Usually requires locally invasive antibiotics
   e. Does not always result in loss of sight

6. Orbital cellulitis may take the form of:
   a. Iridocyclitis
   b. Local oedema
   c. Chorioretinitis
   d. Subperiosteal abscess
   e. Cavernous sinus thrombosis

Case history question

A 42-year-old taxi-driver had failing sight in his right eye because of a cataract and had surgery for this that included insertion of a plastic lens implant. The procedure was uneventful and he was discharged from hospital after the normal length of stay. After 1 week, he was readmitted with a red, discharging right eye. Close examination revealed a crescent-shaped collection of pus in the lower part of the anterior chamber, a cloudy cornea and keratic precipitates. An operative procedure was performed and antibiotic chemotherapy commenced. Despite this, the infection progressed and eventually the eye had to be removed.

1. What is this man's condition called?
2. What organisms might have caused this infection?
3. Can you name the collection of pus?
4. Why was a surgical procedure performed?
5. Give one reason why treatment was unsuccessful

Data interpretation

Three swabs from patients of the eye clinic produce identical results:

   no bacterial growth
   adenovirus isolated

1. Do these results explain why the patients attended clinic?
2. What connection might there be between these patients?
3. How would you establish that connection?
4. What measures would you introduce in the clinic?

Objective structured clinical examination (OSCE)

A 74-year-old man developed a dull ache in his left eye 3 weeks after receiving a lens implant following cataract removal. There was no discharge from the eye, and no chemosis, but there was pericorneal injection. Slit lamp examination revealed a cloudy vitreous and a clear anterior chamber. Vitrectomy was performed, a sample sent for laboratory investigations and antibiotic therapy commenced.

You are asked:

1. Do these features suggest a diagnosis of postoperative endophthalmitis?

2. Is this is a case of panophthalmitis?
3. Would diagnosis be assisted by laboratory procedures commenced in the operating theatre?
4. Would this infection best be treated with intravenous antibiotics?

Short notes questions

Write short notes on the following:

1. How eye infection can impair sight
2. How the laboratory helps to distinguish between the cause of papillary and follicular conjunctivitis

Viva question

What are the problems with antibiotic treatment of eye infections?

Self-assessment: answers

Multiple choice answers

1. a. **True**. The eyelids act as both a physical barrier and a means a clearing particulate matter from the eye surface as they spread the tear film.
   b. **True**. Lacrimal secretions contain lysozyme and other antibacterial substances.
   c. **False**. Phagocytosis in the cornea is inefficient since this is an avascular tissue.
   d. **True**. Trauma of this layer can lead to corneal infection.
   e. **True**. It contains lysozyme and allows particulate matter to be floated to the edge of the eye for removal.

2. a. **False**. Some non-infective conditions also cause a red eye.
   b. **True**. This is a particular indication.
   c. **True**. The redness is in the limbus, the area surrounding the iris.
   d. **False**. Fungal infections can also result in a purulent discharge.
   e. **False**. In uveitis, redness is seen in the vessels immediately surrounding the iris.

3. a. **True**. The most common viral cause in developed countries.
   b. **False**. *S. aureus* is the most common bacterial cause of conjunctivitis.
   c. **True**. *M. lacunata* is a less common cause of bacterial conjunctivitis, associated with angular dermatitis.
   d. **True**. Particularly in children.
   e. **True**. *C. trachomatis* types D–K cause inclusion conjunctivitis.

4. a. **False**. Keratitis is an inflammation of the cornea.
   b. **True**. The most common viral cause.
   c. **True**. This occurs if there is significant pus formation.
   d. **False**. Perforation may occur shortly after the onset of keratitis because of thinning of the cornea. This can occur in some aggressive bacterial infections with pneumococcal or *Pseudomonas* spp.
   e. **True**. It is associated with the use of soft contact lenses.

5. a. **True**. This is a commensal of skin.
   b. **False**. *Bacillus cereus* is the most common bacterial cause of endophthalmitis after corneal trauma.
   c. **False**. The best diagnostic specimen from a patient with endophthalmitis is posterior chamber fluid, i.e. vitreous humour.
   d. **True**. A combination of several agents is often used.
   e. **True**. Prompt treatment is a way of minimising serious sequelae.

6. a. **False**. Iridocyclitis is an infection of the uveal tract caused by, for example, *Toxoplasma gondii*.
   b. **True**. There is proptosis and swollen eyelids.
   c. **False**. Chorioretinitis is an infection of the uveal tract caused by, for example, cytomegalovirus.
   d. **True**. This can develop from cellulitis.
   e. **True**. This is the severe stage that results if cellulitis is not controlled.

Case histories answer

1. This is a case of postoperative endophthalmitis.
2. Although the common agents of infection would be *Propionibacterium acnes* and *Staphylococcus epidermidis*, these organisms usually cause a more insidious infection with a slower onset. The rapid onset suggests either *Staphylococcus aureus* or streptococcal infection, but a fungal species could also cause this picture.
3. 'Hypopyon'
4. The operation was performed to remove the lens implant (a continuing nidus of infection) and vitreous humour for diagnostic purposes. Antibiotics were instilled at the same time.
5. Infection may have progressed too far to arrest it with antimicrobial chemotherapy by this stage, or organisms remaining after the first intravitreal dose may not have been eradicated by subsequent topical, subconjunctival or systemic antibiotics. This patient turned out to have an infection of the filamentous fungus *Fusarium* sp., which only grew after prolonged incubation in the laboratory.

Data interpretation answer

1. They could have been part of a community-wide outbreak of adenovirus conjunctivitis, but they may also reflect infection transmitted in the clinic.
2. Infection may have been passed on in the clinic via an inadequately disinfected device such as a tonometer.
3. By requesting details of the clinic lists, you need to establish if these patients form a sequence who have seen one specialist or been examined with a single

device that contacted the surface of the eye, such as a tonometer. You also need to know what type of disinfection/decontamination procedure was in use.

4. If a link can be established, the device in question has to be disinfected more thoroughly after use. Alcohol surface decontamination is ineffective against adenovirus.

OSCE answer

1. Yes.
2. No. A clear conjunctiva and anterior chamber suggest that infection is restricted to the posterior chamber.
3. Yes. Some centres send laboratory staff to eye theatre to prepare smears for microscopy and inoculate agar plates immediately after collection of vitreous fluid, in order to increase the chances of recovering fastidious or antibiotic-damaged microorganisms.
4. No. The best treatment would be a combination of intravenous and subconjunctival antibiotics. The latter are agents that will be carried backward into the posterior chamber.

Short notes answers

1. Could be tackled either anatomically with examples of specific infections or by exploring the consequences of a single infection in more detail (trachoma would be a good choice because of its worldwide importance).
2. A table of causes of follicular and papillary conjunctivitis is a useful starting point. Remember that tarsal papillae are a feature of bacterial infection, while follicular inclusions are associated with viral and chlamydial disease.

Viva answer

The merits of topical, locally invasive and systemic therapy need to be discussed. The limited range of suitable agents poses problems, and bioavailability is a key issue. Illustrate with specific examples.

13 Bone and joint infections

Overview

Though rare, bone and joint infections are significant because they cause serious disability and even death when they do occur. Early diagnosis and treatment are essential if serious morbidity is to be avoided. Special procedures are required to make a specific diagnosis and guide antimicrobial chemotherapy.

13.1 Pathogenesis

Learning objectives

You should:

- know how infection spreads to bones and joints
- be aware of the lower ability of bone to resist infection.

Bones and joints are normally sterile. In order to cause infection, microorganisms must first gain access to these tissues via the bloodstream by spread from an adjacent focus of infection or by direct inoculation during trauma or surgery. Establishment of infection is favoured by the relatively poor phagocytic capacity of bones and joints. Cortical bone, cartilage and joint capsule may all act as barriers to the spread of infection, but distant spread may still occur via the systemic circulation, resulting in septicaemia.

13.2 Diagnosis

Learning objectives

You should:

- know the features of bone and joint infection
- know the role of imaging and diagnostic microbiology in diagnosis and follow-up.

The principal features of bone and joint infections are local pain, other signs of inflammation and loss of function. Fever, when present, may signify the onset of septicaemia. Imaging techniques are important in the diagnosis and subsequent follow-up of these infections. Technetium bone scan may help to localise the site of bony inflammation early in the course of infection. Radiological changes take longer to develop, and bony erosions may not be evident for several weeks.

It is important to make every reasonable attempt to obtain diagnostic microbiology specimens, even though the site of infection causes practical difficulties. If necessary, orthopaedic surgical or rheumatological help should be sought to obtain subperiosteal pus, bone or synovial fluid, where relevant. Blood cultures should also be obtained if the patient has a fever. The choice of antibiotic depends heavily on the results of microscopy and culture of these specimens.

13.3 Diseases and syndromes

Learning objectives

You should:

- know the major infections of the bones and joints
- know the factors contributing to their occurrence
- understand the basis of their clinical management.

The diseases affecting bones and joints are given in Table 21.

Osteomyelitis

Osteomyelitis is inflammation of bone and adjacent marrow. It usually affects a long bone. It is regarded as an acute condition at the time of first presentation and as a chronic condition if it occurs after completion of at least one course of appropriate antibiotic therapy. Osteomyelitis is also classified according to the most likely means of pathogenesis:

* haematogenous
* contiguous spread
* peripheral vascular disease associated
* prosthesis associated.

Haematogenous osteomyelitis Haematogenous osteomyelitis used to account for the majority of cases but has recently become less prominent, as the other types of osteomyelitis increase in importance. The haematogenous type most commonly affects children, and the primary lesion is usually located in the metaphysis of the femur, tibia or humerus. The most common bacterial species causing the condition is *Staphylococcus aureus*, but *Haemophilus influenzae* may be isolated from children in the preschool age group, especially in non-vaccinated populations. In intravenous drug abusers, Gram-negative bacilli (Enterobacteriaceae) or yeasts may be isolated, and there may be multiple sites of infections in locations such as the sacroiliac joints. Mycobacteria (usually *M. tuberculosis*) can cause osteomyelitis at unusual sites, such as the thoracic spine where vertebral collapse may follow (causing a 'gibbus' or hunchback).

Children are particularly prone to infection of the metaphysis of certain long bones because of the development of the cartilaginous growth plate. There are no vascular anastomoses in the region of the growth plate after infancy. The blood supply is brought close to the growth plate where flow slows down in a network of tightly bent capillary sinuses. Phagocytosis in these vessels is poor and minor trauma occurs easily. Osteomyelitis often follows minor trauma to the adjacent joint. In children, collection of pus following an acute inflammatory response lifts the periosteum and leads to new, circumferential bone formation. The circumferential bone is called 'involucrum' (Fig. 14). In adults, the periosteum is more tightly bound to the bone and does not lift as easily. Instead, infection spreads via the Haversian and Volkmann canal systems. Back pressure on blood vessels causes impaired circulation to living bone and eventually death of bony segments. These segments (called 'sequestrum') may contribute to treatment failure and the development of chronic osteomyelitis by protecting bacteria from antibiotic action. When pus drains via a break in the bone and creates a channel through the overlying soft tissues, a sinus is formed.

Contiguous spread osteomyelitis Direct spread of bacteria from infection in adjacent tissues is called contiguous spread osteomyelitis. Again long bones are a common site of infection, but other sites may be involved, such as the cranial vault following head injury, the sacrum or greater trochanter following decubitus ulceration and the sternum after cardiothoracic surgery. Gram-negative bacilli, anaerobic bacteria and other species are all more commonly isolated than in haematogenous osteomyelitis.

Peripheral vascular disease Osteomyelitis associated with peripheral vascular disease often affects the toes and is commonly caused by streptococci and anaerobic bacteria. It is particularly common in diabetics.

Prostheses Osteomyelitis is being recognised with increasing frequency in association with prosthetic joints and other orthopaedic implants. Infection caused either

Table 21	Infections of bones and joints
Infection	**Features**
Osteomyelitis	Inflammation of bone and adjacent marrow, usually located in one of the long bones
Septic arthritis	Acute inflammation of a joint caused by infection
Reactive arthritis	Inflammation of a joint following a previous infection

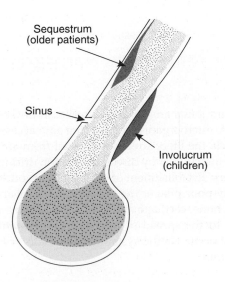

Fig. 14 Osteomyelitis in a long bone.

by perioperative contamination or by haematogenous spread occurs in the postoperative period. The former are more aggressive infections and are caused by staphylococci and other bacteria typical of the indigenous skin flora of the patient or surgeon. An infected prosthetic joint may not unite with surrounding bone. In postoperative prosthesis-associated osteomyelitis, the infection is typically more insidious, perhaps noted only as discomfort in the joint. The causal organisms are usually bacteria such as coagulase-negative staphylococci, streptococci and corynebacteria.

Diagnosis

In acute osteomyelitis, symptoms are usually experienced soon after the onset of infection and include local pain, fever and possibly tenderness and immobility of the adjacent joint. Every attempt should be made to obtain pus, bone and peripheral blood for culture before commencing antimicrobial chemotherapy. Needle aspiration of pus may be possible in some instances. Swabs of wound exudate from patients with infected joint replacements are of little value. X-rays are of limited diagnostic use in the early stages of the disease, but a technetium scan may pinpoint the site of infection. In chronic osteomyelitis, there should be a history of previously diagnosed acute disease followed by a course of antimicrobial chemotherapy. There may also be relevant epidemiological clues such as the patient's age, vascular disease or trauma. Radiological changes will be more obvious in chronic osteomyelitis owing to the prolonged course of the disease.

Chemotherapy

Presumptive treatment of acute osteomyelitis used to be directed almost exclusively against *S. aureus*. Now that other species have become more common causal agents of acute osteomyelitis, greater care must be taken in the choice of presumptive antibiotic treatment. In the preschool child, treatment should be directed against both staphylococci and *H. influenzae* (e.g. flucloxacillin and ampicillin). An antistaphylococcal agent alone may be adequate presumptive therapy in older children and most adults, but treatment may have to be modified according to the results of Gram stain and culture. It is more difficult to specify suitable presumptive therapy for osteomyelitis resulting from contiguous spread, peripheral vascular disease or orthopaedic prosthetic device, since the aetiological agents are much more varied. Gram-negative osteomyelitis is often unresponsive to antimicrobial chemotherapy.

Initial therapy of acute osteomyelitis should be via the intravenous route, but there is disagreement over when and whether to switch to oral agents. Treatment must be continued for several weeks, and long-term follow-up involves repeat X-rays. Treatment of chronic osteomyelitis is problematic. Since prolonged treatment may be required, it is particularly important to obtain suitable specimens for culture before commencing therapy. Agents should be chosen with known activity against the causal pathogen and with good bone and tissue penetration (e.g. clindamycin for Gram-positive bacteria and ciprofloxacin for Gram-negative organisms). Sequestra and sinus tracks will require surgical removal to improve the chances of success.

Septic arthritis

Septic arthritis is acute inflammation of a joint and usually occurs in a single load-bearing joint. The infected joint is hot, swollen and painful, and joint movement is often restricted. A minority of patients are febrile. Some non-infective conditions may mimic septic arthritis. These include gout, pseudogout and rheumatoid arthritis. Infection may be superimposed on these conditions, and patients with inflammatory joint disease are also at increased risk of infection.

Septic arthritis is usually caused by blood-borne bacteria, but occasionally follows contiguous spread and may be caused by viruses or fungi. The arthritis occurring during mumps or rubella is typically mild, short lived and without major impairment of joint function. It may also affect more than one joint. A clinically similar arthritis may occur during hepatitis as a result of deposition of immune complexes. Fungi causing septic arthritis include *Candida albicans*, *Sporothrix schenckii* and other rarer species. The bacterial species causing septic arthritis vary with the age of the patient. The most common species overall is *S. aureus*, which is particularly common in patients with pre-existing joint diseases such as rheumatoid arthritis. *Neisseria gonorrhoeae* is the most common cause in sexually active young adults, particularly women during menstruation and pregnancy. *H. influenzae* is occasionally implicated in preschool children, and streptococci are sometimes found in association with prosthetic joints. Mycobacteria are a rare cause of septic arthritis.

Diagnosis

Joint fluid should be aspirated with care for microscopy and culture. Microscopic examination for crystals should also be requested in order to rule out gout and pseudogout. The results of an urgent Gram stain may confirm the presumptive choice of antibiotic therapy. The joint should be aspirated as thoroughly as possible to improve the prospect of successful therapy. Infection of a prosthetic joint may require removal of the prosthesis to guarantee eradication of infection.

Chemotherapy

Presumptive treatment is determined by the most likely causal pathogen: an antistaphylococcal agent (e.g.

flucloxacillin) is appropriate in most groups, but preschool children should also be given an agent effective against *H. influenzae*, and young adults, particularly menstruating women, should be given benzylpenicillin. Little can be done to prevent the onset of septic arthritis, apart from taking care to follow strict aseptic technique when performing invasive procedures involving the joint, e.g. intra-articular steroid injection and arthroscopy.

Reactive arthritis

Reactive arthritis is an inflammation of the joint(s) following previous bacterial infection. The arthritis is non-infective, usually self-limiting and lasts weeks to months. Bacteria that have been associated with reactive arthritis include *N. gonorrhoeae*, *Chlamydia trachomatis* and *Salmonella*, *Shigella*, *Campylobacter* and *Yersinia* spp. There is increased risk of reactive arthritis in persons with the HLA-B27 locus. The condition is thought to be immunologically mediated.

13.4 Organisms

A checklist of the organisms discussed in this chapter is given in Box 8. Further information is given on the pages indicated.

Box 8 Organisms that infect the bones and joints

Bacteria	see page	Fungi	see page
Staphylococcus aureus	244	*Candida* spp.	269
Streptococci	244–5	*Sporothrix schenckii*	270
Pseudomonas aeruginosa	249–50		
Neisseria gonorrhoeae	252–3	**Viruses**	
Enterobacteriaceae	248–9	Hepatitis A virus	–
Mycobacteria (incl. *M. tuberculosis*)	253–4	Rubellavirus	261
Anaerobic bacteria	247–8, 252	Mumps virus	259
Salmonella spp.	248–9		
Shigella spp.	249		
Campylobacter spp.	251		
Yersinia spp.	249		

Self-assessment: questions

Multiple choice questions

1. Osteomyelitis may develop:
   a. In the toes of diabetics
   b. Because of haematogenous spread
   c. In orthopaedic prosthetic devices
   d. By direct spread from adjacent tissues
   e. In the presence of peripheral vascular disease

2. Osteomyelitis most commonly involves the following sites:
   a. Sternum
   b. Lower femur
   c. Upper tibia
   d. Lower humerus
   e. Thoracic vertebrae

3. Bacteria species that commonly cause acute osteomyelitis are:
   a. *Haemophilus influenzae*
   b. Anaerobic bacteria
   c. *Pseudomonas aeruginosa*
   d. *Staphylococcus aureus*
   e. *Candida albicans*

4. Contiguous spread osteomyelitis occurs following:
   a. Formation of sequestrum
   b. Head injury
   c. Bedsores
   d. Cardiac surgery
   e. Development of involucrum

5. The following investigations are likely to help in the immediate management of acute osteomyelitis:
   a. Needle aspiration of purulent focus
   b. Radiography of affected bones
   c. Bone biopsy
   d. Blood culture
   e. Pus swab

6. Pair the infection with the most appropriate presumptive therapy:
   a. Acute osteomyelitis in a 42-year-old   i. Intravenous benzylpenicillin
   b. Acute osteomyelitis in a 4-year-old child   ii. Intravenous flucloxacillin and fucidic acid
   c. Septic arthritis in a 25-year-old woman   iii. Intravenous flucloxacillin and ampicillin
   d. Osteomyelitis underlying a bedsore   iv. Ciprofloxacin and metronidazole

7. Septic arthritis:
   a. Is most commonly caused by *Staphylococcus aureus*
   b. Is very rarely caused by *Neisseria gonorrhoeae*
   c. Is usually accompanied by fever
   d. Causes local pain, swelling and loss of function
   e. Is not associated with septicaemia

8. Reactive arthritis can follow infection with:
   a. *Chlamydia* sp.
   b. *Salmonella* sp.
   c. *Staphylococcus aureus*
   d. *Streptococcus pyogenes*
   e. *Shigella* sp.

Case history question

> A 54-year-old woman was admitted with a hot, painful right knee. She had been treated for rheumatoid arthritis for over 10 years and recently had been given an intra-articular injection of prednisone. The admitting physician aspirated the joint and then commenced antibiotic treatment. He did not obtain a blood culture first. The pain and swelling subsided over several days without the need for any alteration to the antibiotic regimen.

1. What was the diagnosis?
2. Explain the significance of the prednisone injection
3. What was the value of joint aspiration?
4. Why was no blood culture taken?
5. How did the physician know what antibiotics to use first?

Data interpretation

A 29-year-old man attends clinic with a 1-week history of pain in proximal finger joints and wrists. There are notes from a clinic attendance for diarrhoea 3 weeks previously and the following laboratory report for a faecal specimen in his file:

consistency: fluid
pus, blood not observed
Salmonella typhimurium isolated
Shigella, *Campylobacter* spp. not detected.

1. How does the laboratory result explain his arthropathy?
2. What other infections do you need to exclude in this patient?

3. What non-microbiological laboratory test would you want to request?
4. Is this an indication for antibiotic treatment?

Objective structured clinical examination (OSCE)

A 68-year-old woman who underwent total hip replacement 6 weeks previously has been admitted via the orthopaedic clinic because of discomfort around the prosthesis. On examination she is afebrile and in generally good physical condition for her age apart from the right hip. There is mild tenderness over the hip but no redness or swelling. Radiographs show only the reactive changes expected after elective surgery. The peripheral leucocyte count is within normal limits and the C-reactive protein is 25 (normal range 1–10).

You are asked:

1. Can these features be explained by an infection of the prosthesis?

2. If so, would the most likely bacterial cause be *Staphylococcus aureus*?
3. Will diagnostic imaging at this stage help with subsequent clinical management?
4. Would you view revision arthroplasty as a last resort?

Short notes questions

Write short notes on the following:

1. The principal differences between acute and chronic osteomyelitis
2. The formation of involucrum, sequestrum and sinuses in osteomyelitis
3. The microbiological investigations you would use in the management of a patient with osteomyelitis

Viva question

Why do you think *Staphylococcus aureus* has become less common as a cause of osteomyelitis? What challenges does this pose?

Self-assessment: answers

Multiple choice answers

1. a. **True**. It is associated with peripheral vascular disease.
   b. **True**. This occurs most commonly in children.
   c. **False**. Osteomyelitis develops around the prosthetic device, not in it.
   d. **True**. This can occur after surgery or trauma.
   e. **True**. In this case, streptococci and anaerobic bacteria are often implicated.

2. a. **False**. This is an uncommon site associated with cardiac surgery.
   b. **True**. The metaphysis of long bones is a common site for the primary lesion.
   c. **True**. See b.
   d. **True**. See b.
   e. **False**. This is an uncommon site associated with tuberculosis.

3. a. **True**. Particularly in preschool children.
   b. **False**. Anaerobic bacteria are uncommon causes of osteomyelitis.
   c. **False**. *Pseudomonas aeruginosa* is more commonly associated with chronic osteomyelitis.
   d. **True**. This is the most common species.
   e. **False**. *Candida albicans* is a yeast.

4. a. **False**. Sequestrum is a segment of dead bone inside a long bone with osteomyelitis.
   b. **True**. Damage to the cranial vault leaves it vulnerable to infection.
   c. **True**. These form a source of infectious organisms.
   d. **True**. When the sternum can be infected.
   e. **False**. Involucrum is new bone formed circumferentially after pus separates the periosteum from the outer surface of cortical bone.

5. a. **True**. This provides a sample for diagnostic microbiology.
   b. **False**. Changes that can be detected by radiography may take weeks to develop and are rarely helpful in diagnosing acute osteomyelitis.
   c. **True**.
   d. **False**. Blood cultures should be obtained but will take too long to have a useful impact on immediate therapy.
   e. **False**. Even when pus drains from an osteomyelitis sinus attack, the bacteria isolated are not necessarily representative of those at the site of infection.

6. a. and ii.
   b. and iii.
   c. and i.
   d. and iv.

7. a. **True**. *S. aureus* is the most common overall. *Neisseria gonorrhoeae* is the most common cause of septic arthritis in sexually active young adults, especially women.
   b. **False**. *N. gonorrhoeae* is a common cause.
   c. **False**. Fever is present in only a minority of cases.
   d. **True**.
   e. **False**. Septic arthritis may be either the result of septicaemic spread or the source of a septicaemia.

8. a. **True**.
   b. **True**.
   c. **False**.
   d. **False**.
   e. **True**.

Case history answer

1. Septic arthritis.
2. It may have been the point at which bacteria were introduced into the joint. The steroid injection may also have impaired local defences.
3. For a diagnostic specimen and to improve the chance of successful treatment.
4. If the patient was afebrile, she was unlikely to have a bacteraemia at the time. Only a minority of patients with septic arthritis have a fever.
5. Most patients with septic arthritis superimposed on rheumatoid arthritis have a *Staphylococcus aureus* infection. The admitting physician confirmed his choice of presumptive therapy by asking for an urgent Gram stain on the joint fluid he aspirated, which revealed clusters of Gram-positive cocci.

Data interpretation answer

1. Salmonella infection can be followed by a reactive arthropathy.
2. Sexually transmitted diseases such as *Neisseria gonorrhoeae* infection, and viral infections such as parvovirus B19.
3. HLA typing. The B90 variant is associated with a higher risk of reactive arthropathy.
4. No.

OSCE answer

1. Yes. Postoperative infection of a hip prosthesis can be insidious, making the progression of clinical signs subtle and difficult to detect.
2. No. Skin bacteria such as coagulase-negative staphylococci, corynebacteria or propionibacteria would be more common than *S. aureus*, which would normally cause a more florid, acute infection.
3. Yes. Advanced techniques such as isotope labelled imaging may indicate the location and extent of inflammatory change, although this may be masked in the earlier stages of postoperative repair by normal healing processes. Imaging studies can show whether there has been loosening of the prosthesis, indicating a high probability of failure and a need for revision.
4. Yes, because revision carries a higher risk of subsequent failure.

Short notes answers

1. Explain the pragmatic definition of acute and chronic infection, with reference to aetiology, pathogenesis and management.

2. See p. 152.
3. Best followed in sequence: specimen, urgent microscopy, culture, susceptibility testing, supplementary cultures (i.e. blood, bone biopsy). For full marks, remember unusual pathogens: mycobacteria and fungi.

Viva answer

Better and earlier treatment of staphylococcal infections combined with the rise of other forms, such as prosthesis infection and contiguous osteomyelitis associated with vascular insufficiency. Early diagnosis is more difficult and the wider range of possible pathogens leads to greater difficulty in choosing the right presumptive antibiotic therapy. Underlying co-morbidities such as prostheses and vascular disease increase the risk of treatment failure.

14 Congenital and neonatal infections

Overview

The unborn child and newborn infant are susceptible to infections that do not affect older people or, if they do, have less serious consequences. The infections experienced in the pre-, peri- and neonatal period are largely determined by the nature of the primary encounter with the infective agent, and the degree of immaturity of the immune system. In newborn infants, the presenting features of serious, life-threatening infection may be subtle and apparently innocuous to the inexperienced. For several of these infections, there is still no universally effective treatment, making preventive measures all the more important.

14.1 Pathogenesis

Learning objectives

You should:

- know how the fetus and neonate can become infected
- know the immune capability of the fetus and neonate.

The unborn child occupies an immunologically privileged site in utero, benefitting from the mother's defences against infection and the protective layer of villous trophoblast wall. However, some infections do gain access, either via the uterine cervix (the 'ascending' route) or via the transplacental route from the maternal bloodstream. The unborn child has limited phagocytic capability and cytokine production, making it vulnerable to infection. During delivery, the child encounters an environment densely populated with microorganisms as it passes along the mother's birth canal. Early encounter with organisms in the resident vaginal flora may occur as a result of premature rupture of fetal membranes. Also, maternal infection may cause premature delivery. Microbial colonisation of the neonate's skin, gastrointestinal tract and the respiratory tract occur shortly after delivery. Occasionally, pathogenic bacteria or viruses are acquired this way and, subsequently, cause severe neonatal infection. Premature babies are more compromised than full-term neonates and are often exposed to additional risks of infection during admission to special-care nurseries.

14.2 Diagnosis

Learning objectives

You should:

- know how a neonate responds to infection
- know the problems of laboratory investigations.

The newborn infant does not necessarily respond to systemic infection with a fever. Signs of severe infection may be more subtle: irritability, reluctance to feed, restlessness or non-specific rash. The syndromes caused by congenital infection often have features in common, irrespective of the causal pathogen, so that it may be impossible to make a specific diagnosis without multiple laboratory investigations. It may be necessary to submit multiple cultures and perform multiple antigen detection and serological tests. Collection of blood for culture without contamination by commensal skin bacteria is particularly difficult in newborn infants, yet these same organisms (e.g. coagulase-negative staphylococci) may be the cause of septicaemia. Close liaison with the diagnostic laboratory is essential for effective diagnosis and management.

14.3 Diseases and syndromes

Learning objectives

You should:

- know the major congenital and neonatal infections
- understand the factors contributing to their occurrence
- know the basis of their clinical management.

Infections can be considered as

- congenital
- perinatal
- neonatal.

Congenital infections

The main congenital infections are described in Table 22 and the areas infected in Table 23.

Although exposure to some infective agents shortly before birth results in infection at or shortly after birth, the infections they cause are really perinatal infections. Truly congenital infections are acquired in utero and are usually established by the time of delivery (Table 22). They have other features in common: the mother is usually asymptomatic, different pathogens present similar features, there is a wide range of severity and laboratory diagnosis is principally serological. The causal agents used to be known by the acronym TORCH (toxoplasma, others, rubella,

cytomegalovirus and herpes simplex) but the group has expanded to make this acronym obsolete. An alternative is PoRT HaTCH (parvovirus B19, rubella, *Toxoplasma gondii*, HIV (human immunodeficiency virus), *Treponema pallidum*, cytomegalovirus, herpes simplex)—the vowels have no meaning. (Further details on the specific infective agents mentioned here can be found in Section C.)

The baby is born with a variety of clinical features, any of which may suggest intrauterine infection: rash, hepatosplenomegaly, jaundice, petechiae, microcephaly, cataracts, retinitis, intracerebral calcification or congenital heart disease (Table 23). Deafness or developmental retardation may only be apparent later. Damage is caused by interference with organogenesis, by placental insufficiency and by inflammation. Diagnosis is mainly serological, supplemented by viral culture where appropriate. Since IgG passes across the placenta, single neonatal IgG titres cannot be relied on for diagnosis. Either specific IgM titre or rising IgG titres are required. Effective antimicrobial chemotherapy is only available for syphilis and toxoplasmosis. Prevention is by immunisation and avoiding maternal exposure.

Cytomegalovirus infection

The most common congenital viral infection is with cytomegalovirus. Of those infected in utero, 95% remain asymptomatic. The remainder suffer intrauterine growth retardation (IUGR), jaundice, hepatosplenomegaly, petechiae and pulmonary lesions. Diagnosis is by specific IgM, but the virus can also be cultured from

Table 22 Congenital infections

Infection	Features
Cytomegalovirus	Most common viral infection; 95% asymptomatic; growth retardation, liver, skin and lung lesions
Rubella virus	Teratogenic damage or miscarriage
Toxoplasmosis	Affects the brain, eyes, liver and skin
Human immunodeficiency virus	Infects transplacentally and during delivery; approximately 30% of offspring of infected mothers are HIV positive
Parvovirus	Severe hydrops fetalis
Herpes simplex virus	Rare; disseminated, mucocutaneous or neurological disease
Syphilis	Perinatal death; premature delivery; congenital syphilis syndrome

Table 23 Principal results of intrauterine infection: areas infected

Infective agent	Brain	Eyes	Ears	Heart	Liver	Skin	Bones	Immunity	IUGR*
Cytomegalovirus					+	+			+
Rubella virus	+	+	+	+	+	+			+
Toxoplasma gondii	+	+			+	+			
Parvovirus B19				+					
Treponema pallidum						+	+	+	
Human immunodeficiency virus	?	?							

*IUGR, intrauterine growth restriction.

the baby's throat or urine. There is currently no effective treatment for congenital infection.

Rubella

Rubella virus causes a minor infection in children and adults but can cause major damage to the fetus or embryo.

Transplacental transmission results in miscarriage or teratogenic damage. Common results of intrauterine rubella infection include hepatosplenomegaly, purpura, congenital heart disease, cataracts, hearing loss and mental retardation. Diagnosis is confirmed by viral isolation and specific IgM titres. Congenital rubella is now very rare in developed countries because of immuno-prophylaxis of women of child-bearing age. The vaccine is a live-attenuated strain. Accidental vaccination during pregnancy is uncommon, and experience suggests that the vaccine strain has a lower attributable risk of congenital damage to the unborn child.

Toxoplasmosis

Infection with the sporozoan parasite *T. gondii* in adults usually results in a mild influenza-like illness with lymph-adenopathy. In adults, major complications only arise when there are significantly compromised immune defences. About half of pregnant women who develop toxoplasmosis transmit infection to the fetus. The features of intrauterine infection include petechiae, jaundice and hepatosplenomegaly, retinitis, intracerebral calcification and microcephaly. Diagnosis is by IgM-specific enzyme-linked immunosorbent assay (ELISA; direct fluorescent or indirect fluorescent antibody test; see Ch. 25). Treatment is with pyrimethamine and sulfa-diazine in three courses each of 21 days.

Human immunodeficiency virus

HIV may be transmitted transplacentally. Around 30% of babies born to seropositive mothers develop the acquired immunodeficiency syndrome (AIDS). Of these, 80% sero-convert after 3 years, but serological tests cannot be relied upon in the first few months of life. Nucleic acid amplification (polymerase chain reaction) allows detection of viral RNA in infected neonates before seroconversion

takes place. Disease can be classified in three stages, which has implications for clinical management (Table 24).

HIV culture is available in some teaching centres and is highly specific, but of limited sensitivity. Alternatively, serial Western blot of paired maternal and neonatal serum may be helpful. Zidovudine therapy may prevent or slow progression of HIV disease, but other treatment modalities will be required as T helper cell count diminishes. Immunisations and specific antimicrobial therapy against opportunist infections will be required, and optimal nutrition must be maintained. The social circumstances of the mother may be a significant determinant of outcome.

Parvovirus

Parvovirus causes mild maternal infection but may spread via the placental route causing severe **hydrops fetalis** and possibly fetal death. There is no specific antiviral therapy.

Herpes simplex virus

Intrauterine infection with herpes simplex virus (HSV) I or II is rare. When it does occur, it results in disseminated, mucocutaneous or neurological disease. Diagnosis is serological. Treatment is with aciclovir.

Syphilis

If a pregnant woman is infected with *T. pallidum* and develops primary or secondary syphilis after 16 weeks of gestation, the fetus is liable to infection. The result is peri-natal death, premature delivery or the congenital syphilis syndrome. A smaller percentage is affected if infection occurs in the third trimester. The features include rash on the soles and palms, condylomata lata, polyglandular lymphadenopathy, rhinitis and bony lesions at 1–3 weeks. VDRL (Venereal Diseases Reference Laboratory) and FTA-Abs (fluorescent treponemal antibody, absorbed) tests need to be performed on serum and cere-brospinal fluid with repeat serology at bimonthly intervals, as seroconversion may be delayed. Darkfield microscopy for spirochaetes should also be done on cere-brospinal fluid and nasal discharge. Treatment is with single injection of intramuscular penicillin, but if there is evidence of neurosyphilis, treatment is with penicillin for 10 days. The congenital syndrome is rare in most developed countries because of declining incidence of syphilis and programmes of antenatal screening.

Perinatal infections

Several viruses cause infection either immediately before or after delivery (Table 25). HIV may also be transmitted in this way.

Table 24 Staging of infection with the human immunodeficiency virus in children

Disease stage	Characteristic
P0	Indeterminate
P1	Asymptomatic
P2	Symptomatic: secondary infection, secondary neoplasm, neurological features, respiratory features, others

Table 25 Perinatal infections

Infection	Features
Herpes	Jaundice, bleeding, hepatosplenomegaly; 80% mortality
Varicella (varicella-zoster virus)	Disseminated infection; 30% mortality
Hepatitis B	No immediate effects; long-term hepatic disease
HIV infection	As for congenital infection

Herpes

If the mother has genital herpes at the time of delivery, there is a risk of serious disease in the infant, resulting in jaundice, hepatosplenomegaly and bleeding, the mortality for which is about 80%. Local ophthalmic, skin or central nervous system disease can also occur.

Diagnosis is by viral culture, specific IgM detection or Tzanck smear of vesicle fluid from skin lesions.

Treatment of established infection is with aciclovir. Infection can be prevented by planned delivery via caesarean section.

Varicella

A baby is at greatest risk from varicella-zoster infection during the perinatal period, when disseminated infection has a 30% mortality. Transmission does not occur if the mother does not develop infection more than 5 days before or 4 days after delivery.

Infection is diagnosed clinically and confirmed by smear of skin lesions, viral culture and serology.

Treatment is with aciclovir or vidarabine. Prevention is the main approach to controlling this infection and involves administration of zoster IgG if the baby is born between 5 days before or 4 days after the onset of clinical varicella-zoster infection. Pregnant women known not to have had chickenpox should avoid all contact with persons suffering from varicella, including hospital and clinic staff.

Hepatitis B

The significance of perinatal hepatitis B infection lies in its long-term consequences. The neonate infected with hepatitis B virus is relatively tolerant and therefore unlikely to develop serious disease immediately. However, the failure of infants to mount an effective immune response leads to a high rate of chronic hepatitis, cirrhosis and hepatocellular carcinoma.

Prevention is by administration of hepatitis B immunoglobulin within 12 hours of delivery and hepatitis B vaccine within 2 days whenever the mother is known to be hepatitis antigen positive. In some countries, all babies born to mothers positive for hepatitis B surface antigen are immunised.

Neonatal infections

Exposure to infectious agents during the birth process and in the period immediately following birth can give rise to serious illness in neonates (Table 26).

Septicaemia and meningitis

Septicaemia and meningitis occur spontaneously in newborn infants. In the first week, septicaemia predominates and has a mortality rate of up to 50%. The organisms causing infection are usually acquired from the indigenous flora of the mother's birth canal either during normal vaginal delivery or as a result of premature rupture of membranes and ascending infection. The most common species implicated in neonatal septicaemia are *Escherichia coli*, group B streptococci (*S. agalactiae*) and *Listeria monocytogenes*. The same group of organisms cause late-onset neonatal sepsis, which often presents as a meningitis around 10 days postpartum and has a mortality rate of around 20%.

Diagnosis, whether of early- or late-onset disease requires collection of blood, urine and cerebrospinal fluid for culture and microscopy.

The severity of the condition and the risk of a fatal outcome dictate prompt therapeutic decisions: ampicillin and gentamicin are the usual choice of presumptive antibiotic agents. Attempts to prevent neonatal sepsis by antibiotic prophylaxis of the mother have been unsuccessful. Only a small proportion of maternal carriers of the main agents of infection have babies that go on to develop neonatal sepsis or meningitis; at present it

Table 26 Neonatal infections

Infection	Features
Septicaemia and meningitis	In first week, septicaemia predominates; up to 50% mortality Late-onset (10 days postpartum) meningitis predominates; approximately 20% mortality
Ophthalmia neonatorum	Conjunctivitis, purulent discharge
Omphalitis	Infection of umbilical stump; can disseminate
Necrotising enterocolitis	Loose, blood-stained stools, gas in abdominal tissues
Scalded skin syndrome	Extensive exfoliation of skin caused by *S. aureus* toxin

is not possible to identify those at greatest risk with any certainty. Nevertheless, pre-emptive treatment of babies born following premature rupture of the membranes may be warranted since these children are thought to be at increased risk of infection.

Ophthalmia neonatorum

Ophthalmia neonatorum is an infective inflammation of the neonatal eye, usually appearing as a conjunctivitis or purulent discharge. It is caused by intrapartum infection by agents including *Neisseria gonorrhoeae*, *Chlamydia trachomatis* (serotypes A–K), staphylococci and adenovirus. (Silver nitrate solution used prophylactically in the eyes of neonates sometimes causes a mild, self-limiting inflammation.) Specific diagnosis is made by microscopy and culture, remembering that *N. gonorrhoeae*, *Chlamydia* sp. and adenovirus all require special transport media. Direct immunofluorescence is available for detection of *Chlamydia* sp. The mother should be counselled and investigated as a possible source of infection. Treatment varies widely with the infective agent: for staphylococci, chloramphenicol; for *N. gonorrhoeae*, intravenous and topical penicillin; for *Chlamydia* sp., oral and topical erythromycin. Prevention of gonococcal ophthalmitis is by instillation of silver nitrate drops at birth. Babies born to mothers with known gonorrhoea or chlamydial infection should be treated actively from birth.

Omphalitis

Omphalitis is infection of the umbilical stump. Infection may spread via the umbilical vessels to the abdominal viscera or can develop into septicaemia. It is most often caused by *Staphylococcus aureus* but Gram-negative bacilli and other bacterial species have been implicated. (In some developing countries, it may be the custom to dress the stump with dung or earth, resulting in tetanus; this is not true omphalitis.)

Specific diagnosis is by culture of the inflammatory exudate. Presumptive therapy is with an antistaphylococcal agent, e.g. flucloxacillin. Prevention is by dusting the stump with an antiseptic powder until the stump falls off.

Necrotising enterocolitis

Necrotising enterocolitis is a condition of unknown aetiology that affects premature neonates. The infant typically passes loose, bloodstained stools, has a distended abdomen and gas in the abdominal tissues on X-ray. Various infective agents have been proposed, but as yet there is no consensus on optimal antimicrobial treatment.

Scalded skin syndrome

Extensive exfoliation of skin can occur in infants infected with *S. aureus* (phage group II). The skin manifestations are caused by action of a staphylococcal toxin, exfoliatin, but may be accompanied by invasive disease. Affected surfaces produce an exudate, which may be cultured. Blood culture is also worthwhile.

Treatment is with intravenous flucloxacillin or similar. Outbreaks of scalded skin syndrome have occurred in special care nurseries. These can be prevented by careful hand hygiene among staff and source isolation of infected patients.

14.4 Organisms

A checklist of the organisms discussed in this chapter is given in Box 9. Further information is given on the pages indicated.

Box 9 Organisms involved in congenital and neonatal infections

Bacteria	**see page**	**Viruses**	**see page**
Escherichia coli	248	Rubellavirus	261
Group B streptococci (*S. agalactiae*)	244–5	Cytomegalovirus	257
Listeria monocytogenes	246	Hepatitis B virus	257
Neisseria gonorrhoeae	252–3	Herpes simplex virus	257
Treponema pallidum	255	Human immunodeficiency virus	260
Staphylococcus aureus	243	Parvovirus B19	257–8
		Varicella-zoster virus	257
Parasites			
Toxoplasma gondii	263–4		

Self-assessment: questions

Multiple choice questions

1. The following agents cause intrauterine infection:
   a. Group B streptococci (*S. agalactiae*)
   b. *Staphylococcus aureus*
   c. Rubella virus
   d. Herpes simplex virus
   e. *Toxoplasma gondii*

2. The following agents typically cause infection commencing during the neonatal period:
   a. Group B streptococci (*S. agalactiae*)
   b. *Staphylococcus aureus*
   c. Rubella virus
   d. Herpes simplex virus
   e. *Toxoplasma gondii*

3. The following features may be part of a congenital infection syndrome:
   a. Jaundice
   b. Splenomegaly
   c. Cardiac malformation
   d. Conjunctival inflammation
   e. Mental retardation

4. The following statements apply to neonatal meningitis:
   a. Typically presents in the 2nd or 3rd week postpartum
   b. Recognised by fever, neck stiffness and headache
   c. Caused by *Escherichia coli* and group B streptococci
   d. Treated with oral ampicillin and gentamicin
   e. May be accompanied by septicaemia

5. In neonatal septicaemia:
   a. Mortality rate is around 50%
   b. The most common pathogen isolated is *Listeria monocytogenes*
   c. Organisms from the mother's vaginal flora are the cause of infection
   d. Neonates are only at risk following premature rupture of the membranes
   e. Specific diagnosis only requires blood culture

6. Listeriosis:
   a. May be transmitted to the fetus following maternal infection
   b. Is rarely life threatening
   c. Should be treated with ampicillin or penicillin
   d. Can cause neonatal septicaemia
   e. May be the result of food contamination

7. Ophthalmia neonatorum:
   a. Is only caused by *Neisseria gonorrhoeae*
   b. Can be transmitted to other infants
   c. Is treated with antibiotic eye drops alone
   d. Can be prevented by silver nitrate eye drops
   e. Can be caused by silver nitrate eye drops

Case history questions

History 1

> A 19-year-old drug addict turns up to the antenatal clinic in an advanced state of pregnancy. She is very worried because her boyfriend has just told her that he has AIDS.

1. What laboratory tests would you perform now?
2. What is the risk that the baby will develop AIDS?
3. Does the maternity unit need to know if the mother is HIV positive?

History 2

> A 32-year-old woman gives birth to a full-term, healthy baby boy 48 hours after the fetal membranes were ruptured. Two days later, the baby loses interest in his feeds, is listless and irritable. After developing laboured breathing, diagnostic tests are performed and he is sent to the special care nursery where he is given oxygen and antibiotics.

1. What infections may the child have?
2. What diagnostic microbiology tests were performed?
3. What are the most likely bacterial pathogens?
4. Which antibiotics should have been given?

Data interpretation

An expectant mother, in the 38th week of her pregnancy develops an irritating, vesicular rash on her trunk. Serological tests are performed:

varicella-zoster IgM and IgG: negative
cytomegalovirus IgM: negative
cytomegalovirus IgG: positive
parvovirus B19: negative.

1. What viral infection would have the most serious consequences for the unborn child?

2. How does the serology result help your assessment?
3. What further laboratory test would you use to confirm this infection?
4. What treatment would you use in this case?

Objective structured clinical examination (OSCE)

A 23-year-old woman at 35 weeks of gestation has been admitted in the early stages of labour. As she was booked in by the midwife she was noted to have a vesicular rash extending from the vulva laterally. On questioning, she states that her partner had similar genital lesions recently. You are asked:

1. Is this infection most likely to be varicella-zoster?
2. Should she be given varicella-zoster immunoglobulin immediately and treated with an appropriate antiviral agent?
3. Should she be assessed for a semi-elective caesarean section?

4. If this infection had happened in the first trimester, would the fetus have been at high risk of congenital malformations?

Short notes questions

Write short notes on the following:

1. Why TORCH is no longer an adequate acronym for agents of congenital infection
2. Why some infections cause serious consequences in unborn infants despite multiple barriers against infection
3. Neonatal septicaemia and meningitis

Viva questions

1. Why are there major differences between intrauterine and perinatal infections?
2. What maternal infections present the greatest risk in a maternity unit or special care nursery?

Self-assessment: answers

Multiple choice answers

1. a. **False**. Group B streptococci cause neonatal septicaemia and meningitis.
   b. **False**. *Staphylococcus aureus* may cause outbreaks of scalded skin syndrome in neonates.
   c. **True**. It can cause miscarriage or teratogenic damage.
   d. **True**. This is rare but leads to disseminated infection.
   e. **True**. Approximately 50% of infected mothers transmit the virus transplacentally to the fetus.

2. a. **True**. Can cause neonatal septicaemia.
   b. **True**. The toxin causes scalded skin syndrome.
   c. **False**. Rubella virus causes intrauterine infection.
   d. **False**. Herpes simplex causes intrauterine infection.
   e. **False**. *Toxoplasma gondii* causes intrauterine infection.

3. a. **True**. Cytomegalovirus and *Toxoplasma gondii* cause jaundice.
   b. **True**. Associated with infections with cytomegalovirus, *Toxoplasma gondii* and rubella.
   c. **True**. Rubella and parvovirus B19.
   d. **False**. Conjunctival inflammation is a feature of ophthalmia neonatorum.
   e. **True**. Rubella and toxoplasmosis.

4. a. **True**. Septicaemia is more common in the first week postpartum.
   b. **False**. Fever, neck stiffness and headache are features of meningitis in older children and adults.
   c. **True**. *Listeria monocytogenes* infection also occurs but is less common.
   d. **False**. Treatment should be via the intravenous route.
   e. **True**. The initial presentation is usually meningitis but septicaemia can accompany it.

5. a. **True**. For early-onset septicaemia.
   b. **False**. *L. monocytogenes* is rare compared with *Escherichia coli* and group B streptococci.
   c. **True**. From ascending infection after rupture of membranes or during passage of the fetus down the birth canal.
   d. **False**. Although premature rupture of membranes is a risk factor for neonatal sepsis, infection does occur in other neonates.

   e. **False**. Cerebrospinal fluid and urine should also be cultured.

6. a. **True**.
   b. **False**. Listeriosis may cause stillbirth or neonatal death.
   c. **True**.
   d. **True**.
   e. **True**. *Listeria* spp. can occur in some soft cheeses and pâtés.

7. a. **False**. Also caused by *Staphylococcus aureus*, adenovirus, *Chlamydia* sp. and silver nitrate eye drops.
   b. **True**. *S. aureus* and adenovirus are easily transmissible.
   c. **False**. Ophthalmia neonatorum may require both topical and parenteral antibiotic treatment.
   d. **True**.
   e. **True**. They can cause a mild self-limiting inflammation.

Case history answers

History 1

1. HIV and hepatitis B serology, after counselling.
2. If the mother is HIV positive, around 30–35%.
3. Yes, in order to plan for a high-risk delivery.

History 2

1. Neonatal septicaemia/meningitis.
2. Blood, cerebrospinal fluid and urine culture.
3. *Escherichia coli*, group B streptococci and *Listeria monocytogenes*.
4. Ampicillin and gentamicin.

Data interpretation answer

1. Varicella-zoster.
2. It shows that the mother is non-immune and, therefore, susceptible to infection.
3. Nucleic acid amplification (PCR) for the viral genome in vesicle fluid.
4. A suitable antiviral drug for the mother (e.g. aciclovir) and varicella-zoster immunoglobulin for the infant after delivery.

OSCE answer

1. No. These features are more consistent with a genital herpes infection.
2. No. As it is not likely to be varicella infection, this immune globulin would be without effect.
3. Yes. Congenital herpes infection can be catastrophic. It should be avoided by minimising exposure of the baby to herpes virus and caesarean section prevents exposure to the flora of the birth canal.
4. No. Herpes virus infection of the mother in early pregnancy is not thought to result in major embryo or fetal damage through interference with organogenesis.

Short notes answers

1. State what 'TORCH' stands for, list the infectious agents included under the 'others' category and discuss the changing epidemiology of neonatal infection.
2. Gestational factors—age, organogenesis, immunological immaturity—and maternal infection all need a mention. Give examples.
3. A tabular approach would be adequate.

Viva answers

1. Answer in terms of the pathogens they are likely to encounter, the nature of that encounter and the maturity of host defences.
2. Viral infections, including varicella-zoster, and bacterial infections such as staphylococcal scalded skin syndrome are examples. Remember to indicate what preventive measures can be taken.

15 Infections in older children

Overview

As children grow up, they encounter an increasing variety of social environments, in each of which they are introduced to new infections. As a result, children work their way through a list of common childhood infections, particularly the exanthems and respiratory infections. Some of these infections can be prevented by vaccination. Whether through vaccination or natural immunity, most people have gained resistance to a wide variety of infections by the end of childhood. Diseases reviewed in this chapter are those commonly found in paediatric practice. Some infections are also seen in the adult population and these are dealt with in the appropriate systems chapter.

15.1 Epidemiology and pathogenesis

Learning objectives

You should:

- know what factors contribute to infection in children
- understand the immune system capacity in children
- be aware of the potential for secondary infections.

Epidemiology

Infectious diseases are common in children, increasingly so the younger they are. The exanthems, or rash-causing viral infections, are generally diseases of the preschool age group. Respiratory infections are more common during the winter months in temperate climates, and during the rainy season in the tropics. The main reason for increased risk at this time is the increased time spent indoors, particularly when in crowded, poor housing conditions. The number of siblings and family spacing also contribute to the infection risk. Nutritional status is another important determinant of susceptibility to infection. Malnutrition is both cause and effect of infection in developing countries.

Accurate recording of common childhood infections is needed to assess the effectiveness of vaccination schemes and other preventive measures. There is a statutory requirement to notify the public heath authorities about specific diseases in many countries.

Pathogenesis

A child begins his or her encounter with infective agents with a relatively immature immune system. By 3 to 6 months of age, transplacentally transferred maternal immunoglobulin and the protective effects of breast-feeding have waned. There is then a period of maximum susceptibility to infection with certain agents (e.g. *Haemophilus influenzae*). The child acquires a repertoire of immune-based protective responses to infective agents after recovery from each successive infection, or as a result of vaccination. Immunological immaturity is not always a handicap. Some more common viral infections, such as mumps and chickenpox, are milder in children than in adults. Infections in adults are more likely to have serious consequences. However, this principle does not extend to all infections: the bulk of the mortality and serious morbidity attributed to both respiratory syncytial virus infection and malaria is in children. It is also clear that some infections render the child more susceptible to infection with another microbial pathogen. For example, pneumonia and gastroenteritis may both follow measles infection, especially in developing countries where poor nutrition may already have caused impairment of cell-mediated immunity. Viral infections may be more severe in malnourished children, putting additional pressure on meagre metabolic reserves. Catch-up growth may never be achieved before the onset of further infection.

15.2 Diagnosis

Learning objectives

You should:

- know the signs and symptoms of the exanthems and respiratory infections

- know when to use laboratory tests.

Many of the common infections of childhood have a viral aetiology. The laboratory tests required to make a specific diagnosis are often technically demanding, costly and may not provide a definitive result until after resolution of the infection. These tests are therefore usually reserved for difficult cases. In clinical practice, the diagnosis normally depends on history, signs and symptoms. Fortunately, the exanthems cause fairly clearcut clinical syndromes, but falling incidence resulting from vaccination programmes may reduce overall diagnostic expertise (e.g. for measles). The main features of the important childhood respiratory syndromes are determined by the principal location of the inflammatory insult, but this may not be clear in the early stages of infection. The practical difficulties of paediatric specimen collection often make physicians reluctant to obtain diagnostic specimens. However, every attempt should be made to collect the appropriate specimens from patients with severe, life-threatening disease.

15.3 Prevention

Learning objectives

You should:

- know the vaccination programme used in your community

- be aware of the concept of 'herd immunity' and of the concerns of individual parents

- know why the vaccinations are used in terms of the potential serious sequelae of the infections targeted.

Vaccination schedules

The immunoprophylaxis of common infectious diseases relies heavily on vaccination during childhood in order to confer protective immunity before exposure to infective agents occurs. Sufficiently high levels of immunity in a target population reduce the risk of transmission and can even provide a degree of protection for unimmunised individuals. To achieve this so-called 'herd immunity' it is usually necessary to vaccinate 80–90% of the population. Concerted efforts to achieve high levels of vaccination have had a major impact on the incidence of common infectious diseases in many countries. Almost 80% vaccine coverage was achieved worldwide by 1990. This resulted in a halving of vaccine-preventable deaths and disability despite continued population growth. Smallpox was eliminated by vaccination. Other infectious diseases have now been targeted for elimination by immunisation and other public health measures. It was hoped that, by the year 2000, polio and neonatal tetanus would also have been eradicated. A 95% reduction in deaths from measles is aimed for.

In the UK, the vaccination programme is as follows:

1. diphtheria, tetanus and pertussis (killed) and polio (live attenuated) at 2, 3 and 4 months
2. measles, mumps and rubella (live attenuated) at 12–18 months
3. booster diphtheria, tetanus and polio at 4–5 years before school entry
4. rubella at 10–14 years (females only) (separated from BCG by a 3-week interval)
5. bacillus Calmette–Guérin (for tuberculosis, live attenuated, BCG) at 10–14 years
6. booster tetanus and polio at 15–18 years.

Meningococcal vaccination is used selectively in many countries. In the UK and several other countries where type C *N. meningitidis* is common, a type C meningococcal vaccine has been intorduced for general use.

Haemophilus influenzae type b conjugate vaccine is being used in certain sectors of the population.

In the USA, diphtheria, tetanus, pertussis (DTP) is given at 2-month intervals, and polio vaccine is given only twice. Measles, mumps and rubella are repeated at entry to middle school or junior high.

In other countries, differences in the epidemiology of infectious diseases are the reason for variation in the vaccination schedule. In parts of east Asia where hepatitis B is endemic, hepatitis B vaccination is carried out during early childhood. In areas of high prevalence of tuberculosis, BCG is given in infancy.

A major but often neglected part of vaccination programmes is the efficacy of vaccine at the point of use. For maximum efficacy, any vaccine should be used as directed and within date. The recommended cold storage should have been maintained from packaging, through transport and right up to administration. This is referred to as the 'cold chain' and causes particular difficulties in remote communities in the tropics. It should also be noted that live, attenuated vaccines must not be frozen, while killed whole cell vaccines can be.

15.4 Diseases and syndromes

The common infections of childhood are given in Table 27.

Learning objectives

You should:

- know the major infections of older children
- understand the factors contributing to their occurrence
- know the basis of their clinical management.

Mumps

Mumps is a common childhood infection caused by a paramyxovirus belonging to the parainfluenza group. The mumps virus has a tropism for neural and glandular tissue. Transmission is by droplet infection. The primary viraemia is followed by an incubation period of 15–20 days, after which the characteristic clinical features become evident.

Diagnosis

The clinical features include fever and parotid swelling (which usually displaces the lower earlobe laterally). There may also be signs of mild meningeal irritation and in more severe cases a clinical meningitis. The infection is less common in adults but has serious consequences in a high proportion of adult cases, including unilateral orchitis, oophoritis and pancreatitis. Up to 40% of mumps infections are subclinical. The differential diagnosis includes parotitis, coxsackievirus infection and parotid tumours. Diagnostic tests are unnecessary when the clinical diagnosis is clearcut, but laboratory confirmation of the diagnosis can be made by viral isolation from saliva, cerebrospinal fluid or urine, or antibody detection with complement fixation or enzyme immunoassay.

Chemotherapy

There is no specific treatment. Mumps meningitis has a good prognosis and can be managed with bedrest. Immunity following mumps virus infection is lifelong.

Table 27 Infections of childhood

Infection	Occurrence	Features
Mumps	Common	Fever, parotid swelling
Polio	Rare where there is a vaccination programme (see Table 28)	Meningitis, paralytic encephalomyelitis
Exanthems		
Measles	Rare where vaccination programme has high uptake	Catarrhal cough, conjunctivitis, Koplik's spots on buccal mucosa, rash; can have serious sequelae
Rubella	Common, often subclinical	Fever, rash, lymphadenopathy; has high mortality and morbidity if fetus is infected
Chickenpox	Common	Vesicular rash mainly on thorax and upper limbs, fever
Erythema infectiosum (fifth disease)	Common	Bilateral inflammation of cheeks
Roseola	Most common exanthem	Rash on face and trunk, pharyngitis, cervical lymphadenopathy, fever
Respiratory infections		
Croup	Older infants	Inflammation and obstruction of larynx and large airways
Epiglottitis	Mainly in infants	Acute inflammation of the epiglottis; potential airways obstruction
Bronchiolitis	Seasonal in temperate climates	Cough, fever, breathing difficulties
Whooping cough (pertussis)	Sporadic, mainly in unvaccinated populations	Fever, cough, coryza; cycles of 'whooping' cough paroxysms
Urinary tract infections	More common in girls	Pain on passing urine, frequency, abdominal tenderness, fever
Nappy rash	Common	Contact dermatitis in nappy area
Haemolytic uraemic syndrome	After haemorrhagic colitis	Bloody diarrhoea followed by pallor, oedema and oliguria
Malaria	Common in endemic areas	Recurrent fevers, sweating, shivering; cerebral malaria and severe anaemia can follow
Kawasaki disease	More common in Asian children	Vasculitis, fever, rash, desquamation, cervical lymphadenopathy; carditis can follow

Mumps can be prevented by vaccination with a live attenuated virus during infancy.

Polio (poliomyelitis)

Polio is an infection of the central nervous system caused by a neurotropic enterovirus of the picornavirus group.

In developing countries with no vaccination programme, infection usually occurs during infancy and there is a low incidence of serious sequelae. In more developed countries, better sanitation and general living conditions leads to a peak incidence later in childhood and in early adult life. In this older age group, poliovirus infection causes a meningitis and, in a small proportion, a paralytic encephalomyelitis. Exposure to the virus is through ingestion. This is followed by spread from the intestine, via the bloodstream, to the central nervous system. Most epidemics of polio have been caused by type 1 virus. There are three types altogether. Risk of polio is increased following tonsillectomy and during epidemics by increased physical activity.

Diagnosis
Clinical symptoms are confirmed by isolation of poliovirus from cerebrospinal fluid.

Control
There is no effective antiviral treatment. Prevention is by vaccination either with oral live attenuated virus or with intramuscular killed virus. The oral vaccine colonises the gastrointestinal tract and stimulates mucosal IgA antibody production. It also protects unvaccinated individuals by spreading in communities. Very occasionally, live vaccine strains revert to original pathogenic status and may cause polio. The killed virus vaccine promotes humoral immunity without the intestinal mucosal reaction. Three doses of the oral polio vaccine are usually given in infancy, with single-dose boosters prior to school entry and overseas travel.

Exanthems

The exanthems are a group of diseases common in children and characterised by a rash or exanthem (Table 28). All the exanthems have a viral aetiology.

Measles

Measles is a highly contagious disease of childhood that is caused by a paramyxovirus, the morbillivirus.

In developed countries, measles predominantly affects infants, while in developed countries it is generally a disease of 2–5-year-olds. It is spread by direct contact in the pre-rash stage (and air-borne and droplet spread, to a lesser extent), and has a 90% attack rate among family contacts. Measles is an important cause of mortality and morbidity in developing countries. The measles virus causes the formation of multinucleate giant cells.

Diagnosis
A 4-day period of catarrhal cough and conjunctivitis follows an incubation period of around 10 days. At this time, small white flecks looking like grains of salt (Koplik's spots) can be found on the buccal mucosa. These are characteristic of measles. Koplik's spots disappear at the time of onset of the fine, maculopapular rash.

There are a number of potentially serious sequelae:

- primary measles pneumonia: may occur in immunocompromised children but is rare
- secondary bacterial pneumonia: this is more common, often caused by *Staphylococcus aureus*, and is the most common cause of death in measles
- encephalitis: another serious complication of measles
- post-measles state: includes growth retardation, diarrhoea, corneal ulceration and depressed cell-mediated immunity.

Diagnosis of measles is usually made on clinical findings but may be confirmed by serological tests.

Control
There is no specific antiviral treatment. Secondary bacterial infections require the appropriate antibacterial

Table 28 Viral infections producing rashes in children

Disease	Cause	Incubation period (days)	Rash	Infective period (days)
Measles	Morbillivirus	7–18	Maculopapular	From 5 before to 4 after rash
Rubella	Rubella virus	14–21	Maculopapular, head, upper body	From 7 before to 7 after rash
Chickenpox	Varicella-zoster virus	12–21	Vesiculopustular	From 2 before to 4 after rash
Erythema infectiosum	Parvovirus	4–12	Reticulate, face, limbs	?
Roseola infantum	Human herpes virus 6	5–15	Macular, face and trunk	?

therapy. Vitamin A supplements may help to reduce the incidence of corneal and gastrointestinal complications. In developed countries, measles has been prevented to a great extent by vaccination with a live attenuated virus. Natural infection confers lifelong immunity. Malnourished infants can be given short-lived protection by administration of normal human immunoglobulin. The mortality attributed to measles can also be reduced by breast-feeding, child spacing and vitamin A supplements.

Rubella

Rubella is an exanthematous infection caused by a togavirus; it is notable for its potentially devastating effects on the unborn child.

Rubella is spread by droplets of nasal secretions and becomes established in the upper respiratory tract. A primary viraemia then occurs with spread in lymphocytes.

Diagnosis

After a 2–3 week incubation period, fever, rash and lymphadenopathy develop. The rash is maculopapular like measles, starts on the face and yoke area and spreads to the limbs and trunk. Lymphadenopathy is most pronounced in the cervical, postauricular and occipital nodes. There may be a polyarthralgia. Many rubella infections are subclinical, and the clinical diagnosis is unreliable. The differential diagnosis includes:

- other exanthems
- other viral infection
- acute rheumatic fever.

Serological confirmation of the diagnosis relies on haemagglutination inhibition or complement fixation.

Control

There is no specific antiviral therapy. Prevention is by vaccination with a live attenuated strain of the rubella virus, given at 15–18 months of age with measles and mumps vaccine (MMR) and at 12–15 years for females. All children with rubella should be kept away from pregnant women during the first half of their pregnancy. Unvaccinated individuals are at risk of contracting rubella when they travel to countries without a rubella vaccination programme.

Chickenpox

Chickenpox is an acute, exanthematous infection caused by the varicella-zoster virus, resulting in a pruritic, vesiculopustular rash.

Varicella-zoster virus is a DNA virus and a member of the herpes virus family. It is spread in droplets and gains entry via the upper respiratory tract, after which primary viraemia and spread to distant parts of the body occur.

Diagnosis

Patients are infectious from 2 days before to 5 days after onset of vesicles. After an incubation period of up to 21 days, a pruritic rash develops with a centripetal distribution; i.e. predominantly on the thorax and upper limbs. The rash occurs in crops that go through papular, vesicular, pustular and crusted stages. Fever is in proportion to the severity of the rash. Immunocompromised children and adults are at increased risk of severe disease, including a life-threatening pneumonia. Diagnosis is usually made from the clinical features. The differential diagnosis includes:

- impetigo
- herpes simplex
- enterovirus infection.

Control

Treatment is symptomatic, e.g. codeine for pain relief, but immunocompromised patients may benefit from varicella immunoglobulin.

There is now an effective vaccine against varicella-zoster virus.

Shingles Chickenpox is a disease of non-immune individuals that results in lasting immunity. However, the virus is capable of remaining dormant in dorsal sensory root ganglia and causing disease at a later stage through reactivation. When this happens, there is a unilateral, intensely pruritic, vesicular rash distributed over one or more dermatomes. This is shingles or **herpes zoster**. It is less infective than chickenpox, but transmission of the virus can occur.

Diagnosis is clinical. Strong analgesics may be required. Intravenous aciclovir may help to reduce severe pain but its use requires hospital admission. Treatment does not have a useful effect on latent virus and therefore does not prevent further reactivation.

Erythema infectiosum (fifth disease)

Erythema infectiosum is caused by a single-stranded DNA virus or parvovirus B19. Infection is transmitted by the respiratory route and results in a bilateral inflammation of the checks (hence its informal name of 'slapped cheek syndrome'). The inflammation becomes a lacy, reticulate rash on cheeks and limbs. There may also be a pancytopenia, which resolves spontaneously, although in individuals with the sickle cell trait a haemolytic crisis may occur.

Diagnosis is mainly clinical but can be confirmed by IgM or rising IgG titre.

There is no specific treatment or vaccine.

Roseola infantum (exanthem subitum)

Roseola infantum is a febrile, exanthematous infection caused by human herpes virus 6. It is the most common exanthem in children under 12 years and its features include a macular rash on the face and trunk, fever, pharyngitis and cervical lymphadenopathy. The rash characteristically begins after the short-lived fever subsides. The diagnosis is therefore made only after the child has begun to recover, but it can be confirmed serologically. No specific treatment or vaccine is available.

Respiratory infections

Children are prone to some of the respiratory infections seen in adults and to others that are more common or more severe in the child.

Croup

Croup is inflammation and obstruction of the larynx and large airways caused by viruses of the 'respiratory group' most often the parainfluenza viruses. It occurs in older infants.

Diagnosis

Croup is a self-limiting infection in which a sudden onset, hoarse, barking cough occurs, with no evidence of spread outside the respiratory tract. The child may be restless, breathless and have inspiratory stridor. Rib retraction, cyanosis and increased breathing rate are all features of severe infection. The diagnosis is based on clinical findings.

Control

Management is directed to preventing worsening respiratory obstruction. The use of night-time humidification, cool mist and fluid replacement may halt the progression of the disease in more severe cases; however, there is some debate over the value of humidification in croup.

The main differential diagnosis is epiglottitis.

Epiglottitis

Epiglottitis is an infection of the upper respiratory tract by *H. influenzae* that causes acute inflammation of the epiglottis. The child is at risk of sudden airway obstruction. Type b *H. influenzae* is responsible for almost all cases of epiglottitis, which occurs mainly in infants.

Diagnosis

The child has a fever and is restless, leans forward, drools and resists swallowing. Oral examination should be avoided where there are no facilities for immediate intubation or tracheostomy. The differential diagnosis includes:

- croup
- foreign body
- laryngeal diphtheria.

Blood cultures should be taken, since septicaemia is common in epiglottitis. A lateral neck radiograph may reveal epiglottic swelling.

Chemotherapy and control

Treatment is usually with intravenous ampicillin. Epiglottitis and other invasive *H. influenzae* infections can be prevented with Hib conjugate vaccine.

Bronchiolitis

Bronchiolitis is an inflammatory condition of the smaller airways caused by infection with respiratory syncytial virus (an RNA paramyxovirus). Other 'respiratory viruses' can cause a similar clinical picture. In temperate climates, bronchiolitis is a seasonal disease that causes significant mortality and morbidity in children under 1 year of age. Infection is transmitted in droplets of nasal secretions from affected individuals. The virus then spreads along the respiratory mucosa, causing fusion of cell membranes in infected cells.

Diagnosis

Bronchiolitis has an insidious onset, starting with cough and a low fever. It then progresses to laboured, rapid, shallow breathing. There is wheezing, hyperexpansion of the lungs and air trapping. The infection is self-limiting in most cases, but severe cases require respiratory support in a paediatric intensive care unit. The diagnosis can be confirmed rapidly by viral antigen detection with enzyme immunoassay or indirect immunofluorescence.

Chemotherapy

In addition to respiratory support, children with severe disease may benefit from aerosolised ribavirin, if given early enough. Humidification of inhaled air is also required. Attempts to develop a vaccine have been unsuccessful so far.

Whooping cough (pertussis)

Whooping cough is an upper respiratory infection caused by *Bordetella pertussis* in which there are recurrent paroxysms of coughing. *B. pertussis* is a small Gram-negative bacillus with fastidious growth requirements. The bacterium produces adhesins and several toxins, including a lipopolysaccharide and a tracheal cytotoxin. The infection is transmitted in droplets of respiratory secretions.

Diagnosis

Three stages of the infection are recognised: prodromal, catarrhal and paroxysmal. Fever, cough and coryza develop after an incubation period of around 10 days. There is tracheal irritation and production of thick, viscous mucus, which leads after about another 10 days to the cycles of coughing, which reach a crescendo with the characteristic inspiratory whoop. Other results of coughing paroxysms include subconjunctival haemorrhages, sublingual frenal ulcer and, in rare cases, respiratory distress and hypoxic brain damage. Deaths from whooping cough may occur during epidemics. When older children and other family contacts contract the disease, it usually takes a milder form, resembling a common upper respiratory tract infection.

The diagnosis can be confirmed by passing a thin, wire-mounted pernasal swab and asking the patient to cough. This is then used to inoculate a selective agar (Bordet–Gengou) for *B. pertussis*.

Control

By the time a diagnosis has been made, antibiotic treatment is of little value to the patient, but treatment with erythromycin may help to reduce the risk of transmission. Prevention is by vaccination of infants with a killed bacterial cell preparation (part of DPT). Controversy has surrounded the use of pertussis vaccine, since some cases of encephalitis have been attributed to vaccine administration. However, it is now clear that the risk of lasting neurological sequelae from pertussis vaccination is substantially less than that from the disease itself.

Pulmonary infection in cystic fibrosis

Respiratory failure is the most common cause of death in cystic fibrosis, and bronchiolitis and pneumonia are important contributory factors. Patients with cystic fibrosis have impaired clearance of respiratory secretions and are prone to chronic infection with bacteria such as *S. aureus*, *Pseudomonas aeruginosa* and the more recently recognised *Burkholderia cepacia*. It is not easy to distinguish between bacteria causing chronic infection and those merely colonising an abnormal lower respiratory tract. Antibacterial treatment does not necessarily result in clinical improvement and may lead to further colonisation with more resistant bacterial species. Appropriate diet and regular physiotherapy may be as important as antibiotic therapy for long-term survival of these patients.

Other diseases

Urinary tract infection

Children contract acute infections of both the bladder and kidney. Prompt diagnosis and initiation of treatment are required to reduce the risk of permanent renal damage. Urinary tract infection (UTI) in children is usually caused by *Escherichia coli*. Other Enterobacteriaceae cause a small proportion of cases, and haemorrhagic cystitis is sometimes caused by adenovirus infection. UTI is more common in females, after the newborn period. Bacteria gain access via the 'ascending' route, i.e. by the urethra. Around a third of these infections recur within a year.

Symptoms include:

- pain on passing urine
- urinary frequency
- abdominal tenderness
- fever.

Children with pyelonephritis may also have perilumbar pain and tenderness, but pyelonephritis cannot be reliably distinguished from cystitis in children. Asymptomatic bacteriuria also occurs in children and requires careful evaluation. A good-quality urine specimen must be obtained for laboratory confirmation of the diagnosis. Midstream specimens of urine are only possible in some older children and in teenagers. In infants, suprapubic aspiration is the ideal approach. Failing this, a 'clean catch' specimen can be obtained by a parent collecting some of the urine flow during micturition. As a last resort, perineal urine collection bags are available, but these are prone to contamination by perineal bacteria. Specimens will require evaluation of cellular content, quantitative bacterial culture and antibiotic susceptibility testing. After completion of treatment, a follow-up specimen should be obtained. A high proportion of children with urinary tract infection have anatomical abnormalities of the urinary tract. It is therefore necessary to follow up UTI in children with radiological investigations, including intravenous pyelogram and micturating cystogram. Some authorities recommend radiological studies following a first UTI in all boys, in girls younger than 3 years and following UTI with fever. Treatment is with antibiotics effective against local Enterobacteriaceae, particularly *E. coli*. The difficulty in distinguishing pyelonephritis from cystitis in children makes it unwise to rely on short-course therapy. 10 days of treatment is recommended.

Nappy rash

Nappy rash is a common complication of perineal contact dermatitis in nappy-wearing infants. The condition usually starts with dermatitis caused by a combination of moisture, friction and ammonia. The affected area rarely extends further than the point of contact between apposed skin surfaces. Secondary infection is most often with yeasts, particularly *Candida albicans*. When this occurs, there is further inflammation, which may extend beyond the apposed skin surfaces. There are often discrete areas of inflammation, called 'satellite' lesions.

The diagnosis can be confirmed by microscopic detection of yeasts in a potassium hydroxide smear of scrapings from the affected area.

Treatment is with topical nystatin or miconazole, but drying out of the lesion is equally important.

Haemolytic uraemic syndrome

Haemolytic uraemic syndrome is a postinfective condition occurring after haemorrhagic colitis. It is associated with shiga-like toxin-producing strains of *E. coli* O157 (and other serotypes of enterohaemorrhagic *E. coli* (EHEC), or verotoxin-producing *E. coli*) and *Shigella* spp., which cause enterohaemorrhagic colitis; evident as a bloody diarrhoea. Up to a week after the diarrhoea, the child becomes pallid, oedematous and oliguric. Stool culture should be performed using a specialised medium (sorbitol MacConkey agar) to detect *E. coli* O157. Shiga-like toxin (also known as **verotoxin** because of its cytotoxic effect on Vero cell monolayers) can then be detected by latex agglutination or cytotoxic effect on cell culture. The absence of enterohaemorrhagic *E. coli* O157 does not exclude a diagnosis of haemolytic uraemic syndrome.

Antibiotic treatment is of doubtful benefit and the child may require haemodialysis until the acute renal failure resolves. Enteric precautions should be continued for at least 10 days to prevent secondary spread.

Malaria

Malaria is an infection caused by sporozoan protozoa of the genus *Plasmodium* and is transmitted by the bite of female anophelene mosquitoes. It is a common disease in the tropics and is becoming increasingly common in international travellers from temperate climates. In endemic areas, mortality is common in young children and diminishes with increasing age because of acquired immunity. Deaths are mainly from cerebral malaria and severe anaemia. Most severe and fatal malaria is caused by *Plasmodium falciparum*, but malaria may also be caused by *P. vivax*, *P. ovale* and *P. malariae*. The pathogenesis of malaria and its complications is still not fully understood. Infection follows inoculation of malaria sporozoites in the saliva of anophelene mosquitoes during a blood meal.

Diagnosis

In acute malaria, there are recurrent episodes of fever, sweating and shivering, corresponding to bursts of parasites released into the bloodstream. Coma, convulsions and respiratory arrest may ensue in severe cases, where the differential diagnosis includes:

- septicaemia
- meningitis
- hypoglycaemia
- intracranial space-occupying lesions.

The diagnosis is confirmed by microscopy of a Romanowsky-stained blood film. Maximum sensitivity is obtained by staining at higher than normal pH (7.0), preparing blood films on at least two separate occasions and making at least one thick film (the sensitivity of which is about 25 times greater than a thin film).

Control

Malaria is treated with one or more of chloroquine, quinine and other antimalarials, the choice depending on the species of parasite and the prevalence of drug resistance in the area. A repeat blood film after about 12–24 hours of treatment is valuable in severe disease. These patients often require intensive care during the initial stages of management.

Prevention is by reducing mosquito breeding, avoiding contact with mosquitoes and by chemoprophylaxis. The choice of prophylactic agent depends on the area to be visited and may change from year to year. Expert advice should be sought (further details in Ch. 19).

Kawasaki disease

Kawasaki disease is a life-threatening condition of unknown aetiology, thought to be infective in nature. It was originally known as **mucocutaneous lymphadenopathy syndrome**. Asian children are at greatest risk of the condition, but it does occur rarely in non-Asian children. The case fatality rate is around 2%. There have been several epidemics of Kawasaki disease, but there is no evidence of true person-to-person spread. There is an extensive vasculitis, and there have been reports of high rates of carriage of streptococci and staphylococci producing the toxic shock syndrome toxin in patients with Kawasaki disease, suggesting an aetiological role for a 'superantigen'.

Diagnosis

The disease causes a fever in all cases. Most patients have a rash, mucosal and conjunctival inflammation, desquamation and cervical lymphadenopathy. The differential diagnosis is extensive and includes:

- Scarlet fever
- toxic shock syndrome
- the exanthems
- Stevens–Johnson syndrome.

The mortality results from carditis.

At present there is no laboratory confirmation of the diagnosis.

Control

Treatment with aspirin and human normal immunoglobulin reduces the risk of mortality and severe disease.

15.5 Organisms

A checklist of the organisms discussed in this chapter is given in Box 10. Further information is given on the pages indicated.

Box 10 Organisms that cause infections in children

Bacteria	see page	Viruses	see page
Staphylococcus aureus	243	Measles virus	259
Haemophilus influenzae	251	Rubellavirus	261
Bordetella pertussis	–	Varicella-zoster virus	257
Pseudomonas aeruginosa	249–50	Parvovirus	257–8
Burkholderia cepacia	250	Human herpesvirus 6	257
Escherichia coli/E. coli O157	248	Mumps virus	259
Shigella spp.	249	Poliovirus	259–60
Other Enterobacteriaceae	248–9	Parainfluenza viruses	259
Corynebacterium diphtheriae	246–7	Respiratory syncytial virus	259
Clostridium tetani	247		
		Parasites	
		Plasmodium falciparum	263
Fungi		*P. vivax*	263
Candida albicans	269	*P. ovale*	263
		P. malariae	263

Self-assessment: questions

Multiple choice questions

1. In the following conditions a diagnosis is usually made without laboratory investigation:
   a. Mumps in a school child
   b. Chickenpox in a preschool child
   c. Whooping cough in a teenager
   d. Kawasaki disease in a Japanese child
   e. Haemolytic uraemic syndrome

2. The exanthems include:
   a. Measles
   b. Mumps
   c. Rubella
   d. Fifth disease
   e. Varicella

3. Features of measles infection include:
   a. A low attack rate within families
   b. A fine maculopapular rash
   c. Conjunctivitis
   d. White spots inside the mouth
   e. Short-lived natural immunity

4. Populations at particular risk of rubella include:
   a. International travellers
   b. Young children
   c. Unborn children
   d. Adult males
   e. Pregnant women

5. Measles can be prevented by:
   a. Vitamin A supplements
   b. Human normal immunoglobulin
   c. Contraception
   d. Breast-feeding
   e. Killed virus vaccine

6. Infection with the mumps virus causes:
   a. Fever
   b. Parotitis, which may be unilateral
   c. Orchitis, which is usually bilateral
   d. Self-limiting meningitis
   e. A characteristic rash

7. The consequences of respiratory syncytial virus (RSV) infection include:
   a. Epiglottitis
   b. Croup
   c. Meningitis
   d. Upper respiratory tract infection
   e. Bronchiolitis

8. In whooping cough, damage is caused by:
   a. Hyalauronidase
   b. Lipopolysaccharide
   c. Cytotoxin
   d. Adhesin
   e. Paroxysmal coughing

9. The following bacteria commonly cause chronic lung infection in cystic fibrosis:
   a. *Pseudomonas cepacia*
   b. *Pseudomonas aeruginosa*
   c. *Haemophilus influenzae*
   d. *Staphylococcus aureus*
   e. *Streptococcus pneumoniae*

10. Pair up the patient and the most appropriate urine specimen collection method:
    a. Toddler   i. Midstream urine
    b. Infant   ii. Clean catch
    c. Teenage girl   iii. Suprapubic aspirate
                         iv. Perineal bag

11. Features of haemolytic uraemic syndrome include:
    a. Onset within a week of haemorrhagic colitis
    b. Association with *Escherichia coli* O157
    c. Always possible to confirm by stool culture
    d. Damage caused by a salmonella-like enterotoxin
    e. Antibiotic treatment assists recovery

12. Acute malaria should be diagnosed:
    a. Serologically
    b. By microscopy of routinely stained blood film
    c. By microscopy of thin blood film
    d. By microscopy of thick blood film
    e. By microscopy of several blood films

13. Treatment of malaria in children:
    a. Should always include chloroquine
    b. Should avoid the use of quinine
    c. Requires intensive care in severe cases
    d. Depends on the identity of the parasite
    e. Can be evaluated by repeat blood film

14. Kawasaki disease:
    a. Does not occur outside Asia
    b. Causes fatal heart disease in children
    c. Is transmitted from person to person
    d. Causes a rash and desquamation
    e. Responds to aspirin and immunoglobulin

Case history questions

History 1

> A 2-year-old girl is brought into your surgery by her mother, who says that the child has been going to the toilet very often and cries while on her potty. The mother adds that her daughter had a 'urine infection' earlier in the year that was treated with antibiotics.

1. What is the likely cause of the girl's symptoms?
2. What microbiology investigation would you request?
3. What other investigations should be performed?
4. Where did the infecting organisms come from?
5. What advice would you give the mother regarding antibiotics?

History 2

> A 5-year-old boy is brought into the paediatric ward. He has become lethargic and has lost his appetite after a bad bout of diarrhoea, when a lot of blood was seen in his stools. You notice that he looks rather pale and has a puffy appearance round his face, which his mother says is 'not his usual self'. She is worried that he has not passed any urine at all for at least 24 hours. The boy's sister also had diarrhoea about 10 days ago but is now well.

1. What is the condition called?
2. What organisms are associated with it?
3. What laboratory test(s) would help confirm your diagnosis?
4. Is there any risk of transmission from the boy, or from the sister?
5. Would you give the patient antibiotics?

Data interpretation

An 8-year-old child presents with a low-grade fever, a loss of appetite and a swollen left cheek. Examination reveals an area of tenderness in the left parotid region.

The serology results are:

measles:	IgG and IgM, negative
mumps:	IgG, negative.

1. Which of the two above infections is most likely to cause these clinical features?
2. Why is the serology result negative?
3. What other laboratory test might help to complete an aetiological diagnosis?
4. What complications of this infection can follow?
5. Has this child been vaccinated?

Objective structured clinical examination (OSCE)

A 7-year-old child of an immigrant family has presented with fever, listlessness and a fine maculopapular rash. There was no past medical history of note but the child's older sibling had had a short febrile illness with a similar rash recently. Closer examination reveals mild suffusion of both conjunctivae and a few white spots on the buccal mucosa inside each cheek. The maculopapular rash is extensive and most marked over the trunk. Serological studies have been performed. You are asked:

1. Are these features most likely to be caused by rubella?
2. Could this infection be caused by a wide range of infective agents?
3. Would a vaccination history contribute to your aetiological diagnosis?
4. Should serodiagnostic tests be requested on other family members?
5. Would you keep the child under observation in a general paediatric ward?

Short notes questions

Write short notes on the following:

1. The relationship between impoverished living conditions and infection
2. Roseola infantum
3. The pathogenesis of polio
4. The clinical course of *Bordetella pertussis* infection and its diagnosis
5. Malaria as an important disease of childhood

Viva questions

1. Compare chickenpox and shingles
2. Compare croup and epiglottitis
3. In your view, what are the most important components of the vaccination schedule?

Self-assessment: answers

Multiple choice answers

1. a. **True**. Investigation is unnecessary if the clinical diagnosis is clear.
   b. **True**. The clinical features are clear.
   c. **False**. Whooping cough usually causes a mild upper respiratory infection in teenagers that requires laboratory confirmation.
   d. **True**. No laboratory test is available.
   e. **False**. Haemolytic uraemic syndrome can be diagnosed clinically but isolation of *Escherichia coli* O157 or *Shigella* spp. is usually attempted for confirmation.

2. a. **True**. There is a maculopapular rash.
   b. **False**. Mumps does not cause a rash and is therefore not an exanthematous infection.
   c. **True**. The rash is like measles and spreads from face and yoke to the trunk and limbs.
   d. **True**. The rash on the cheeks gives rise to the name 'slapped cheek syndrome'.
   e. **True**. Chickenpox has a distinctive vesiculopapular rash.

3. a. **False**. The attack rate for family contacts is around 90%.
   b. **True**. Appears after 4 or 5 days.
   c. **True**. This is an early sign.
   d. **True**. These are known as Koplik's spots.
   e. **False**. Immunity after infection is lifelong.

4. a. **True**. If the travellers visit countries without a vaccination programme.
   b. **True**.
   c. **False**. The fetus is not at increased risk of infection; however, when infection does occur as a result of transplacental spread, it may have devastating consequences.
   d. **True**. Many adult males will not have been vaccinated against rubella.
   e. **False**. The pregnant woman is at no greater risk of rubella infection and may be at reduced risk because of prior vaccination.

5. a. **False**. Vitamin A does not prevent measles but does prevent some of the consequent epithelial damage.
   b. **True**. This gives short-lived protection.
   c. **False**. This does not *prevent* measles but spacing of children does reduce the mortality and morbidity.

d. **True**. Breast-fed children are less vulnerable to infection and to the serious sequelae.
   e. **False**. The vaccine is a live attenuated strain of the virus.

6. a. **True**. This is an early sign.
   b. **True**. This usually displaces the lower earlobe laterally.
   c. **False**. Mumps orchitis is usually unilateral and only rarely causes infertility.
   d. **True**.
   e. **False**. Mumps is not an exanthem.

7. a. **False**. This is caused by *Haemophilus influenzae*.
   b. **True**. RSV occasionally causes croup-like illness.
   c. **False**. Infections are of the respiratory tract only.
   d. **True**.
   e. **True**. This is seasonal in temperate climates and can be serious in children under 1 year of age.

8. a. **False**. Hyalauronidase is produced by invasive streptococci, not *Bordetella pertussis*.
   b. **True**. This is a bacterial product.
   c. **True**. *B. pertussis* produces a tracheal cytotoxin.
   d. **False**. The adhesin assists in colonisation but is not a direct cause of damage.
   e. **True**. It can cause haemorrhages, frenal ulcer and, rarely, brain damage.

9. a. **True**.
   b. **True**.
   c. **False**. *H. influenzae* may cause acute pulmonary infection but is not a common cause of chronic lung infection in cystic fibrosis.
   d. **True**.
   e. **False**. *S. pneumoniae* may cause acute pulmonary infection but is not a common cause of chronic lung infection in cystic fibrosis.

10. a. and ii.
    b. and iii.
    c. and i.

11. a. **True**. It is caused by toxins produced by the initial infective organisms.
    b. **True**. *Shigella* spp. can also be a cause.
    c. **False**. Not always possible; culture with a specialised medium can detect *E. coli* O157.
    d. **False**. The toxin is a shiga-like verotoxin.
    e. **False**. Antibiotics are not helpful.

12. a. **False**.
    b. **False**. Romanowsky staining is required.
    c. **True**.
    d. **True**. Sensitivity is approximately 25 times greater than with a thin film.
    e. **True**. To detect the parasite at different stages in the life cycle.

Diagnosis is best achieved by several blood films, including both thick and thin films, which should be stained at higher pH than is routine in haematology practice.

13. a. **False**. Chloroquine-resistant falciparum malaria is becoming increasingly common.
    b. **False**. Because chloroquine-resistant falciparum malaria is becoming increasingly common, quinine is an important component of treatment for severe malaria.
    c. **True**. Particularly in the initial stages of severe infection.
    d. **True**. The species affects the choice of drug.
    e. **True**. To determine the effect on the proliferation of the parasite.

14. a. **False**. The disease occurs outside Asia, occasionally in people of non-Asian origin.
    b. **True**. Carditis causes deaths.
    c. **False**. Kawasaki disease has occurred in epidemics, but no evidence for person-to-person spread has been found.
    d. **True**.
    e. **True**. This reduces the risk of severe disease and death.

Case history answers

History 1

1. Recurrence of urinary tract infection.
2. Urine microscopy, quantitative culture and antibiotic susceptibility testing. Clean catch specimen required.
3. Intravenous pyelogram and micturating cystogram to exclude possible urinary tract abnormalities.
4. The perineum or lower gastrointestinal tract.
5. Antibiotics need to be continued for a full 10 days to ensure the best chance of cure.

History 2

1. Haemolytic uraemic syndrome (HUS).
2. *Escherichia coli* O157 and *Shigella* spp.
3. Culture for the organisms mention under 2 above, followed by latex agglutination test or cell cytotoxicity test for verotoxins.

4. Organisms may be transmitted for up to 10 days after the diarrhoea, so the patient is still a potential infection hazard. The girl is now unlikely to develop HUS and is no longer an infection risk.
5. Antibiotic treatment is of no benefit since this is a postinfective syndrome.

Data interpretation answer

1. Mumps is more likely.
2. IgG seroconversion may take several weeks after the onset of clinical signs.
3. Mumps IgM and viral culture.
4. Mumps meningitis. Orchitis and pancreatitis can occur but are normally restricted to adults with mumps infection.
5. Unlikely.

OSCE answer

1. No. The spots on the buccal mucosa (Koplik's spots) are features of measles.
2. Yes. Although the features are those of measles, the rash could be caused by a variety of other infective agents including rubella virus and some enteroviruses.
3. Yes. If a vaccination record or history is available, it is possible that this might exclude measles. Conversely, a lack of measles vaccination would support a presumptive diagnosis.
4. Yes. Measles is a notifiable disease in many countries. A sibling with a recent similar illness may have been the source for this patient. There is a higher probability that the sibling will have seroconverted because of the longer period since time of onset.
5. No. Measles is highly transmissible and requires additional respiratory infection control precautions to prevent hospital staff and other patients from contracting the disease. The child should not be nursed in a general ward, even if all the patients there may have been immunised.

Short notes answers

1. You could mention four factors: crowded dwellings, inadequate sanitation, malnutrition and inadequate primary health care. Refer to examples to show effect on transmission and consequences of infection.
2. See p. 174.
3. Remember age-related severity and viral neurotropism.
4. Three stages of disease: prodromal, catarrhal and paroxysmal to be described. Diagnosis by pernasal/cough swab.

5. Cause of childhood death in tropics; preventable mortality increasing in children who travel internationally.

Viva answers

1. Mention the differences in clinical presentation, treatment and epidemiology.
2. Refer to the different aetiology, clinical course and treatment. A comment about the effect of Hib vaccination would be useful.
3. Difficult choice. You could pick a disease that is part of a worldwide eradication programme (e.g. polio or measles), an infection that has come back to prominence because of falling vaccination (e.g. pertussis) or a new addition that has made a big impact on major morbidity (e.g. *Haemophilus influenzae*). Whatever you choose, give your reasons.

16 Infections in hospital patients

Overview

Infections arising in hospital patients after the time of hospital admission are referred to as hospital-acquired or nosocomial infections. These infections are unsought consequences of medical technology. Hospital infections are often caused by antibiotic-resistant microorganisms. This chapter reviews selected issues in hospital infection.

16.1 Epidemiology and pathogenesis

Learning objectives

You should:

- know the factors that increase the risk of infection in patients
- know the potential sources of cross-infection and endogenous infection
- understand the routes of infection.

Epidemiology

Around 10% of hospital patients develop a nosocomial infection. In general, risk of infection increases with the duration of stay in hospital, the severity of illness and the number of interventions (e.g. surgical procedures, therapeutic agents). Urinary tract infection (UTI) is the single most common type of nosocomial infection. Other common infections include pneumonia and surgical wound infection. Infections associated with intravascular cannulas are also becoming common. The type of nosocomial infection most often associated with death of the patient is pneumonia. The microorganisms most frequently implicated as a cause of nosocomial infections include *Staphylococcus aureus*, *Pseudomonas aeruginosa*, *Klebsiella pneumoniae*, *Enterococcus faecalis* and *Acinetobacter baumannii*.

Pathogenesis

There are many locations in the inanimate hospital environment that may be contaminated with potential microbial pathogens. Despite the recognition of this potential source of infection over a century ago and the subsequent introduction of antiseptic techniques, the hospital environment remains an important source of infection. Potential environmental sources of infection include any permanently moist area (water bacteria, e.g. *Pseudomonas* spp.), inanimate surfaces soiled by organic material (e.g. human body fluids, mucosal flora), used surgical or anaesthetic equipment (mucosal flora, tissue- or blood-borne organisms), hospital bedding and protective clothing.

Although the hospital environment may possess an abundant microbial flora, it is the staff and patients that serve as the principal source of hospital-acquired infection. Infection involving organisms transmitted from one patient to another is referred to as 'cross-infection'. This process is commonly assisted by medical, nursing and domestic staff. When the source of microorganisms is the patient's own resident microbial flora, infection is said to be of an 'endogenous' origin, which probably accounts for the majority of hospital-acquired infections.

Microorganisms can be transmitted to patients by a variety of routes, including direct contact (e.g. hands of staff), indirect contact (from one patient to another on a piece of equipment), by the air-borne route in droplet nuclei, by ingestion (e.g. contaminated hospital food) or by inoculation (via blood transfusion). Organisms causing hospital-acquired infection invade and spread with the assistance of medical procedures and the impairment of host defence systems caused by underlying diseases (i.e. primary reason for hospital admission). Any invasive medical device will, by definition, penetrate an epithelial barrier. The breach in the epidermis provides a route of entry for infecting organisms. If the device remains in the patient for a prolonged period (an 'indwelling device'), a layer of bacteria embedded in polysaccharide slime, known as 'biofilm', will form. The biofilm layer provides protection against antibiotic penetration, and the bacteria it contains grow more slowly than usual. Antibiotics that depend on rapid cell turnover for their bactericidal action therefore have a relatively poor effect on medical device-associated infections. It is often necessary to remove the device to guarantee antibiotic efficacy and eradication of infection.

16.2 Diagnosis

Learning objectives

You should:

- be aware of surveillance and targeted sampling
- be aware of the use and limitations of epidemiological investigations.

The diagnosis of hospital-acquired infections is generally the same as in community-acquired infections, the principal epidemiological clue being that the patient must have been in hospital long enough not to have contracted the infection prior to admission.

Much emphasis is placed on the detection of hospital outbreaks or common-source incidents. The investigation of such an incident aims to establish a source and means of transmission so that appropriate action can be taken to prevent further cases from occurring. Two main investigative approaches are used: surveillance and targeted sampling. Surveillance requires the regular submission of specimens and clinical information from a particular hospital unit. Laboratory results and other data are scrutinised regularly in order to identify common-source incidents early enough to intervene before the problem gets out of hand. This approach is costly and labour intensive and only rarely helps with specific outbreaks. However, surveillance techniques can be used to good effect in providing additional information once a given problem has been recognised.

Most epidemiological investigations are conducted in response to a perceived infection problem (e.g. increase in wound infections or an outbreak of diarrhoea). Diagnostic and possibly environmental specimens are collected from patients and relevant members of hospital staff, along with epidemiological information (such as location, surgical procedures or food consumed). The aim of laboratory investigations is to help to identify a common microbial pathogen and find its source. Once this has been done, it may be possible either to remove the source or to interrupt the means of transmission. The methods used by the microbiology laboratory to establish the co-identity of an organism isolated from a patient and its putative source depend on the genus concerned. Methods employed include antimicrobial susceptibility pattern, plasmid type, bacteriophage susceptibility, serum agglutination reactions and a variety of molecular methods such as DNA macrorestriction analysis (pulsed field gel electrophoresis).

The value of newer molecular epidemiological methods should not be overestimated, e.g. by using results to attribute responsibility for an outbreak of nosocomial infection. It must be remembered that unless a sequence of samples was taken from patient and presumed source, it is not possible to be absolutely sure in which direction transmission occurred. Moreover, in certain instances, the source may turn out to be a third site from which both the patient and the presumed source were contaminated. If a single type has spread widely, molecular typing is less able to discriminate or distinguish outbreak from background isolates.

16.3 Management

Learning objectives

You should:

- be aware of the problem of antibiotic resistance
- know the basis on which a suitable therapy is chosen
- be aware of basic preventive strategies.

Chemotherapy

The antimicrobial chemotherapy of nosocomial infections poses a number of problems. Bacterial hospital-acquired infections are more likely to be caused by antibiotic-resistant strains, making failure of presumptive therapy more likely. Even if the optimal agents are given by the best route, patients may take longer to respond to antimicrobial treatment because of compromised host defences, or possibly the presence of an indwelling medical device. The empirical choice of agent(s) must, therefore, be based on an up-to-date knowledge of the organisms most likely to cause the infection in question, and their local antibiotic susceptibility pattern. It is also important to obtain the appropriate diagnostic specimens before presumptive therapy has begun, so that treatment can be modified according to susceptibility results. The more commonly reported nosocomial pathogens can often be isolated from the body surfaces of hospital patients. The presence of the organism without clinical evidence of infection should not be accepted as sufficient reason for antimicrobial treatment. If it is, unnecessary treatment with 'broad-spectrum' agents can result in increasing the promotion of antibiotic resistance and the risk of toxic or allergic reactions.

Prevention

The range of preventive strategies is a reflection of the high prevalence of hospital infections. Endogenous source infections, which constitute the majority of nosocomial infections, are the most difficult to prevent and require an approach specific to the type of infection. In theory, common-source incidents are easier to prevent, since the transmission of infection can be interrupted and the source eradicated. In practice there are regular reports of hospital outbreaks, some of them caused by well-recognised problems. There are many reasons for this, including the introduction of new medical devices, new types of antibiotic or antiseptic resistance or even renovation work in hospital wards and operating theatres. But more often the precipitating factor in a hospital outbreak lies in the actions of staff, e.g. a lapse in hand-washing technique, failure to institute appropriate isolation procedures, inadequate maintenance of equipment or poor hygiene in the hospital kitchens.

The protection of vulnerable patients against hospital-acquired infection is the responsibility of every member of the hospital staff, particularly those who have direct physical contact with the patient, irrespective of their status within the organisation. It only requires one careless action to negate the preventive efforts of all the other staff attending to the patient. Those with responsibility for the patient's care should promote an interest in hospital hygiene among their staff and provide an example for their junior colleagues.

Hand washing, preferably with a disinfectant preparation, before and after contact with a patient or their body fluids is probably the single most effective means of preventing transmission of microorganisms between hospital patients. A pair of clean latex gloves should be worn whenever there is deliberate contact with moist body surfaces, body fluids, faeces or blood, and the gloves should be discarded as contaminated waste immediately afterwards. This precaution will protect patients from cross-infection and protect staff against viral infection (hepatitis B and human immunodeficiency virus (HIV)). A more thorough hand wash with disinfectant and the use of sterile latex gloves is required before operative procedures, invasive investigations or contact with any sterile equipment (disinfection and sterilisation is covered in Ch. 6).

The following services provide essential, though often forgotten, support in the maintenance of hospital hygiene and prevention of hospital infection:

- the sterile supplies department (sterilised equipment ready packed for use in the operating theatre
- the hospital laundry (decontamination of soiled or infected bed linen)
- the kitchen (a diet free from food-borne pathogens)
- the waste-disposal service (safe disposal of hazardous waste).

All of these hospital support services require supervisory input from infection control staff.

Infection control teams
In many hospitals, the prevention of hospital-acquired infection is supervised by an infection control team, which reports to an infection control committee. The infection control team will typically consist of a medical microbiologist or other specialist in infectious diseases, a specialist infection control nurse and, where resources permit, a member of the microbiology laboratory staff. The infection control team will arrange regular surveillance activities, periodic inspection of hospital support facilities and the investigation of any suspected outbreak. The infection control doctor (usually a microbiologist) is the first source of advice when an outbreak occurs. He will take executive responsibility for initiating additional investigations and preventive measures, such as arranging for the isolation of patients, or even the closure of a ward to new admissions. He will probably set up an action team, consisting of the infection control team and any other hospital staff essential to the control of the current outbreak.

Infection control procedures
A patient known to be a potential source of infection may be placed in 'isolation'. The term is not meant to imply a total exclusion of the patient from all forms of human contact. Rather, it refers to additional precautions that reduce the risk of transmitting infection by placing barriers in the way. These may be physical barriers, such as walls, impervious plastic aprons or latex gloves, or chemical barriers such as disinfectants. Two main types of isolation may be encountered: source and protective isolation (where the protection refers to the patient, who is usually immunocompromised or otherwise susceptible to infection). These terms were replaced along with 'barrier' and 'reverse barrier' nursing. Since the purpose is to restrict the spread of

infection, precautions are applied to interrupt the most likely routes of transmission. For example, a patient with smear-positive pulmonary tuberculosis and a productive cough needs to be nursed in a single side ward by BCG-vaccinated staff away from other patients. By comparison, an HIV-positive patient does not require isolation in a single side ward providing that blood and body secretions can be effectively contained. This should be possible by use of what were originally called 'universal precautions'—application of preventive methods to all patients and their body products on the assumption that anyone could be a potential source. Patients with diarrhoea necessitate very careful disposal of faeces and protection of the hands of attending staff with gloves and disinfectant wash to prevent infection by the faecal–oral route. The regular application of a set of standard hygiene measures in everyday practice now comes under the umbrella term 'standard infection control precautions'. The extra measures applied to prevent enteric, droplet or contact routes of transmission in hospitals are now referred to as 'additional precautions'.

16.4 Issues in hospital infection

Learning objectives

You should:

- know the major infections of hospital patients
- know the factors contributing to their occurrence
- understand the basis of their clinical management.

Nosocomial urinary tract infection

Patients at greatest risk of nosocomial UTI are those admitted by the urological service and other units where urinary catheterisation or urethral instrumentation is commonly employed (Table 29). Older adult males are more at risk than adult females. The risk increases with increased duration of catheterisation. The bacteria that cause these infections include *P. aeruginosa*, *Klebsiella* spp., *E. faecalis* and coagulase-negative staphylococci. These organisms are found in and around the perineum and are introduced during catheterisation or instrumentation of the urethra. Even if bacteria do not gain access at this stage, they may ascend the urethra later on, either along the outer surface of a urinary catheter or via the fluid column it contains. Once organisms have colonised the inner catheter surface, they are difficult to eradicate. While antibiotic treatment may alleviate the symptoms of invasive UTI, bacteria that remain on the surface of the catheter act as a focus for reinfection when treatment is stopped. The presence of bacteria in a catheter specimen of urine, especially in the absence of pyuria, does not always indicate a need for antimicrobial chemotherapy. Removal of the catheter increases the chance of eradicating the infection. Patients with long-term indwelling catheters (e.g. those with multiple sclerosis) are particularly prone to infection. Aseptic technique should be used during catheter insertion or urological instrumentation to help to prevent nosocomial UTI. Urinary catheters should be taped to the patient's inner thigh and should be connected to sterile closed urine collection systems, with non-return valves. Urinary catheters should be used for the shortest time possible, and their use should be avoided where an alternative solution is practical.

Surgical wound infection

Infection of surgical wounds is common in hospital practice (see also Ch. 7) and is usually caused by one of a small group of bacterial species. The most commonly implicated bacteria are *S. aureus*, *P. aeruginosa*, the Enterobacteriaceae (*Escherichia coli*, *Klebsiella* spp., *Enterobacter* sp., etc.) and anaerobic bacteria.

Contributory factors can be considered in relation to the surgical procedure, i.e. pre-, peri- and postoperative. Common preoperative risk factors include:

- obesity
- diabetes mellitus
- steroid therapy
- infection at a distant site or prolonged hospital stay.

Perioperative risk factors include:

- shaving the skin surface
- large incisions
- lengthy operations
- poor haemostasis

Table 29 Common device-associated infections

Medical device	Infection	Infective agents
Urinary catheter	UTI	*Klebsiella, Pseudomonas, Proteus, Candida* spp.
Tracheal tube	Pneumonia	*Pseudomonas, Staphylococcus aureus*, Enterobacteriaceae, *Acinetobacter* spp.
Intravenous cannula	Phlebitis	Coagulase-negative staphylococci, corynebacteria, *Candida* spp.

- incomplete debridement
- foreign bodies (e.g. invasive medical devices)
- spillage of microorganisms (e.g. large bowel surgery or drainage of deep abscesses)
- large numbers of unscrubbed staff in the operating theatre.

Postoperative risk factors include:

- exposed deep tissues
- persistently moist surfaces
- ischaemia
- foreign bodies or haematomas.

The source of infection is often the patient's own skin or mucosal flora. Occasionally, infecting microorganisms are transmitted during or after the surgical procedure from a staff, patient or environmental source.

Diagnosis

The most common types of wound infection are superficial and easily diagnosed if the wound site is inspected regularly. An offensive smell or purulent discharge should be regarded as suspicious. A thin serous discharge is common during wound healing and does not indicate a need for further action when other features of infection are absent. Early discharge of patients from hospital means that some surgical wound infections can be expected to present after hospital discharge. Deep soft tissue infections, such as subphrenic abscesses, may be particularly difficult to diagnose when they present after hospital discharge.

Laboratory confirmation of the diagnosis is by microscopy and culture of purulent discharge, best done by sending a specimen of exudate on a portion of the dressing. Failing that, wound exudate on a cotton swab is a less satisfactory alternative. Deep soft tissue infection requires collection of either a substantial pus specimen or tissue from the affected site.

Treatment and control

Treatment of superficial surgical wound infections should include an antistaphylococcal agent such as flucloxacillin, but deep infections following abdominal surgery or those associated with arterial surgery may also require an anti-anaerobic agent, such as metronidazole, and an agent effective against local aerobic Gram-negative bacilli. Isolation of Gram-negative bacilli from surgical wounds may indicate no more than colonisation of a moist surface and should not necessarily be taken as an indication for antibiotic treatment.

A variety of approaches can be taken to prevent surgical infection.

Pre-existing infection. Infection of a distant site diagnosed preoperatively should be treated before the procedure begins. Shaving of the operation site should be avoided if at all possible (clipping excessive hair is a preferable alternative).

Prophylaxis. Patients who are requiring surgical procedures that carry a high risk of infection and for which the value of antibiotic prophylaxis has been established should be given antibiotics prior to the start of the procedure. The antimicrobial agents chosen should differ from those used to treat established infection in the same hospital. The initial dose should be timed to peak at the time of the procedure. Normally only a single dose is given, but for lengthy procedures a further dose may be required. Prophylactic regimens should not be continued after the operation. If a therapeutic regimen is required, different agents should be chosen, according to the most likely microbial pathogens and their antimicrobial susceptibility pattern.

Operative procedure. The operation site should be prepared with a suitable antiseptic, e.g. chlorhexidine or povidone iodine. All opening staff should follow a thorough surgical scrub hand-washing procedure and, after drying their hands on sterile towels, put on sterile gowns and latex gloves. All equipment, sutures, drapes and other materials that may come in contact with the operation site should be sterile. Thorough haemostasis, debridement, closure and other aspects of surgical technique all help to reduce the risk of infection.

Postoperative care. The wound site is at increased risk of infection and is a potential source of infection postoperatively. Staff should take care to follow hand hygiene precautions reviewed above whenever they expose the wound. Dressings should be discarded as contaminated waste and discarded safely.

Infection associated with intravascular cannulas

The plastic cannulas used to provide vascular access provide a potential route for microbial invasion of a normally sterile body space (see Table 29). Risk factors for intravascular cannula-related infection include:

- prolonged use (greater than 48 hours for peripheral vein cannulas)
- diabetics
- neutropenia
- 'broad-spectrum' antibiotic use
- parenteral nutrition
- heavy bacterial colonisation at the cannula insertion site.

The source of infection may be the patient's or the doctor's skin at the time of insertion, but it could also be connection points with intravenous fluid-giving sets, or even haematogenous spread from a distant focus within the patient.

Diagnosis

Infection may be evident as superficial inflammation around the insertion site, blockage of the cannula or sometimes fever and other signs of systemic infection. Laboratory confirmation of diagnosis is by culture of the cannula tip once it has been removed (light growth of skin organisms can be caused by contamination during removal and is not considered significant). If cannula removal is not practically possible, culture of blood drawn through the cannula may provide some evidence of a cannula-related infection. The commonest cause of these infections is coagulase-negative staphylococci, which are usually resistant to the more commonly used antistaphylococcal antibiotics. Other organisms isolated from these infections include *S. aureus* and yeast species such as *C. albicans*.

Treatment and control

Removal of peripheral cannulas is often sufficient management in patients who do not have significantly compromised host defences, but if antimicrobial chemotherapy is required, vancomycin or other antimicrobial agents may have to be given. Cannula-related infection can be prevented by sterile insertion technique, replacement of peripheral cannulas after a maximum of 48 hours and meticulous handling of the insertion site and giving set. In some hospitals, a specialist multidisciplinary team manages all intravascular cannulas—a strategy that has been shown to substantially reduce the cannula infection rate.

Infection associated with blood transfusion

Transfusion of blood and blood products carries a risk of transmitting blood-borne microorganisms. Infection was common in the early days of blood transfusion, when reusable collection sets were in use and blood was not routinely screened for viral agents. The patients now at greatest risk of transfusion-associated infection are either patients who have had multiple units of blood (e.g. during cardiac surgery) or those who require blood products pooled from many donors (e.g. haemophiliacs). The microorganisms most commonly implicated are either bacteria or viruses. Bacteria may cause overwhelming systemic sepsis, usually within minutes to hours of the onset of transfusion. There is a high mortality rate when this occurs. Viral infection, by comparison, has a much longer incubation period and may only become clinically apparent months after transfusion. Bacterial infection is usually the result of contamination at the time of donation, poor storage, contaminated equipment or a combination of these. Viral infection in the recipient is usually caused by the presence of viral infection in the donor. Bacteria include *Citrobacter* spp., *Pseudomonas* spp. and *Yersinia enterocolitica*. Viruses include hepatitis B and C viruses, HIV and cytomegalovirus. A severe acute transfusion reaction resulting from infection may take the form of septicaemia. Shock is a poor prognostic indicator.

The only immediately useful microbiological investigation is a Gram stain of any remaining blood (but remember non-infective causes that require haematological investigation). Culture takes too long to help to determine immediate clinical management.

Treatment and control

The single most important action in an acute transfusion reaction is to stop the transfusion. If bacterial infection is suspected, antimicrobial chemotherapy should be commenced immediately, with intravenous agents effective against Gram-negative bacilli. As viral transfusion-associated infections are often well established by the time of diagnosis and cannot be treated with currently available agents, the emphasis is on prevention.

Prevention relies on a combination of selecting low-risk donors and screening donated blood for blood-borne pathogens. Many countries screen donated blood units for HIV, hepatitis B and C viruses, syphilis and cytomegalovirus, in selected instances. The withdrawal of financial incentives for blood donation has further reduced the risk of blood-borne infection in some countries. Collection of donated blood into single use, sterile plastic collection sets that can be used for storage and subsequent transfusion also reduces the risk of transfusion-associated infection.

Sharp injury

Needle-stick and other sharp injuries are the most common means of transmitting hospital-acquired HIV infection and hepatitis B. These injuries are frequently the result of recapping hypodermic syringe needles after completion of venesection, but other reasons include encounter by domestic staff with discarded needles hidden in bed linen and pricking by sutures or scalpel blades during surgical procedures. The common site of injury is the thumb and forefinger of the non-dominant hand. Sharps injuries should be reported to supervising staff. Serum should be taken from the patient and the staff member. The patient's serum is then tested for evidence of hepatitis B and C and, when permission is given, for HIV infection. The staff serum is stored for comparison with a further serum specimen to demonstrate seroconversion, or for further testing if the patient's serum is hepatitis B positive. Staff will normally require counselling regarding the risk of hepatitis and HIV infection. Transmission of hepatitis B virus occurs far more readily than HIV. If the patient is hepatitis B positive, the staff serum should be checked for antibodies to hepatitis B surface antigen. The staff member has satisfactory protection only if they have already been vaccinated and have a high antibody titre. If the titre is low or absent, a booster dose of vaccine is required, along with a dose of hepatitis B immunoglobulin. Staff, particularly those working in high-risk areas (e.g. renal dialysis units or accident departments), should be vaccinated against hepatitis B.

Hospital-acquired diarrhoea and vomiting

Outbreaks of diarrhoea and vomiting occur from time to time in hospitals, particularly on paediatric and geriatric wards. The cause, if established, is found to be bacteria, bacterial toxins or viruses. Transmission is by the faecal–oral route or by droplet spread, and the incubation period is short, often less than 24 hours. The incubation period has important implications for the duration of infection control precautions and may narrow the range of causal agents to be searched for. A careful food history should be taken and, if hospital food is a potential source, specimens may have to be sought from the hospital kitchens. Diagnosis is confirmed by electron microscopy of diarrhoea stool, and culture for bacterial causes of gastroenteritis. Rotavirus, which may cause this type of infection, can be detected rapidly by enzyme-linked immunosorbent assay (ELISA). There is no specific antimicrobial treatment. Patients with diarrhoea and vomiting should be nursed away from unaffected patients, but the rapid spread of these infections may necessitate the closure of the ward to admissions. Nursing staff who develop symptoms of infection should be encouraged to take sick leave until well again. Elderly patients with community-acquired diarrhoea and vomiting should not be admitted to acute geriatric units if it can be avoided.

Nosocomial respiratory infections

In addition to those patients who are vulnerable to infection in hospital simply because they are there or their treatment makes them susceptible, certain pre-existing conditions also pose a risk for the hospitalised patient; for example, *Burkholderia cepacia* causes chronic respiratory infection in patients with cystic fibrosis. Strains of *B. cepacia* with a 'cable' pilus can be easily spread from patient to patient.

Nosocomial pneumonia
Pneumonia is the third most common hospital-acquired infection and the most common one to cause death. Pneumonia is covered in detail in Chapter 7.

Nosocomial tuberculosis
Nosocomial tuberculosis can occur, particularly when there are patients in open hospital wards with pulmonary tuberculosis caused by multidrug-resistant strains.

Nosocomial Legionnaire's disease
Hospital-acquired infections with *Legionella* sp. occur sporadically through contamination of hospital air-conditioning.

Antibiotic resistance in hospital

Acquired resistance to antimicrobial agents is more common in microorganisms isolated from hospital patients than in organisms causing community-acquired infections. Hospitals provide an environment in which antibiotic-resistant strains collect, concentrate and are maintained by a higher level of antibiotic usage than is normally found in the community.

Multiple-resistant strains of nosocomial pathogens may be endemic, especially in large teaching hospitals. These strains may be transmitted from patient to patient in mini-outbreaks, or present in the hospital environment in a reservoir that maintains the overall level of antibiotic resistance at a high level. Moreover, the higher rates of antibiotic usage in hospital practice provide these resistant organisms with an ecological survival advantage. Sometimes, resistant strains enter the hospital as part of the patient's indigenous flora at the time of admission. When these patients are given antimicrobial agents (e.g. surgical prophylaxis), susceptible species are eradicated and their place taken by the remaining organisms, whether carrying acquired resistance mechanisms or intrinsic resistance.

Probably the most important factors selecting acquired antibiotic resistance are:

- the widespread use of antibiotics to treat self-limiting upper respiratory tract and gastrointestinal infections
- the use of topical agents to treat minor soft tissue infection
- the extensive use of cephalosporins in both community and hospital practice.

Commonly encountered resistant species include *K. pneumoniae*, *P. aeruginosa*, *Enterococcus* spp., *A. baumannii* and methicillin-resistant *S. aureus* (MRSA).

The presence of intrinsic or acquired antibiotic resistance is demonstrated by susceptibility testing of clinical isolates. Many centres monitor the susceptibility patterns of important species in order to detect the emergence of new kinds of acquired resistance.

There is no reliable means of eradicating acquired resistance once it has become established. The ingenuity of pharmaceutical companies has in the past allowed us to believe that there will always be a new antimicrobial agent when the current choice of compounds ceases to be effective. Sadly, confidence has given way to realism as microorganisms demonstrate their limitless ability to devise new strategies for evading the antimicrobial action of whole families of antimicrobial agents.

Multiple-resistant *Mycobacterium tuberculosis*, MRSA and extended-spectrum β-lactamase-carrying Enterobacteriaceae are just a few examples of infective agents edging towards untreatability.

Attempts to prevent the spread of antibiotic resistance in hospital combine hospital infection control with antimicrobial pharmacology. Numerous approaches have been tried, none of them entirely successful. They include isolation of patients with resistance organisms (e.g. MRSA), stepping up hand-hygiene precautions, promoting short-course antimicrobial chemotherapy, use of narrow-spectrum antimicrobial agents, rotating the range of agents available and restricted reporting of susceptibility results. No approach is likely to succeed without the willing cooperation of hospital medical staff.

16.5 Organisms

A checklist of the organisms discussed in this chapter is given in Box 11. Further information is given on the pages indicated.

Box 11 Organisms involved in hospital-acquired infections

Bacteria	see page	Fungi	see page
Staphylococcus aureus	243	*Candida albicans*	269
Coagulase-negative staphylococci	243		
Enterococcus faecalis	245	**Viruses**	
Escherichia coli	248	Hepatitis B and C virus	257
Klebsiella pneumoniae	248	Human immunodeficiency virus	260
Enterobacter spp.	248–9	Cytomegalovirus	257
Citrobacter spp.	188	Rotavirus and small round structured	260
Pseudomonas aeruginosa	249–50	virus group	
Acinetobacter baumannii	250		
Yersinia enterocolitica	249		
Treponema pallidum	255		
Mycobacterium tuberculosis	253–4		

Self-assessment: questions

Multiple choice questions

1. The overall nosocomial infection rate would be expected to rise as a result of:
   a. Increasing numbers of operations on elderly patients
   b. An increase in patients requiring a shorter hospital stay
   c. New invasive surgical procedures
   d. Promotion of a new hand-washing agent
   e. Reducing the numbers of nursing staff

2. Important sources of organisms causing nosocomial infections include:
   a. The patient's indigenous flora
   b. Hands of hospital staff
   c. Single-use medical devices
   d. Food from hospital kitchens
   e. Used endoscopes

3. Pair up the following means of transmitting hospital infection with the appropriate example:
   a. Direct contact
   b. Indirect contact
   c. Droplet infection
   d. Inoculation

   i. Patient with productive cough
   ii. Unwashed staff hands
   iii. Blood transfusion
   iv. Unwashed bed linen

4. Disposable medical devices help the development of infection by:
   a. Penetrating epithelial barriers
   b. Enabling direct access to sterile tissues
   c. Providing a site for biofilm development
   d. Promoting rapid bacteria cell turnover
   e. Allowing the persistence of microorganisms despite antimicrobial use

5. Match the infection with the best type of isolation procedure:
   a. Pulmonary tuberculosis
   b. AIDS
   c. Septicaemia
   d. Diarrhoea

   i. Blood/body fluid precautions
   ii. Single side ward
   iii. Enteric precautions

6. Among the factors increasing the risk of hospital-acquired urinary tract infection (UTI) are:
   a. Male sex
   b. Prior history of community-acquired UTI
   c. An indwelling urinary catheter
   d. A cystoscopic procedure
   e. Antiseptic cleansing of the urinary meatus

7. Surgical wound infection can be prevented by:
   a. Antiseptic application to incision site
   b. Strict hand hygiene among operating staff
   c. Thorough haemostasis
   d. Antibiotic prophylaxis
   e. Keeping wound moist after surgery

8. The following factors predispose to infections associated with intravascular cannulas:
   a. Use for less than 24 hours
   b. Diabetes mellitus
   c. Leaving insertion site undressed
   d. Parenteral nutrition
   e. Hospital admission for carcinoma

9. The following infections can be transmitted as a result of transfusion of blood or blood products:
   a. HIV
   b. Hepatitis C
   c. Syphilis
   d. Malaria
   e. *Candida albicans*

10. Sharps injury:
    a. Refers only to skin puncture caused by a hypodermic needle
    b. Occurs most often during recapping of hypodermic needles
    c. Should prompt collection of serum from both patient and staff member
    d. Most often affects the finger and thumb of the dominant hand
    e. May result in transmission of HIV

11. Outbreaks of diarrhoea and vomiting:
    a. Occur on geriatric wards
    b. Are often caused by small round structured viruses
    c. Are best diagnosed by serological methods
    d. May result in closure of the ward
    e. Are uncommon in modern hospitals

Case history questions

History 1

In a 2-hour period, seven patients develop diarrhoea and vomiting on your ward. Your consultant and the control of infection officer cannot be contacted since it is a public holiday.

1. What diagnostic tests would you arrange?
2. Are there any therapeutic measures that might be of use?
3. How would you prevent further cases from occurring?

History 2

> After major abdominal surgery, a 52-year-old insulin-dependent diabetic required intravenous nutrition. One week later, he developed an intermittent fever (temperature maximum of 38°C). His antibiotic regimen was changed to give cover against staphylococci, but with no effect. Eventually, the feeding cannula ceased to work. There was no inflammation around the cannula insertion site.

1. What factors contributed to the cannula-related infection?
2. How would you confirm the presence of infection?
3. Why was there no benefit from antibiotic treatment?

Data interpretation

Enterococcus faecalis isolates from five patients are tested in a reference laboratory by DNA macrorestriction analysis (pulsed field gel electrophoresis) and the results are given in Table 30.

1. Is this an outbreak?
2. What additional information would help you to establish a connection between these patients?
3. What is 'vanB' resistance in *E. faecalis*?
4. What does 'identical' mean?
5. How useful do you think the information from surveillance rectal swabs was?

Objective structured clinical examination (OSCE)

During resuscitation of a suspected heroin abuser, you miss your target and accidentally stick a hypodermic needle into your left hand.

1. Should you complete an accident report before you do anything else?
2. Will pre-exposure vaccination give you adequate protection against infections that might be contracted in this type of accident?
3. Will the patient's infection status help to determine further action?
4. Should your serological status for blood-borne infections be determined right away?
5. Will you need antiviral treatment within the next 48 hours?

Short notes questions

Write short notes on the following:

1. How 'cross-infection' occurs in a hospital and its prevention
2. The role of the microbiology laboratory in the investigation of a hospital outbreak with reference to an example known to you
3. The methods that are available to control acquired antibiotic resistance in hospital

Viva questions

1. How would you improve compliance with hand-hygiene measures in your hospital?
2. What would you do to change a poor infection control record in a hospital where you have just been appointed as infection control officer?

Table 30 DNA analysis of *Enterococcus faecalis* isolates

Patient	Ward	Date	Specimen	Resistance	Molecular typing
A	Dialysis	November	Intravenous access	VanB	Identical
B	Dialysis	January	Blood	VanB	Identical
C	Dialysis	February	Rectal	VanB	Identical
D	Dialysis	February	Rectal	VanB	Identical
E	Geriatric	March	Urine	VanB	Identical

Van, vancomycin.

Self-assessment: answers

Multiple choice answers

1. a. **True**. Elderly patients are often frail and have concomitant disease.
   b. **False**. Risk of nosocomial infection increases with duration of hospital stay.
   c. **True**.
   d. **False**. Promotion of a novel hand hygiene agent, such as an antiseptic hand wash, should only serve to increase interest in hospital hand hygiene.
   e. **True**. Reduced numbers of nursing staff increases the risk of nosocomial infection by putting the remaining staff under greater pressure, and by increasing the number of patients any individual nurse cares for.

2. a. **True**. This gives rise to 'endogenous' infections.
   b. **True**. Hand hygiene is the single most effective means of preventing transmission of organisms between patients.
   c. **False**. Single-use medical devices are not a significant source of infection if they are sterilised before use and only used once, as intended.
   d. **True**. These provide for a large population, both staff and patients.
   e. **True**. Endoscopes are difficult to decontaminate under clinic conditions and may be the cause of hospital-acquired infection.

3. a. and iv.
   b. and ii.
   c. and i.
   d. and iii.

4. a. **True**. The break in the epithelium allows a route of entry.
   b. **True**. Again a route of entry is established.
   c. **True**. If the device remains in the body for any length of time.
   d. **False**. Bacteria in biofilms responsible for device-associated infections have a slow rate of turnover; this makes them relatively resistant to antibiotics that require rapid metabolism or cell division.
   e. **True**. See d.

5. a. and ii.
   b. and i.
   c. None of these; does not require isolation
   d. and iii.

6. a. **True**. Older adult males are at increased risk.
   b. **False**.
   c. **True**. It provides a source of infection with perineal organisms both at insertion and while inserted.
   d. **True**. This can introduce perineal organisms to the urethra.
   e. **False**. However, there is no evidence that antiseptic application to the meatus (meatal toilet) significantly reduces the incidence of nosocomial UTI, though the practice still goes on in many centres.

7. a. **True**. To reduce skin microflora.
   b. **True**. A vital factor in reducing all nosocomial infections.
   c. **True**. This reduces perioperative infection.
   d. **True**. Both superficial and deep wounds should be treated.
   e. **False**. A moist wound surface encourages the growth of bacteria. Deliberate wetting of the wound surface should therefore be avoided as much as possible.

8. a. **False**. Peripheral venous cannulas are at increased risk after more than 48 hours of use.
   b. **True**. Natural neutrophil defences are reduced in diabetics.
   c. **False**. Dressing the insertion site may actually increase the risk of the infection, depending on the type of dressing.
   d. **True**. This provides the ideal site for bacterial growth.
   e. **False**. Carcinoma is not particularly associated with intravenous cannula infections, though neutropenia (e.g. chemotherapy) is.

9. a. **True**. The virus can be detected by screening blood.
   b. **True**. See a.
   c. **True**. Screening can detect *Treponema pallidum*.
   d. **True**. Malaria sporozoites can be transmitted in transfused blood in endemic areas.
   e. **False**. *Candida albicans* is associated with intravenous cannula infections, but not with blood transfusion.

10. a. **False**. Sharps injuries can be caused by all sorts of other items including sutures, scalpel blades and intravenous cannulas.
    b. **True**. Usually of the thumb or forefinger of the non-dominant hand.
    c. **True**. This enables the potential for infection to be assessed (patient) and gives a baseline comparison for seroconversion (staff).
    d. **False**. It most often affects the non-dominant hand, since the sharp item is held in the dominant hand.
    e. **True**.

11. a. **True**. Elderly patients are vulnerable as are paediatric patients.
    b. **True**. Rotavirus is the most common agent in outbreaks in both the elderly and the very young.
    c. **False**. Electron microscopy of diarrhoea stool is the single most useful investigation.
    d. **True**. The outbreaks spread rapidly.
    e. **False**. Outbreaks of diarrhoea and vomiting are regrettably common in hospitals.

Case history answers

History 1

1. Electron microscopy for small round structured viruses and rotavirus; ELISA (enzyme-linked immunosorbent assay) and culture for bacterial enteric pathogen.
2. Fluid and electrolyte replacement as oral rehydration salts is possible.
3. Separate the affected patients from others on the ward; institute enteric isolation precautions (specify); stop movement of nursing staff between the two groups of patients; and stop further admissions to the ward if possible.

History 2

1. The presence of the cannula, his diabetes, parenteral nutrition and possibly the continuation of antibiotics after surgery.
2. Ideally by removing the cannula and sending the tip for bacterial culture, but if this is not possible, draw blood via the cannula (if not blocked) and at the same time from an uncannulated peripheral vein.
3. Several reasons are possible. If infection was caused by a coagulase-negative staphylococcus, it may have been resistant to standard antistaphylococcal agents (e.g. flucloxacillin) and would require vancomycin. Bacteria may have been present in a biofilm around the cannula tip and therefore protected against

antibiotic action. Or the infection may have been with *Candida* sp. and therefore resistant to antibacterial agents. Once established, it is usually necessary to remove a parenteral nutrition cannula to guarantee eradication of infection.

Data interpretation answer

1. At most, there have been three infections (rectal swabs are for infection control surveillance purposes) spread over 5 months and two different units. At face value, this does not appear to be a case cluster in terms of either time or place.
2. Did patients A–D spend any time on the geriatric ward or did patient E visit the dialysis unit? Were there any other patients with vancomycin-resistant *E. faecalis* infection in the hospital during this period? Why were rectal swabs being collected on the dialysis unit? How do other *E. faecalis* infections compare with these isolates by molecular typing?
3. A type of vancomycin-resistant *Enterococcus* sp. that may remain susceptible to teicoplanin.
4. 'Identical' probably means 'indistinguishable by DNA macrorestriction', which compares around 10% of the DNA from each isolate. Unless more is known about the population structure of *E. faecalis* in this hospital and the surrounding community, it is difficult to be certain that this typing result helps much.
5. The rectal swab results neither determine a common source for a case-cluster nor suggest any useful infection control interventions. However, by contributing two additional isolates, they may have unintentionally added ascertainment bias to the process of case finding. Many institutions avoid non-contributory infection control investigations of this kind.

OSCE answer

1. No. The first priority is to wash the needle-stick site and encourage blood flow to clean out the track. Paperwork has its place but does not come before first aid.
2. No. Vaccination against hepatitis B is important for all health-care staff engaged in exposure-prone procedures but vaccination will not protect against hepatitis C or HIV.
3. Yes. If the patient is known to be positive for HIV or hepatitis C, more intensive postexposure management and follow-up are required.
4. Yes. This will demonstrate that seroconversion could not have happened prior to the accident.
5. Yes. Antiretrovirus agents are used in many centres for postexposure prophylaxis following an accident

involving a high-risk patient. The treatment should be commenced as soon after the needle-stick injury as possible. This patient would be regarded as high risk and the exposure medium-to-high risk since a hollow bore needle was involved.

Short notes answers

1. Could be answered in tabular format; cover routes of transmission and ways these can be interrupted. Examples would be helpful.
2. Two main areas: identification of causal microorganisms and subsequent typing (e.g. phage, sero- or plasmid type) and tracking down a potential source (staff, patients and environmental screening). An example of the way these results can be used to identify source and route of transmission would be

useful.
3. Can be classified as laboratory-, pharmacy- and educationally based methods. Some idea of their respective limitations would be helpful.

Viva answers

1. No single measure has been universally effective. Behaviour modification and educational initiatives are worth discussing but be critical in your appraisal of these. Role models, educational aids and provision of good hand-washing facilities all have their place.
2. You would probably want to discuss briefly how to assess the factors likely to contribute to the poor record. The most important single change would be hand-hygiene measures (see answer to 1).

17 Infections in immunocompromised patients

Overview

Impaired host defences directly cause an increased risk of infection. The infections that develop in immunocompromised patients may be caused by unusual microorganisms. This can cause problems in diagnosis and treatment. Allowances have to be made in both laboratory diagnosis and antimicrobial chemotherapy for immunocompromised status. However, knowledge of the nature of the patient's compromised immune defences helps to narrow the range of possible microbial pathogens. Four specific categories of compromised host defence are considered.

17.1 Pathogenesis

Learning objectives

You should:

* understand the effects of immune defects on the types of infection that occur
* be aware of the unusual infections that are seen in the immunocompromised.

Defects in the immune defences can be either congenital (rare, since they are often incompatible with a life long enough to produce offspring) or acquired. Defences against specific infections constitute the humoral and cellular arms of the immune system, complement and phagocytic cells. While deficient neutrophil function (either quantitative (neutropenia) or qualitative, e.g. caused by diabetes) is not an impairment of specific immune function, neutropenia is usually considered alongside forms of specific immune compromise. The defect can be very specific, such as in deficiency of a specific complement component, or it can be more generalised, such as impaired T lymphocyte function. A deficiency in the immune system can affect the type of infection in several ways

* determining the type of pathogen that will successfully infect
* allowing infections by organisms that would not normally succeed (opportunist pathogens)
* allowing multiple infections to occur more often
* allowing dormant, or latent, infections to activate.

Whatever form of compromised defence exists, the deficit determines which infections the patient will contract. Conversely, the type of infection encountered points to the type of immune compromise (Table 31). So, while patients with a cell-mediated immune defect are at greater risk of viral, fungal and intracellular bacterial infections, a patient who develops *Pneumocystis carinii* pneumonia (PCP) is likely to have impaired cell-mediated immunity.

Immunocompromised patients are at greater risk of infection with organisms that would not normally cause infection or that would require a much larger inoculum to cause infection. These are sometimes referred to as opportunist pathogens. In addition, immunocompromised patients are more likely to develop two or more infections at the same time, further complicating the clinical picture. Finally, some types of compromise (particularly impaired cell-mediated immunity) also put the patient at risk of infection with organisms that lie dormant, such as herpes viruses, mycobacteria and some protozoa. These are sometimes called 'latent' infections. As a general rule, the risk of infection is in proportion to the extent of compromise.

Table 31 Common infections associated with immune defects

Defect	Infecting organisms
Humoral immunity	Bacteria
Cell-mediated immunity	Viruses, yeasts, intracellular bacteria
Phagocytes	Bacteria
Complement	*Neisseria* spp., *Streptococcus pneumoniae*

17.2 Diagnosis

Learning objectives

You should:

- be aware that the responses to infection will be atypical

- understand the necessity to consult the laboratory to ensure the likely (unusual) pathogens are sought.

The diagnosis of infection in the immunocompromised patient poses a number of problems. The response to infection is, by definition, impaired. This means that the features of infection that depend on a host response may not be present. For example, a neutropenic patient will not develop an accumulation of pus in an abscess, and a patient with impaired cell-mediated immunity may not develop classical granulomas at the site of mycobacterial infection. The iatrogenic compromise caused by glucocorticosteroid treatment can even dampen the febrile response, so that a patient with systemic infection may not develop a fever. Localising the site of focal involvement can therefore be difficult, causing problems with microbiological and biopsy specimen collection. Prior communication with the diagnostic laboratory is necessary to ensure that the full range of expected opportunist pathogens is searched for. Failure to state the nature of the patient's compromised defences can lead to potentially important findings being discarded (along with the specimen) on the grounds that they are of doubtful clinical significance.

17.3 Management

Learning objectives

You should:

- be aware of the greater need for extended or multiagent therapy in the immunocompromised

- understand the techniques used to choose treatment regimens

- be aware of the importance of infection control procedures and the possibility of protective measures before an immunocompromising event.

Chemotherapy

The treatment of infections in the immunocompromised patient presents further problems. While patients with normal host defences may only require a single antibiotic (monotherapy) for a relatively short period, immunocompromised patients rely more heavily on chemotherapy totally to eradicate viable microorganisms. They are therefore more likely to require prolonged treatment with a combination of agents. Moreover, the usual indicators of a favourable response to treatment may be less pronounced. In addition, it is necessary to choose empirical treatment without the results of specific diagnostic tests. One response to these problems has been to develop a standardised approach to chemotherapy, based on the results of multicentre clinical trials. When new antimicrobial agents become available they can be assessed against established agents in a trial programme, and the effect on variables such as post-treatment survival measured. Another approach is to base presumptive chemotherapy on the organisms most commonly encountered in a given group of patients in the centre concerned. In practice, choice of agents is often based on a combination of the two approaches. Some infections cannot be fully eradicated in immunocompromised patients, in which case the patient may benefit from prolonged periods of 'maintenance' chemotherapy.

Prevention

The increased risk of death from infection in immunocompromised patients has led to an interest in preventive measures. Clearly, these will vary with the type of infection. If the source of the infective agent is external to the patient, infection can be prevented either by eradicating the source or by stopping transmission to the patient. Simple infection control procedures, such as putting the patient in a single-bedded side ward or rigorous hand hygiene, take on an even greater importance than usual. When the source is endogenous (e.g. latent infections) this approach is of little use, and chemotherapy is used to prevent disease progression. In some situations, it may even be possible to vaccinate prior to an expected immunocompromising event (e.g. pneumococcal vaccine before splenectomy).

17.4 Common infection problems

Learning objectives

You should:

- know the major infections of immunocompromised patients

- understand the factors contributing to their occurrence

- know the basis of their clinical management.

Infections in the immunocompromised can be considered in four groups based on the cause of failure in the immune system:

- patients with human immunodeficiency virus (HIV) infection
- neutropenic patients with fever
- organ transplant recipients
- splenectomy and sepsis.

Infections in HIV-positive patients

HIV-1 and HIV-2 cause a variety of sequelae, which include an initial acute retroviral disease, polyglandular lymphadenopathy (PGL), the acquired immunodeficiency syndrome (AIDS) and the AIDS-related complex (ARC). HIV is transmitted by sexual contact, the parenteral route and perinatally. There are three major epidemiological patterns recognised in countries throughout the world.

Pattern I (industrialised countries) in which most HIV-positive persons are homosexual, bisexual or intravenous drug abusers

Pattern II (sub-Saharan Africa), where spread is predominantly heterosexual and perinatal

Pattern III (North Africa, Asia, Eastern Europe) where spread has been more recent but rapid.

As we amass more data on the variety of disease attributable to HIV, it has become clear that the formal definitions and staging used for epidemiological purposes have limited use in the management of individual patients. There are important geographical and racial variations in the presentation of disease in HIV-positive persons. The initial acute retroviral disease often goes unnoticed by the patient and even if noted has many of the non-specific features of acute viral infection including fever, adenopathy and a fine maculopapular rash. The main presenting features of HIV-related disease are infection and neoplastic disease. HIV has a tropism for CD4 T (helper subset) lymphocytes, which are required for an effective cell-mediated immune response. Infection of these cells causes a depletion of helper T lymphocytes and a corresponding polyclonal rise in immunoglobulins.

Diagnosis of HIV infection

Diagnosis of HIV infection is by detection of antibodies (enzyme-linked immunosorbent assay; ELISA), and it is confirmed by Western blot for antibodies to viral proteins and glycoproteins. However, in some countries, tests for HIV may only be performed after obtaining the consent of the patient, which can, of course, be refused. Suspicion of HIV-related disease in the first place is usually because of the occurrence of an unusual infection, some of which are so unusual that they are referred to as AIDS-defining illnesses (i.e. diagnosis means that the patient has AIDS). There are other infections that are either more common or have an unusual presentation in HIV-positive persons. It is now recognised that more typical bacterial infections occur with higher than expected frequency during the period between the acute retroviral illness and the onset of AIDS. The risk of infection is in proportion to the extent of T helper cell depletion and probably also to the distortion of the helper to suppressor cell ratio. When the helper cell count falls below to below 200×10^6 cells/l, the patient is at significantly increased risk of an AIDS-defining infection. However, counts higher than this figure do not mean that the patient has no risk of opportunistic infections at all (Fig. 15). Commonly encountered infections include those involving the lungs, the gastrointestinal tract, the skin and the central nervous system.

Immune function in HIV infection

The risk of progressive deterioration of immune function and thus the risk of secondary infections in HIV-positive patients can be reduced by treatment with a combination of antiretroviral agents. These are complex drug regimens and require a high degree of motivation to ensure compliance. An example would be ritonavir plus saquinavir plus zidovudine plus lamivudine.

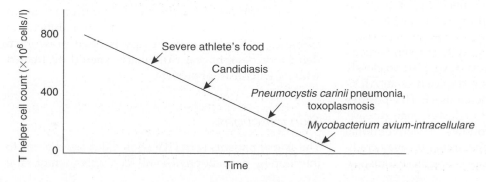

Fig. 15 The risk of severe opportunistic infections increases as the T helper cell count falls in HIV infection.

Pulmonary infection

Pneumocystis carinii pneumonia

The most common initial diagnosis in AIDS is PCP. *P. carinii* is a protozoan parasite (though some believe this organism to be fungal). PCP results in a progressive breathlessness and diffuse bilateral shadowing on chest radiograph. Blood gas analysis provides a useful index of severity. There is no or little sputum production. Diagnostic specimens are therefore obtained either by inducing sputum production with instilled saline or by bronchoscopic bronchoalveolar lavage. *P. carinii* is detected by silver stain or with an immunofluorescent monoclonal antibody stain. Treatment is with either high-dose co-trimoxazole or pentamidine. Prophylaxis for patients with a CD4 T cell count of less than 200×10^6 cells/l or a previous episode of PCP is with co-trimoxazole or aerosolised pentamidine. There is a high incidence of adverse reactions, especially with co-trimoxazole.

Cytomegalovirus

Cytomegalovirus has been associated with a pneumonitis in HIV-positive patients. It is diagnosed by viral culture or nucleic acid amplification. Treatment with ganciclovir or foscarnet is of uncertain benefit. There may be co-infection with both of the above microorganisms.

Atypical mycobacteria

Another group of agents causing pulmonary infection in these patients is the mycobacteria. 'Atypical' mycobacteria, particularly *M. avium* and *M. intracellulare*, can be recovered from the lungs, blood, lymph nodes and faeces of patients with severely depleted CD4 T lymphocytes. These mycobacteria are usually resistant to conventional antituberculous agents and require combinations of conventional and other agents. Maintenance treatment is also required, usually to the end of the patient's life. The advanced state of the patient's immune compromise means that treatment may contribute little to survival.

Tuberculosis

Mycobacterium tuberculosis infection is also more common in HIV-positive patients, because of reactivation of latent infection (e.g. a Ghon focus), and does not require such severe depletion of CD4-lymphocytes for its occurrence. In many developed countries, the incidence of tuberculosis has stopped falling and may even be rising again because of the effect of AIDS. In sub-Saharan Africa, pulmonary tuberculosis and AIDS are so closely interlinked that tuberculosis is recognised as an AIDS-defining illness. Pulmonary tuberculosis in HIV-positive patients is more often diffuse or lower zone disease. Diagnosis and treatment follows a conventional approach, and a full course of chemotherapy may eradicate infection. Since tuberculosis is the most transmissible AIDS-related infection, additional respiratory infection control precautions should be practised for all patients requiring hospital admission. Prophylactic administration of isoniazid (for 12 months) to newly recognised HIV-positive persons has been successful in preventing subsequent tuberculosis.

Gastrointestinal tract infection

Infective diarrhoea

The gastrointestinal tract is another important site of infection in HIV-positive patients. Diarrhoea lasting longer than 4 weeks, accompanied by a weight loss of 10% body mass is regarded as an AIDS-defining illness. In Africa, this is very common and is referred to as 'slim'. The high incidence of slim is probably a reflection of the prevalence of gastrointestinal infections in these countries.

One of the common causes of HIV-related diarrhoea is the sporozoan parasite *Cryptosporidium muris*. The diarrhoea is profuse and watery and can resemble that in cholera. Diagnosis is by microscopy of faeces treated with a modified version of the Ziehl–Neelsen stain. There is no effective antimicrobial chemotherapy.

Other parasites, e.g. microsporidia and *Isospora belli*, bacteria such as *Salmonella* spp. and *M. avium* and *M. intracellulare*, and viruses including cytomegalovirus, may also cause diarrhoea. A cause is found in only approximately 50% of patients. Unlike cryptosporidiosis, isosporiasis may benefit from treatment with co-trimoxazole. Salmonella infection is more likely to result in invasive disease and should therefore be treated more aggressively than in immunocompetent individuals. There is some evidence for an AIDS enteropathy, which is thought to be caused by HIV itself.

Candidiasis

Candidiasis is common at the other end of the gastrointestinal tract. In fact, candidiasis in the oesophagus occurring in the absence of another form of immune compromise or antibiotic treatment should raise suspicion of HIV-related illness. The presenting symptoms are dysphagia and retrosternal pain. Diagnosis is by microscopy of a potassium hydroxide or Gram-stained preparation of white plaque scraped from the affected mucosa. Treatment is with an oral antifungal agent (e.g. nystatin, miconazole). The condition is difficult to eradicate and continuous therapy is often prescribed. Refractory oesophageal candidiasis should be treated with parenteral amphotericin.

Skin infections

The skin of patients with HIV-related disease is prone to infection by dermatophytes and to reactivation of viral infection. Severe athlete's foot and shingles may be seen in these patients. If the patient has not already been diagnosed as HIV positive, the unusually severe presentation of these infections may make them difficult to recognise. Scrapings for microscopy, culture or biopsy should be collected if there is any doubt.

Central nervous system infections

Infections of the central nervous system and eyes are less common in HIV-positive patients but when they do occur, can cause serious neurological or visual damage.

Toxoplasmosis

The most common focal intracranial lesion in patients with HIV-related disease is caused by *Toxoplasma gondii*, a protozoan parasite that causes a mild influenza-like illness with lymphadenopathy in immunocompetent adults. In HIV-positive persons, infection is caused by reactivation and results in multiple abscesses in the brain. These can cause epileptic seizures and focal neurological signs. Diagnosis is supported by computed tomographic or magnetic resonance scan. Serological investigations are not diagnostic but absence of detectable anti-toxoplasma IgG suggests an alternative aetiology. Treatment is with sulfadiazine and pyrimethamine.

Cryptococcosis

The yeast *Cryptococcus neoformans* causes meningitis in HIV-positive patients that can be diagnosed by examination of cerebrospinal fluid (CSF). Microscopy of an India ink preparation or latex agglutination can produce a rapid diagnosis. The yeast can also be cultured from CSF. Treatment with amphotericin and flucytosine has been only moderately successful. Alternative antifungal agents such as fluconazole have been tried.

HIV encephalopathy

HIV is neurotrophic and can cause an encephalopathy by itself. This is a diffuse process that results in impaired motor function and dementia. Magnetic resonance imaging may show cerebral atrophy, but CSF findings are non-specific. There is no effective specific treatment.

Cytomegalovirus

Cytomegalovirus causes an encephalitis that can progress rapidly and a progressive haemorrhagic retinitis, which can permanently impair vision or cause total blindness. The diagnosis of retinitis is mainly on fundoscopic appearance. Treatment of both conditions is with ganciclovir or foscarnet.

Neutropenic patients with fever

Whether caused by primary disease (e.g. acute leukaemia) or treatment (cytotoxic therapy), neutropenia puts the patient at increased risk of bacterial and yeast infection. The risk of infection increases with a decreasing neutrophil count, so relative neutropenia is less risky than absolute neutropenia.

Diagnosis

Fever in a neutropenic patient should lead to a thorough review, looking for signs of:

- pneumonia
- urinary tract infection
- skin sepsis (particularly around intravascular catheter insertion sites)
- oral and perianal infection
- septicaemia.

It should be remembered that as collections of neutrophils are unlikely to form, signs of focal inflammation may be absent. The organisms most often implicated are bacteria and yeasts which often originate from the patient's gastrointestinal tract. Thus Gram-negative bacilli including Enterobacteriaceae, *Pseudomonas aeruginosa*, *Stenotrophomonas maltophilia*, enterococci and *C. albicans* are often isolated from blood cultures in these patients. Infections associated with intravascular catheters are more often caused by skin bacteria such as *Staphylococcus aureus*, coagulase negative staphylococci and coryneform bacteria (such as *Corynebacterium jeikeium*). The increasing use of indwelling intravenous cannulas (Hickman) for delivery of cytotoxic chemotherapy has led to an increase in infections in neutropenic patients at the insertion site, along the catheter tunnel or at the tip. Each of these may give rise to septicaemia. Bacterial or yeast infections can be confirmed by culture of the infecting agent.

Treatment

The impaired defences against infection cause a more rapid deterioration in the patient's condition; it is therefore important to commence empirical antimicrobial chemotherapy as quickly as possible after collecting diagnostic specimens. A standard antimicrobial protocol would begin with an aminoglycoside and a β-lactam effective against *Pseudomonas* spp. (e.g. gentamicin and piperacillin). If the patient has a cannula-related infection, an antistaphylococcal agent such as flucloxacillin would be chosen to start with. Failure to respond to initial empirical therapy should result in a review of preliminary laboratory results and ward charts. Antimicrobial resistance (either intrinsic or acquired) is common in organisms isolated from this group of patients. Antifungal therapy should be considered if there is no response to empirical therapy within 48 hours of onset of fever.

As yet, there is no completely successful means of preventing infection in the neutropenic patient. In fact, as chemotherapy regimens for treating leukaemia become more aggressive, infection has become a common cause of death and major morbidity during treatment. However, some precautions can substantially reduce the risk of infection. Patients should avoid contact with visitors and staff who have known infections. They should also avoid food liable to contamination with large numbers of bacteria, e.g. fresh fruit, raw vegetables, salads, cook-chilled foods and soft cheeses. They can benefit from being nursed in a single-bedded side ward with air under positive pressure, but there is little additional benefit from laminar flow beds and rigorously enforced protective isolation. Some centres use oral antibiotic prophylaxis, though the preventive benefit has been marginal in some trials and there is a risk of promoting antibiotic resistance. It may be possible to reduce the patient's degree of compromise in some cases by stimulating neutrophil production with granulocyte-macrophage colony-stimulating factor.

Infection in organ transplant recipients

Solid organ transplants are becoming more common. Although renal, cardiac and hepatic allografts would appear to be very different procedures, they result in a similar pattern of transplant-related infection. The reason for this apparent paradox is that the risk of infection is largely the result of immunosuppressive treatment given to prevent graft-versus-host disease. This treatment is in principle standardised for all solid organ transplants. Ciclosporin, glucocorticosteroids and anti-lymphocyte globulin combine to produce a comprehensive, broad-spectrum immune compromise. The risk of infection increases with the extent and duration of compromise; consequently, infections can be related to the time of organ transplant.

During the first month. Bacterial and nosocomial infections predominate. These are infections that were incubating at the time of transplant, infected the allograft or infected the blood transfusion (hepatitis C).

Between 1 and 6 months post-transplant. There is a risk of infection with members of the herpes virus group (particularly cytomegalovirus), *M. tuberculosis*, *T. gondii* and *P. carinii*, all of which reflect deficient cell-mediated immunity.

After 6 months. The patient is at increased risk of mainly community-acquired infections.

Management

Management of infection during the first 6 months post-transplant requires accurate aetiological diagnosis and aggressive treatment. The response is particularly poor if there is continuing graft-versus-host disease. Prevention is by careful screening of the patient and donor prior to transplant. Cytomegalovirus status of donor, recipient and blood for transfusion during the operation are of particular concern. PCP can be prevented by administration of prophylactic co-trimoxazole.

Splenectomy and sepsis

Patients may lose their spleen through abdominal trauma or elective surgery; they may also become functionally asplenic through various diseases. Loss of splenic function puts them at risk of infection with capsulated bacteria (particularly *Streptococcus pneumoniae*, *Haemophilus influenzae* and *Neisseria meningitidis*). The greatest risk is in children, patients with malignant disease and in the 2 years following splenectomy.

Since the most common cause of infection in *S. pneumoniae*, vaccination (preferably more than 2 weeks prior to elective splenectomy) with the 23-valent vaccine has been used to prevent ensuing septicaemia, peritonitis and other severe pneumococcal infections. Long-term prophylaxis with penicillin has been employed, but there is some doubt as to its efficacy, especially where vaccination has already been given. Patients should be advised that they are at increased risk of infection and should seek medical advice quickly during any febrile illness.

17.5 Organisms

A checklist of the organisms discussed in this chapter is given in Box 12. Further information is given on the pages indicated.

Box 12 Organisms involved in infections of the immunocompromised

Bacteria	see page
Streptococcus pneumoniae	245
Mycobacterium tuberculosis	253–4
Mycobacterium avium and *M intracellulare*	254
Salmonella spp.	248–9
Enterobacteriaceae	248–9
Pseudomonas aeruginosa	249–50
Stenotrophomonas maltophilia	250
Enterococcus spp.	245
Staphylococcus aureus	243
Coagulase-negative staphylococci	243
Corynebacterium jeikeium	247
Haemophilus influenzae	251
Neisseria meningitidis	252–3

Viruses	
Human immunodeficiency virus 1 and 2	260
Cytomegalovirus	257
Varicella-zoster virus	257
Hepatitis C virus	–

Fungi	see page
Candida albicans	269
Dermatophytic fungi	269–70
Cryptococcus neoformans	269

Parasites	
Pneumocystis carinii	264
Cryptosporidium sp.	264
Microsporidia	264
Isospora belli	264
Toxoplasma gondii	263–4

Self-assessment: questions

Multiple choice questions

1. The following strategies might be used to prevent endogenous infection in an immunocompromised patient:
   a. Prophylactic chemotherapy
   b. Rigorous hand washing
   c. Minimising the use of invasive procedures
   d. Protective isolation
   e. Pre-exposure vaccination

2. The human immunodeficiency virus (HIV) may cause:
   a. An acute viral syndrome
   b. Polyglandular lymphadenopathy
   c. AIDS-related complex (ARC)
   d. AIDS (acquired immunodeficiency syndrome)
   e. Asymptomatic infection

3. AIDS-defining illnesses include:
   a. Pulmonary tuberculosis
   b. Diarrhoea
   c. Dementia
   d. *Pneumocystis carinii* pneumonia
   e. Oral candidiasis

4. Increased susceptibility to infections in AIDS results from:
   a. Impaired defences against mainly bacterial infection
   b. Reduced neutrophil production
   c. Reduced helper T lymphocytes
   d. Increased sensitivity to microbial toxins
   e. Decreased IgG production

5. In HIV-positive persons, pneumonia can be caused by the following:
   a. *Pneumocystis carinii*
   b. *Toxoplasma gondii*
   c. Cytomegalovirus
   d. *Mycobacterium tuberculosis*
   e. *Streptococcus pneumoniae*

6. Diarrhoea in HIV-positive persons:
   a. May be caused by no specific microbial agent
   b. Can result in severe wasting
   c. Caused by *Cryptosporidium* sp. should be treated with antibiotics
   d. Caused by *Isospora belli* cannot be treated with antibiotics
   e. Caused by *Salmonella* spp. can result in invasive infection

7. In neutropenic patients, infections:
   a. Are mainly caused by fungi
   b. Are often caused by bacteria from the gastrointestinal tract
   c. Associated with intravascular cannulas cause fever
   d. Should be treated initially with a single intravenous antibiotic
   e. Causing fever lasting longer than 48 hours are often caused by fungi

8. Postsplenectomy sepsis:
   a. Is usually within 2 years of splenectomy
   b. Is more common in adults following abdominal trauma
   c. Can best be prevented by long-term antibiotic prophylaxis
   d. Is caused most often by *Haemophilus influenzae*
   e. Can be prevented by vaccination at the time of splenectomy

Case history questions

History 1

A 23-year-old African truck driver is brought in by relatives, severely wasted and with a prolonged history of profuse watery diarrhoea. He has a non-productive cough and is afebrile.

1. What infections is he likely to have?
2. How would you investigate his diarrhoea?
3. Is there any treatment you can offer?
4. What is the significance of his occupation?

History 2

A 28-year-old woman with acute myeloid leukaemia undergoing induction chemotherapy for her disease had just reached the threshold for absolute neutropenia when she developed a fever. Careful physical examination and chest radiograph revealed no obvious focus of infection. Midstream urine specimen and blood cultures were collected and she was commenced on intravenous gentamicin and piperacillin. After 24 hours, she remained febrile despite antibiotic treatment.

1. What site(s) of infection has yet to be excluded?
2. How could a specific aetiological diagnosis be achieved?
3. What are the most likely organisms to cause this infection?
4. Outline what presumptive antimicrobial chemotherapy should now be given

Data interpretation

A 44-year-old leukaemic man developed a fever peaking at 38°C 10 days into a course of chemotherapy. Neutrophil count was $200 \times 10^6/l$ (normal range, $3000-11\,000 \times 10^6/l$). C-reactive protein was 55 mmol/l (normal range, 0–10). Peripheral venous blood cultures were negative after incubation for 48 hours. One blood culture collected via the Hickmann line yielded coagulase-negative staphylococci in one of the two bottles after 48 hours. The patient was treated with intravenous ticarcillin/clavulanic acid combination, gentamicin and vancomycin shortly after collection of blood cultures but still has an intermittent fever.

1. Do the results of culture explain the failure of therapy?
2. What further laboratory investigations would you organise now?
3. What would be your next choice of antimicrobial agent?
4. How does the neutrophil count relate to this infection?
5. Why are blood cultures collected via the Hickmann line and a peripheral vein?

Objective structured clinical examination (OSCE)

A single 32-year-old man has attended the clinic for the fourth time in as many months with the same complaint: a watery diarrhoea. On his first and second visits, the stool specimen he provided was fluid and contained *Cryptosporidium* sp. oocysts. On the third occasion he had not improved but he declined further investigation of his illness. You are asked the following

1. Is diarrhoea caused by *Cryptosporidium* sp. usually self-limiting? How long would you expect it to last?
2. Could this presentation herald the onset of HIV infection?
3. Is there any suitable specific antiparasite therapy?
4. Is there any useful therapy that you can offer this patient?
5. Would most other intestinal parasitic infections respond to specific therapy equally badly in this type of clinical setting?

Short notes questions

Write short notes on the following:

1. Diagnosis of infection in immunocompromised patients
2. Central nervous system infections in HIV-positive patients
3. Infections following solid organ transplant

Viva question

What are the key determinants of infection in immunocompromised patients?

Self-assessment: answers

Multiple choice answers

1. a. **True.**
   b. **True.** Hand washing helps to prevent exogenous infections.
   c. **True.** Invasive procedures like vascular cannulation provide a portal of entry for organisms in the indigenous flora.
   d. **True.** Isolation helps to prevent exogenous infections.
   e. **True.** Vaccination helps to prevent exogenous infections.

2. a. **True.** This occurs in the period immediately after infection and often goes unnoticed.
   b. **True.** As a consequence of the changes in CD4 T cells.
   c. **True.** This is a combination of intermittent fever, weight loss, diarrhoea, fatigue and night sweats.
   d. **True.** Time from infection to the development of AIDS varies and can be extended with antiretroviral drugs.
   e. **True.** Many patients are unaware of the initial acute viral syndrome and are only identified when they develop an AIDS-defining illness.

3. a. **True.** Tuberculosis is an AIDS-defining illness in sub-Saharan Africa.
   b. **False.** Only diarrhoea lasting longer than 4 weeks and accompanied by wasting of more than 10% body mass counts as an AIDS-defining illness.
   c. **False.** Dementia is a feature of AIDS encephalopathy but by itself is not specific to AIDS.
   d. **True.** This is the most common initial diagnosis in AIDS.
   e. **False.** To be an AIDS-defining illness, candidiasis must be oesophageal and in the absence of other immunosuppression or antibiotic therapy.

4. a. **False.** Defences are impaired against viruses, yeasts and intracellular bacteria.
   b. **False.** Falling CD4 T cells occurs.
   c. **True.** The primary defect in host defences caused by HIV infection is a reduction in T helper subset (CD4) lymphocytes.
   d. **False.** There is no change in sensitivity to toxins although HIV-positive individuals may be more prone to infections including with toxin-producing organisms.
   e. **True.** In advanced disease, there is impairment in IgG production.

5. a. **True.** This is the most common AIDS-defining illness.
   b. **False.** *T. gondii* does not cause a pneumonia.
   c. **True.** It causes a pneumonitis.
   d. **True.** Reactivation of latent infection may occur; tuberculosis is an AIDS-defining illness in sub-Saharan Africa.
   e. **True.** *S. pneumoniae* causes pneumonia more commonly than in HIV-negative people even before the CD4 cell count has fallen below 200×10^6 cells/l.

6. a. **True.** It is a component of the AIDS-related complex (ARC).
   b. **True.** It is only considered as AIDS-defining if accompanied by wasting of more than 10% of body mass.
   c. **False.** There is no effective antimicrobial treatment for cryptosporidiosis in HIV-positive individuals.
   d. **False.** *Isospora belli* infection can be treated successfully with co-trimoxazole.
   e. **True.** This is more common than in immunocompetent individuals.

7. a. **False.** Although fungi may cause infection in the febrile neutropenic patient, bacteria are more common.
   b. **True.** This is the most common source.
   c. **True.** Sepsis is common around cannulas and leads to fever.
   d. **False.** Empirical treatment of the febrile neutropenic patient usually requires at least two agents to start with, e.g. aminoglycoside and an anti-pseudomonal β-lactam antibiotic.
   e. **True.** Initial empirical therapy is usually not antifungal.

8. a. **True.** This is the period of greatest risk.
   b. **False.** Postsplenectomy sepsis is more common in children and following malignant disease.
   c. **False.** Antibiotic prophylaxis (e.g. with long-term oral penicillin) is of unproved benefit, especially after vaccination.
   d. **False.** The single most common organism causing infection is *Streptococcus pneumoniae*.
   e. **True.** Vaccination is best given 2 weeks before splenectomy but still has some benefit if given at the time of operation.

Case history answers

History 1

1. 'Slim', possibly pulmonary tuberculosis or even *Pneumocystis carinii* pneumonia; underlying all this, HIV infection.
2. Microscopy, for parasites, modified Ziehl–Neelsen stain for cryptosporidia, ordinary Ziehl–Neelsen stain for *Mycobacterium avium* and *M. intracellulare*, plain smear for *Isospora belli* and if available electron microscopy for microsporidia. The stool should also be cultured for bacterial pathogens, particularly *Salmonella* spp.
3. Yes; co-trimoxazole for isosporiasis and an appropriate antibiotic (e.g. a quinolone) for invasive salmonellosis, subject to results of laboratory tests.
4. In Africa, truck drivers have been an important means of transmitting HIV infection via prostitutes along the main trucking routes.

History 2

1. Intravascular cannulas (e.g. peripheral and central veins), the mouth and the anal margin. Of these, intravascular cannulas are probably the most common. Another explanation might be systemic infection with an antibiotic-resistant bacterium or a yeast, e.g. *Candida albicans*.
2. Culture from the relevant site. Repeat blood culture is worth performing, despite the antibiotic treatment. This should be done via the vascular cannula and via a peripheral vein at about the same time so that comparison of results will help to distinguish skin contaminants from cannula infection-associated bacteraemia.
3. Coagulase-negative staphylococci, *Staphylococcus aureus* and coryneform bacteria (e.g. *Corynebacterium jeikeium*); also Gram-negative bacilli and yeasts such as *Candida albicans* are possibilities.
4. An agent effective against Gram-positive bacteria, probably vancomycin is the preferred choice, possibly with a change of Gram-negative antibiotic (e.g. a quinolone such as ciprofloxacin). If there is no response within a further 24 hours, addition of systemic antifungal therapy should be considered.

Data interpretation answer

1. No. They raise more questions than answers. The coagulase-negative staphylococci could be incidental contamination of the blood culture with skin flora during specimen collection, or it could be a clinically significant result.

2. Repeat the blood cultures during a febrile episode, collect bacteriological specimens from any site of possible focal infection (e.g. urine) and repeat the C-reactive protein to see whether the inflammatory marker has been trending up or down while on therapy.
3. Addition of an antifungal agent, because a proportion of febrile episodes in these patients may be caused by culture-negative fungaemia.
4. The neutropenia, whether caused by the leukaemia or the chemotherapy, is a key compromise in the patient's defences against infection. The risk of bacteraemic infection is roughly proportionate to the extent of neutropenia.
5. Hickmann lines are an important site of device-related infection. Paired blood cultures will help to establish whether the cannula is colonised by bacteria (and therefore a potential source of bloodstream infection) or there is detectable peripheral bacteraemia.

OSCE answer

1. Yes. It usually lasts 2–6 weeks.
2. Yes. This is a common cause of diarrhoea in HIV-positive individuals.
3. No. Many compounds have been tried but so far none has been found to have any convincing or lasting benefit.
4. Yes. The patient will need fluid and electrolyte replacement. Improvement of cellular immunity by radical antiretroviral therapy may help to increase mucosal defences.
5. No. There are effective therapies against most other intestinal parasites even when the patient has moderately impaired cellular immunity.

Short notes answers

1. Remember the altered clinical presentation of infectious diseases, the wider range of potential pathogens and the need for rapid results. Examples required for this answer.
2. Epidemiology, presenting features, diagnosis and treatment where applicable in each of cryptococcal meningitis, cytomegalovirus encephalitis, AIDS encephalopathy, cerebral toxoplasmosis (there is a list of less-commonly encountered agents in specialist texts).
3. Emphasise the relationship between time of transplant and onset of infection. It is possible to answer this in a tabular form.

Viva answer

The nature and extent of the defect in host defences. Give examples to illustrate your points. HIV is probably the best to use now that so much is known about the inter-relationship of disease progression and secondary opportunistic infection.

18 Infection in international travellers

Overview

The dramatic increase in international travel in recent years has brought with it a corresponding increase in travel-related infections, particularly in those who travel from temperate to tropical climates. Most of the infections acquired by international travellers belong to a relatively small group of diseases, the risk of which can be reduced by simple preventive precautions before and during travel. Despite this, many people travel abroad without even basic travel health advice. Moreover, travel health recommendations from medical sources are often dangerously inaccurate.

18.1 Pathogenesis

Learning objective

You should:

- know the factors increasing risk of infection in travellers.

Whatever the principal reason for travelling, whether for business or pleasure, the international traveller is exposed to sources of microorganisms not experienced in the home environment. Differences in climate, accommodation, diet and behaviour all contribute to an increased risk of infection. A warmer climate means a greater variety of insect life (some of which may be important disease vectors) and faster deterioration of food. Sewage disposal is inadequate in many popular international destinations; consequently water and uncooked foods become a common source of infection. Local customs can also play a role in exposure to infection. For instance, personal hygiene practices may be very different, or rules of hospitality may demand consumption of a high-risk food. The degree of exposure determines the probability of infection, so overland trekkers may be at very high risk of a variety of infections. However, staying in a five star hotel does not guarantee freedom from gastrointestinal or insect-borne infections. It is perhaps surprising that international travellers suffer from the more exotic parasitic tropical infections relatively rarely. The most common infections they contract during their travels are gastrointestinal, vaccine preventable or malaria.

18.2 Diagnosis

Learning objectives

You should:

- be aware of the importance of a travel history in the last year

- know the approach required for diagnosis in patients with diarrhoea and with fever.

A history of recent travel (up to a year ago in some cases) should be sought in the investigation of any infectious disease. Although the fact that the patient has travelled abroad is probably the single most important piece of information, the destination, duration of stay and details of accommodation, diet and daily activities are also valuable. It is essential to make tactful enquiries about sexual activity abroad if a sexually transmitted disease is a possibility.

The two most common problems encountered in returning travellers are diarrhoea and fever. The investigation of diarrhoea is reviewed below and discussed in more detail in Chapter 9. It is safest to assume that fever in someone who has just returned from the tropics is most likely to be malaria until proved otherwise. The mortality from travel-related infections is greater in countries that have relatively little experience of diseases such as malaria. The long list of possible causes of fever in someone just returned from the tropics dictates a comprehensive diagnostic work-up for fever of unknown origin. Remember that these patients can also contract infections seen in temperate countries while overseas.

18.3 Prevention

Learning objectives

You should:

- know the basic pretravel counselling

- be aware of the dangers of change in sexual behaviour

- know the vaccination recommendations for major destinations.

The majority of people travelling abroad for business, pleasure and other reasons do not take adequate advice about maintaining health while travelling. Only a small minority make use of facilities such as travel medicine or vaccination clinics. Moreover, the advice given to prospective international travellers by doctors, nurses, pharmacists and other health-care workers is often inaccurate; sometimes dangerously so.

The first step in preventing travel-related infections is to persuade prospective travellers to assess the potential risks of travel. This is particularly important if they are embarking on a particular type of travel for the first time. Their risks can be assessed on a rule-of-thumb basis from the changes they are likely to experience in climate, accommodation, diet and behaviour. If there is little difference between current and destination lifestyle, there is little to be gained from elaborate health precautions. However, expected differences on all four points would be a good reason to seek detailed professional advice.

Pretravel counselling has become increasingly popular in recent years. Much of the advice given by doctors relates to simple precautions against diarrhoea and malaria, and the need for specific vaccinations. It may be awkward to raise the issue of sexual behaviour in this setting, but the growing importance of human immunodeficiency virus (HIV) infection in popular travel destinations, combined with the greater promiscuity of many adult travellers, makes this a priority issue for preventive counselling. Although advice has to be tailored to the needs of each individual, it is helpful to give the traveller a written summary of key points to act as an *aide memoire*. Some countries publish a general guide to travel health and make this available through travel or ticketing agencies.

International travellers should make sure that their routine vaccinations are kept up to date. This includes diphtheria (now prevalent in the former Soviet Union), tetanus, and polio (prevalent in some developing countries). Yellow fever vaccination is required for entry to many countries in tropical Africa and South America, supported by a vaccination certificate. Most other vaccinations are not mandatory, but the possibility of exposure to infection makes vaccination a preferable alternative. The advisability of vaccination may be marginal in some cases. Many of these additional vaccinations require more than one inoculation, so that a vaccination programme needs planning weeks to months before the date of travel. However, persons who have to travel at short notice are usually better to leave with the partial protection of an incomplete course, than to leave with no vaccine-based protection at all.

18.4 Diseases and syndromes

Learning objectives

You should:

- know the major infections of international travellers

- know the factors contributing to their occurrence

- understand the basis of their clinical management.

The infections most often encountered in international travellers are listed in Table 32 and the precautions that can be taken to prevent them in Table 33.

Diarrhoea

Up to 50% of people travelling from temperate climates to the tropics develop diarrhoea. In the majority of these cases the period of acute, watery diarrhoea lasts for 2 to 5 days and is a self-limiting process. Enterotoxigenic *Escherichia coli* is the cause in up to 70% of cases. The remainder of acute diarrhoeas are caused by rotavirus, adenoviruses, salmonellas, shigellas, campylobacters and other organisms. The short-lived nature of most cases means that medical assistance is often not sought, so the cause often goes undiagnosed. Treatment is usually limited to oral replacement of fluids and electrolytes. Bismuth subsalicylate and an antimotility agent (e.g. loperamide) may provide some symptomatic relief in more severe cases.

The most common reasons for seeking medical attention for traveller's diarrhoea are prolonged symptoms, the presence of blood or pus in the stools or the

Table 32 Infections associated with international travel

Infection	Features
Diarrhoea	Usually an acute, watery diarrhoea lasting 2–5 days; can be prolonged, with blood or pus in stools and accompanied by fever
Malaria	Intermittent bouts of fever, shivering and sweating
Enteric fever	Fever, headache, chest pain, constipation; sometimes small pink macules ('rose spots'); erosion of the gut can cause ulceration and haemorrhage
Hepatitis A	Fever, sickness, jaundice, dark urine, abdominal pain
Hepatitis B	Uncommon: headache, fever, chills, weakness, jaundice
Yellow fever	Short-lived fever, headache; can be followed by jaundice, bleeding, renal failure
Rabies	Fatal encephalitis; initial paraesthesiae at site of bite, hydrophobia, muscle spasms
Japanese encephalitis	Mostly mild; a few develop fever, meningeal irritation, cerebral dysfunction (25% of these die)
Human immunodeficiency virus	In many countries HIV is prevalent and associated with heterosexual sex
Sexually transmitted diseases	Travellers changing to risky sexual behaviour can become infected

Table 33 Travel-associated infections and precautions

Infection risk	Precautions
Diarrhoea	Safe water, no ice, cooked food, only self-peeled fruit, pack oral rehydration salts
Malaria	Stay inside at dawn and dusk, cover arms and legs, bednet at night, insect repellent, appropriate antimalarial prophylaxis
Enteric fever	Typhoid vaccine
Infectious hepatitis	Hepatitis A vaccine
Yellow fever	Vaccine, avoid exposure to mosquitoes
Japanese encephalitis	Vaccine if high risk, avoid exposure to mosquitoes
Rabies	Pre-exposure vaccine if high risk; if bitten, postexposure vaccine, wound toilet
Human immunodeficiency virus, other sexually transmitted diseases	Avoid promiscuous intercourse, condoms provide some protection

development of a fever. Prolonged diarrhoea in travellers is most often caused by disaccharidase deficiency following an initial microbial insult to the small intestinal mucosa. This will resolve in time but may take up to several months before normal function is restored. Less commonly, prolonged diarrhoea may be caused by *Giardia lamblia* infection, or by tropical sprue. Opinion is divided on whether to treat all cases presumptively with metronidazole or to investigate first with microscopy of stools for giardia cysts, stool pH and if necessary intestinal function tests. The appearance of blood or pus in stools from a patient with pain on defaecation suggests a diagnosis of dysentery. Specimens should be collected for bacterial culture, looking for *Shigella* spp., and a warm stool specimen should be sent for immediate microscopy for trophozoites of *Entamoeba histolytica*. Amoebic dysentery is common in many developing countries, but the patient need not have travelled outside Western Europe or strayed out of a five star hotel to be exposed to infection with this organism. Treatment of bacillary dysentery is with trimethoprim in the first instance, but antibiotic resistance may necessitate a change of therapy when susceptibility results are known. Amoebic dysentery is treated with metronidazole. Patients with diarrhoea and fever need a blood culture and systemic antimicrobial therapy. They may have

enteric fever (see below), although typhoid does not usually present with diarrhoea in the early stages of disease.

The risk of enteric infection can be reduced by careful selection of food and drink. Tap water, ice and diluted drinks should be avoided, even for brushing teeth. Bottled water is not always safe. Milk should be pasteurised and goats' milk should be avoided. Fresh vegetables, fruits and salads should also be avoided. Only fruit that can be peeled immediately before consumption is safe. Care should be taken to avoid seafood, particularly shellfish, which are highly efficient at filtering enteric pathogens from sewage-contaminated water. The safest foods are the dishes that are served piping hot immediately after they have been cooked. Antibiotic prophylaxis is not recommended.

Malaria

Malaria is characterised by intermittent bouts of fever, shivering and profuse sweating. It is caused by sporozoan parasites of the genus *Plasmodium*, which are transmitted to humans by the bite of an anophelene mosquito (see also Ch. 15).

The incubation period for malaria varies from 2 days to several months (some cases have been reported after a year or more of last possible exposure). Cases of malaria have been climbing steadily in countries where the disease is not endemic because of the increasing volume of international travel. Many travellers embark on their journeys with little or no knowledge of the precautions they should take. Moreover, air travel enables a traveller to return home before the end of the incubation period. As a result, the traveller is likely to seek assistance from a physician who has had relatively little experience in the diagnosis of malaria.

Diagnosis

The single most important diagnostic issue in malaria is making the distinction between an infection caused by *Plasmodium falciparum* and one caused by the other three *Plasmodium* species, since *P. falciparum* causes the majority of fatal infections. Severe complications of infection include:

- coma caused by cerebral malaria
- severe haemolysis
- renal failure (blackwater fever).

This species is also more likely than the other three to be resistant to chloroquine.

Diagnosis is made by examining a Giemsa stain of peripheral blood. Both thick and thin blood films should be examined, and they should be repeated on at least a second occasion to avoid missing the diagnosis through the cyclical nature of the parasitaemia.

Treatment

Treatment is with chloroquine, unless chloroquine resistance is suspected, in which case quinine should be used or possibly atovaquone-proquanil. Infection with *P. vivax* or *P. ovale* should also be treated with primaquine (except in those with glucose 6-phosphate deficiency) to avoid late recurrence caused by the hypnozoite forms.

Control

Prevention of malaria is by a combination of personal precautions aimed at reducing exposure to malaria-carrying mosquitoes (long sleeves, trousers, staying inside after dusk, insect repellent and mosquito netting over beds) and chemoprophylaxis. Unfortunately the rapid spread of chloroquine-resistant *P. falciparum* and the occurrence of resistance to other agents has made the choice of chemoprophylaxis very complex. Expert advice should be sought, since the epidemiology of resistance is changing. Travellers should be advised that they will gain maximum benefit from malaria prophylaxis by starting 1 week prior to departure and continuing for 4 weeks after their return. Although chemoprophylaxis is advisable for anyone travelling to an endemic area, it does not give 100% protection. Fever occurring after return should be assumed to be malaria until proved otherwise.

Enteric fever

Enteric fever refers to typhoid and related infections. These are febrile systemic infections caused by *Salmonella typhi* or *paratyphi*. Although the infection is acquired by ingestion, and the causal agent is *S. typhi* or *S. paratyphi*, the early stages of disease are typified by systemic and constitutional symptoms rather than diarrhoea.

Diagnosis

The incubation period is up to around 10 days and is followed by fever, headache, chest pain, constipation and, in some cases small pink macules called 'rose spots'. At this stage, stool culture may be negative for the causal pathogen, but the majority of patients will have a positive blood culture. The organism can also be isolated by needle aspiration of bone marrow or even from the rose spots. In the small intestine, *S. typhi* invades the gut-associated lymphoid tissue, which may ulcerate or even cause intestinal perforation. Stool cultures become positive later in the disease in most cases. A small proportion of those affected become chronic carriers when *S. typhi* settles in the gall bladder.

Laboratory confirmation of the diagnosis is by culture of blood, stool or needle aspirate. This organism is a non-lactose fermenter, but unlike other salmonellas, *S. typhi* may be O-antigen negative on initial testing because of the masking effect of the Vi (virulence) antigen. This may cause a delay in the definitive identification of blood culture isolates.

Control

The patient needs to be treated in hospital and may require additional infection control precautions. Treatment is with chloramphenicol or ampicillin intravenously. Increasing antibiotic resistance in some regions has necessitated the use of alternatives such as ciprofloxacin. The aminoglycosides and cephalosporins are unsuitable for treatment of enteric fever despite apparent susceptibility results on disk diffusion testing.

The only reservoir of infection by *S. typhi* or *S. paratyphi* is the human population, particularly asymptomatic and convalescent carriers. Once identified, these people should be excluded from handling food until consistently clear of *S. typhi*, as documented by repeated stool culture. A very small percentage remain persistent carriers despite prolonged antibiotic treatment, often because of the presence of gallstones. Cholecystectomy may resolve the problem.

Overseas travellers can reduce the risk of typhoid by pretravel vaccination with either several doses of a live attenuated oral strain (Ty21a) or intramuscular purified killed typhoid vaccine. The protective effect is around 50–70% and lasts up to 5 years. Vaccine against *S. paratyphi* A and B is ineffective.

Hepatitis

Hepatitis is discussed in greater detail in Chapter 9. Travellers are at risk of infective hepatitis in many developing countries, especially if they consume shellfish and uncooked seafood. Careful choice of food and drink can help to reduce the risk, but a killed virus vaccine is now available for adults and is a worthwhile precaution for those who have not already had hepatitis A. In Asia, hepatitis B is endemic. Those intending to stay for a prolonged period may benefit from pretravel vaccination with killed virus vaccine or gammaglobulin.

Yellow fever

The condition known as yellow fever is endemic throughout tropical parts of Africa and South America. Infection is transmitted by mosquito bite. In the urban setting, the main vector species is *Aedes aegypti*, but in rural and jungle settings a variety of non-anophelene species can act as vectors.

Diagnosis

Infection results in a spectrum of clinical disease, from a short-lived fever and headache to the less common but more severe biphasic disease. In this latter form, the initial viraemic stage is followed by an afebrile period. The patient then becomes jaundiced, prone to bleeding and may develop renal failure. Up to half those with the severe form die.

The diagnosis should be considered in all persons with fever and jaundice who have returned from tropical Africa or America. The virus can be isolated from serum during the initial stage of the disease. IgM antibodies are detectable within a week of onset of disease. A variety of serological methods have been used to detect antibodies. Anicteric disease does occur and may be confused with other viral haemorrhagic fevers such as Lassa, Ebola and Marburg fevers. Patients with yellow fever should be kept away from mosquitoes under mosquito netting.

Control

Prevention is by avoiding contact with biting mosquitoes and by vaccination with a live attenuated virus strain. The vaccine is highly effective and protection lasts for at least 10 years. Vaccination is regulated by the World Health Organization and is a statutory requirement for travellers entering certain countries.

Rabies

Rabies is a uniformly fatal encephalitis caused by a bullet-shaped RNA virus of the rhabdovirus family. Infection is endemic in animals of the dog family, bats and other species throughout many parts of the world.

Transmission is usually through the bite of a rabid dog, but contact with saliva from a rabid animal can cause infection. The incubation period is between 20 and 90 days but may be as short as 4 days after facial or cerebral bites.

Diagnosis

The first sign of disease is the development of paraesthesiae at the site of the bite. Rabies should be suspected whenever neurological symptoms develop a week or more after being bitten by an animal. After a variable interval, the patient begins to respond to swallowing with characteristic spasms of neck and facial muscles, accompanied by unexplained terror (hydrophobia). Hallucination, mood change and eventually coma ensue. This form of the disease is called 'furious' rabies. There is also a paralytic variant called 'dumb' rabies. Diagnosis is by immunofluorescent stain of the skin or brain biopsy, but detectable antirabies antibodies in cerebrospinal fluid (CSF) or serum are diagnostic if the patient has not been vaccinated.

Control

Although the prognosis is dismal once the disease is established, postexposure vaccination with repeated doses of intramuscular tissue culture vaccine over 4 weeks commencing immediately after the injury has been very successful. Antirabies immunoglobulin should also be given if the patient has not been vaccinated prior to exposure. Wound toilet, antibiotic treatment and tetanus prophylaxis following an animal bite should not be forgotten.

Prevention is by pre-exposure vaccination with a tissue culture vaccine (e.g. human diploid cell) in repeated intradermal doses. Those travelling to rural parts of countries where rabies is endemic, or in occupations likely to bring them into contact with dogs, should be vaccinated. Control of stray dogs and more recently mass vaccination of the dog population has been effective in controlling canine rabies in some countries.

Japanese encephalitis

Japanese encephalitis is an arbovirus infection of the central nervous system endemic throughout south and southeast Asia. It is caused by a neurotropic flavivirus transmitted by the bite of a culicine mosquito. The majority of infections are mild or subclinical. Only a small minority go on to develop fever, meningeal irritation and cerebral dysfunction. Around 25% of those with encephalitis die from the disease.

Diagnosis

Diagnosis is by detection of specific IgM in CSF. Detection of the virus in brain or CSF by culture or immunofluorescence is a poor prognostic indicator.

Control

There is no specific antiviral treatment. Prevention is by administration of an inactivated virus in repeated doses to school-age children in endemic areas. People travelling for prolonged periods in rural parts of an endemic area should be considered for pretravel vaccination. During epidemics of Japanese encephalitis, the insect vector can be controlled by widespread insecticide spraying.

HIV infection

HIV infection is reviewed in detail in Chapter 17. Travellers are at increased risk of HIV-related disease since many alter their patterns of sexual behaviour away from their home environment, exposing themselves to HIV and other sexually transmitted infections. Persons leaving developed countries with temperate climates for destinations in the developing tropics may perceive AIDS and other HIV infections as a problem of other groups (e.g. homosexual/bisexuals, or haemophiliacs).

Yet in many developing countries, AIDS is transmitted by heterosexual intercourse and a high proportion of prostitutes are HIV positive. The practice of sexual tourism is particularly risky. Single travellers are also prone to casual sexual encounters that may be just as risky. The full impact of HIV disease on international travellers has not been accurately measured, but it is becoming increasingly important to take a sexual history in the investigation of unexplained disease in returning travellers. The only reliable form of prevention is to limit sexual intercourse abroad to an accompanying, lifelong partner. Condoms obtained locally in some developing countries can be unsafe.

18.5 Organisms

A checklist of the organisms discussed in this chapter is given in Box 13. Further information is given on the pages indicated.

Box 13 Organisms that infect international travellers

Bacteria	see page	Viruses	see page
Enterotoxigenic *Escherichia coli* (ETEC)	248	Yellow fever virus	–
Salmonella spp.	248–9	Japanese encephalitis virus	–
Salmonella typhi	249	Hepatitis A virus	–
Salmonella paratyphi	249	Hepatitis B virus	257
Shigella spp.	249	Human immunodeficiency virus	260
Campylobacter spp.	251	Rabies virus	260–1
Vibrio cholerae	250	Rotavirus	260
Parasites			
Plasmodium falciparum	–		
Plasmodium vivax, malariae and *ovale*	–		
Giardia lamblia	–		
Entamoeba histolytica	–		

Self-assessment: questions

Multiple choice questions

1. All of the following are common infections in international travellers:
   a. Tuberculosis
   b. Japanese encephalitis
   c. Traveller's diarrhoea
   d. Hepatitis B
   e. Malaria

2. The following travel-associated infections can be prevented by pretravel vaccination:
   a. Diarrhoea caused by enterotoxigenic *Escherichia coli* (ETEC)
   b. Typhoid fever
   c. Cholera
   d. Hepatitis A
   e. Cerebral malaria

3. Traveller's diarrhoea is most often caused by:
   a. *Salmonella* spp.
   b. *Salmonella typhi*
   c. *Shigella* spp.
   d. Enterohaemorrhagic *Escherichia coli*
   e. Enterotoxigenic *Escherichia coli*

4. Features associated with diarrhoea in a recently returned traveller that should prompt further investigation include:
   a. Liquid stools for more than a month
   b. Bloody stools
   c. Watery stools
   d. Pus in or on the stools
   e. Pale, bulky, offensive stools

5. In many tropical countries high-risk foods or drinks include:
   a. Raw fish
   b. Salad, lettuce
   c. Canned fruit
   d. Recently roasted beef
   e. Goats' milk

6. Prevention of malaria:
   a. With chemoprophylaxis causes more harm than the disease
   b. Is not necessary for travellers to urban destinations
   c. Need only begin when the traveller reaches the destination
   d. Is never 100% reliable
   e. Is not necessary in people who have already lived in the tropics

7. In enteric fever:
   a. Diarrhoea is not the most common presenting feature
   b. Blood culture is often positive in the first week of the disease
   c. A pruritic, urticarial rash often develops on the trunk
   d. Cough and headache may be present
   e. An aminoglycoside should be used for presumptive therapy

8. Yellow fever:
   a. Is endemic in Asia
   b. Can be treated effectively with antiviral agents
   c. Is spread by mosquitoes of the genus *Anopheles*
   d. May result in an anicteric infection (i.e. without jaundice)
   e. Can be prevented by pretravel vaccination with a live attenuated virus

Case history questions

History 1

> A 30-year-old veterinary worker comes to see you for advice. He has just been told that he has to fly out tomorrow to start a project in remote rural part of central Africa. He has never been to the tropics before, but he is up to date with all the routine vaccinations.

1. What advice would you give him regarding diarrhoeal disease?
2. Is it too late to start malaria chemoprophylaxis?
3. Are there any vaccines he might benefit from?
4. What other precautions are important enough to mention in a 5-minute consultation?

History 2

> A 25-year-old woman presented with an infected dog bite 2 days after returning home from a holiday in India. She said that the dog was destroyed because it had turned on its owner. The accident occurred 5 days previously. On removal of the makeshift dressing, a small puncture wound was found from which a small amount of serous exudate had leaked.

1. What infections is the patient at risk from?
2. What would you do about the wound?
3. Is there anything to be gained by vaccination?

Data interpretation

Blood film examination on a patient who has just returned home after several years working overseas showed the following:

> malaria parasites: scanty organisms seen
> parasitaemia < 0.5% red blood cells
> predominantly schizonts of *Plasmodium vivax*
> detected few ring forms, occasional gametocytes

These results do not exclude a mixed infection.

1. Does this result suggest the early stages of a potentially life-threatening infection?
2. Why might this be a mixed infection?
3. If this infection had been treated overseas, what explanation can you provide for these results?
4. What additional laboratory investigations would you perform at this stage?

Objective structured clinical examination (OSCE)

A 39-year-old mining engineer complained of fever, mild headache, irritating cough and disturbed bowel habit 10 days after returning home from West Africa. He had been taking chloroquine and paludrine malaria prophylaxis throughout his stay and only stopped 3 days ago. A blood smear for malaria was negative and a routine stool specimen sent to the laboratory by his general practitioner last week was normal apart from scanty cysts of *Entamoeba coli*. On examination his temperature was 38.5°C, and there were a few fine crackles at both lung bases. There was mild central abdominal tenderness. He had been admitted to hospital for observation and further laboratory investigations. You are asked:

1. Is the most likely infection clear from these features?
2. Can you exclude a diagnosis of malaria?
3. Does another type of bacteriological culture need to be performed?
4. Can the illness be explained, at least in part, by the stool result?
5. Is it possible that this patient may have more than one infection?

Short notes questions

Write short notes on the following:

1. Why infections are common in international travellers
2. The relationship between AIDS and international travel

Viva question

What travel health resources are available to support the general practitioner? How can these be used to best effect?

Self-assessment: answers

Multiple choice answers

1. a. **False**. Tuberculosis is uncommon as a travel-associated infection.
   b. **False**. Japanese encephalitis is a vaccine-preventable disease that is uncommon even in travellers to endemic areas.
   c. **True**. Up to 50% of travellers from temperate to tropical climates develop diarrhoea.
   d. **False**. Hepatitis B is a vaccine-preventable disease that is uncommon even in travellers to endemic areas.
   e. **True**. Precautions are often neglected by travellers.

2. a. **False**. It causes 70% of cases of travellers' diarrhoea.
   b. **True**. Vaccination is not effective for paratyphoid.
   c. **True**. Cholera can be prevented by vaccination: the old injectable vaccine provides only partial protection for a few months, but new subunit oral vaccines appear to be more effective in field trials.
   d. **True**.
   e. **False**. Various candidate vaccines for malaria are at various stages of evaluation, but none is available for widespread use, as yet.

3. a. **False**. *Salmonella* spp. can be a cause but in less than 20% of cases; it is more common in returnees than in travellers.
   b. **False**. *S. typhi* causes fever, headache, constipation and rash.
   c. **False**. *Shigella* spp. is an uncommon cause.
   d. **False**. These cause gut and kidney mucosal damage (e.g. *E. coli* 0157).
   e. **True**. This causes 70% of cases. It produces a toxin causing fluid secretion and, hence, diarrhoea.

4. a. **True**. This can be caused by a disaccharidase deficiency, which will resolve, or by *Giardia lamblia* or tropical sprue.
   b. **True**. This suggests dysentery.
   c. **False**. Watery stools per se are not a sign of serious intestinal infection and are common in traveller's diarrhoea.
   d. **True**. This is suggestive of dysentery.
   e. **True**.

The signs listed in a, b, d, and e may indicate the presence of infection that might respond to specific chemotherapy, e.g. bacillary or amoebic dysentery, giardiasis or tropical sprue.

5. a. **True**. Water is often contaminated and raw food is a risk in itself.
   b. **True**. Uncooked food that may have been washed in contaminated water.
   c. **False**. Unlike fresh fruit, canned fruit is relatively safe, but the aspic or ice it is served with may not be.
   d. **False**. Properly cooked meat is usually safe. In the case of roast beef, the meat should not be red.
   e. **True**.

6. a. **False**.
   b. **False**.
   c. **False**.
   d. **True**.
   e. **False**.

All the above reasons have been given at some time for not bothering with malaria chemoprophylaxis. None is adequate reason for avoiding precautions against a potential preventable cause of death or severe morbidity.

7. a. **True**. The patient may actually present with constipation rather than diarrhoea.
   b. **True**. Stool culture may, however, be negative.
   c. **False**. The rash appears as widely dispersed, fine macules ('rose spot').
   d. **True**. Fever, chest pain, rash and constipation can also occur.
   e. **False**. Aminoglycosides are relatively ineffective since they have little action against intracellular bacteria.

8. a. **False**. Yellow fever is only endemic in tropical Africa and South America, despite the presence of the major vector species in Asia.
   b. **False**. There is no effective antiviral treatment.
   c. **False**. The vectors are *Aedes aegypti* and other non-anophelene mosquitoes.
   d. **True**. Although most are jaundiced.
   e. **True**. Protection then lasts 10 years.

Case history answers

History 1

1. Basic precautions with food and water and the use of oral rehydration salts.
2. No, although starting a week previously would have been better. Note that chloroquine resistance is likely to be a problem where he is going. An up-to-date

source of advice on chemoprophylaxis should be consulted.

3. Yes, rabies vaccine, which can be given in these circumstances on one occasion in multiple sites; also yellow fever may be required, depending on the destination. If so vaccination should be completed before leaving—possibly a good excuse to delay departure until more comprehensive travel health precautions have been taken. A vaccination certificate will be required for yellow fever.

4. How to avoid insect contact, particularly mosquitos, and precautions against HIV disease and other sexually transmitted infections. If he has time to stop in a bookshop before departure, he could purchase a copy of *Traveller's Health* (Dawood R or similar) to read on the flight.

History 2

1. The patient is at risk from rabies (endemic in India), bacteria from the dog's mouth, such as *Pasteurella multocida*, and tetanus. The dog's change of behaviour (i.e. turning on its owner) might be the result of canine rabies. Unfortunately, it would be impractical to obtain brain tissue from the dog at this stage.

2. The wound should be thoroughly cleaned and any necrotic tissue removed; antibiotic treatment would be prudent.

3. Yes. The patient should be given full courses of both rabies and tetanus vaccines. If she has had neither before, she should also be given rabies and tetanus immunoglobulins.

Data interpretation answer

1. No. These are the features of an established infection with *P. vivax* and possibly another *Plasmodium* species. They do not suggest early *P. falciparum* infection.

2. If only a few parasites are seen, some of the *Plasmodium* species may be difficult to tell apart, e.g. *P. vivax* and *P. ovale*.

3. *P. vivax* may persist unless the extra-erythrocytic part of the life cycle is eradicated. This requires an agent effective against the hypnozoite form: primaquine.

4. A repeat set of thick and thin films to be sure that this is not part of a rapidly changing picture, and a *P. falciparum* rapid antigen test if there is any doubt.

OSCE answer

1. No. There is a wide differential diagnosis and the investigations that have been performed so far are potentially confusing.

2. No. A single blood film, particularly if it was a thin film, will miss a proportion of cases of malaria. Malaria prophylaxis is not 100% effective but may mask the diagnosis if blood films are prepared at an early stage.

3. Yes. This patient may have typhoid. Blood culture is more sensitive than stool culture in the early stages of enteric fever.

4. No. *Entamoeba coli* is a non-pathogenic inhabitant of the human intestine, but it may reflect exposure to other enteric pathogens.

5. Yes. Travellers to high-risk locations in developing countries often return with more than one infection.

Short notes answers

1. Increasing travel to distant parts, climate, diet, insects, inadequate purification of potable water supply and poor sewage/refuse disposal all need to be included in the answer.

2. There is a high rate of HIV in populations of many developing countries that are popular as tourist destinations. Particularly high rates occur in prostitutes. Single adult travellers are prone to risky patterns of sexual behaviour.

Viva answer

There are excellent information sources available via the Internet (e.g. MASTA, CDC, WHO), in hard copy (travel and tropical medicine journals) and specialist travel health agencies. In some countries, travel and ticketing agencies provide printed health information advice to adventure travellers. The basic health advice and vaccination needs of the majority of international travellers are usually fairly straightforward and can be handled effectively in either a standard clinic session or with the support of appropriate printed fact sheets. Overland travellers, those with complicated itineraries or professional people with specific high-risk exposures often need a more detailed case-by-case approach. These are the ones who should be referred to a specialist travel health service, if available, for a tailor-made preventive health plan.

19 Orphan infections

Overview

When infectious diseases are considered under the major organ systems or clinical specialties, a number of important diseases and syndromes are left out. These clinical entities neither belong to one particular system nor present to one particular type of specialist. The conditions reviewed in this chapter cause significant morbidity and mortality as a result of systemic spread or multisystem disease. Their clinical presentation also contributes to difficulties in arriving at a presumptive, working diagnosis.

19.1 Pathogenesis

Learning objectives

You should:

- understand the term 'orphan infection' and its common features
- be aware of the consequences of dissemination of the pathogen via the systemic circulation
- know the effects of direct invasion, immune complex deposition and embolism.

A common feature of the orphan infections is the dissemination of the infective agent via the systemic circulation. Invasion of the vascular space is required at an early stage of infection. This may result from:

- focal infection
- inoculation during penetrating trauma (including invasive surgical procedures)
- arthropod inoculation
- an unknown source or means of acquisition.

Systemic spread also results in the development of fever in a large percentage of those affected. In Gram-negative bacterial infections, the fever is the result of endotoxin (lipopolysaccharide) release, but other bacterial cell wall components (e.g. teichoic acids from Gram-positive bacteria) can also trigger a febrile response. In fact, the collection of clinical features referred to as 'septic shock' can be caused by products of bacteria, viruses, fungi and protozoa.

Dissemination of microorganisms via the bloodstream results in rapid establishment of infection at distant sites and embolic phenomena if the particles are large enough. Damage to the vascular endothelium may also arise from direct invasion or immune complex deposition. Internal organs with a high blood flow are at special risk of embolic, vasculitic or immune complex damage.

19.2 Diagnosis

Learning objectives

You should:

- know the common causes of pyrexia of unknown origin (PUO)
- know the important features to look for in a history
- know the laboratory tests that can help to reach a diagnosis.

Clinical features

As fever is a common feature in this group of infections, all may present initially as pyrexia of unknown origin (PUO). Some of the orphan infections are among the common causes of PUO (Table 34), while others are only common in people who have had some form of high-risk exposure. It is therefore important to obtain a detailed travel, occupational and food history, and to ask about animal contact. Many of the clinical features of a specific

Table 34 Causes of pyrexia of unknown origin (PUO)[a]

Category	Examples
Infectious	Tuberculosis, infective endocarditis, hidden abscess
Neoplastic	Hepatoma, renal carcinoma
Connective tissue disease	Systemic lupus erythematosus
Other	Factitious (false) fever

[a]For complete list refer to text on infectious diseases.

aetiological diagnosis are non-specific and do not by themselves help towards a specific aetiological diagnosis. However, careful examination may uncover signs of a primary focus or secondary spread. These will in turn help in the choice of laboratory investigations. An unusually large battery of investigations may be required in patients with one of the orphan infections, but in most cases blood cultures will be needed.

Laboratory tests

Blood culture technique is important if reliable results are to be obtained. Two bottles should be used in each set: one for aerobic organisms and the other for anaerobes. The probability of obtaining a positive result is increased by using additional sets—two or three are often used— but these should be inoculated at intervals of at least 30 minutes. They should be inoculated with 5–10 ml blood each, using a no-touch technique and following careful skin disinfection to avoid contamination by bacteria. Ideally, blood cultures should be taken just before the fever peaks, but as this is obviously not practical, they are usually taken at or near the peak as possible. Some of the orphan infections are caused by non-cultivatable microorganisms. Since these cannot be recovered in the laboratory, it is necessary to use other methods (e.g. antigen or antibody detection) to make a specific diagnosis.

In difficult cases, where the diagnosis cannot be confirmed easily, it is worth saving a baseline serum sample for future serological investigations and possibly even inoculating a laboratory animal.

19.3 Management

Learning objectives

You should:

- understand the use of empirical therapy and the problems that it can cause in diagnosis

- be aware of preventive measures, particularly in occupational and zoonotic infections.

Chemotherapy

There may be a significant delay to diagnosis in many of these infections, while in the more severe cases the patient's condition may deteriorate rapidly. It is therefore necessary to start empirical therapy based on clinical impression and epidemiological clues. Since some of these infections are caused by obligate or facultative intracellular pathogens, the physician may find it necessary to use antibiotics such as tetracycline or chloramphenicol. In cases where no specific diagnostic tests produce positive results yet there are grounds to believe that systemic infection is present, a trial of therapy may be required. Though this may be in the patient's immediate interest, a trial of therapy can interfere with any remaining diagnostic tests.

Prevention

Various measures can be taken to prevent orphan infections. Avoiding contact with the primary source is effective, but only when the source is clearly defined. This approach applies particularly to occupational and zoonotic infections. Some of the orphan infections can be prevented by vaccination, either of the human population or even by vaccination of the animal reservoir where this is a domesticated species. Other preventive measures include pasteurisation of milk and chemoprophylaxis of high-risks groups.

19.4 Diseases and syndromes

Learning objectives

You should:

- understand the common features of orphan infections

- know the basis of their clinical management

- be aware of which infections constitute a medical emergency requiring rapid therapy.

This group of diseases will not necessarily have features in common. Most affect multiple organ systems and most are spread via the bloodstream (Table 35).

Septicaemia

Septicaemia is a clinical syndrome in which microorganisms actively multiply in the bloodstream. Many species of bacteria, fungi, viruses and parasites have been implicated; however, the majority of cases are caused by bacteria from a small number of genera. Gram-negative

Table 35 Orphan infections

Infection	Features
Septicaemia	Microorganisms multiply in the bloodstream; fever, increased pulse and respiratory rate, raised leucocyte count, reduced blood pressure, clotting dysfunction
Infective endocarditis	Infection of the endocardium; usually with systemic features: fever, night sweats, lethargy, weight loss, haemorrhages in distal limbs, cardiac murmur
Syphilis (tertiary)	
Benign	Granulomas in soft tissues, bones, internal organs
Cardiovascular	Vasa vasorum, ascending aorta affected, aneurysms
Neurosyphilis	General paresis, manic depression, tabes dorsalis, encephalitis
Lyme disease	Spreading annular erythematous rash, polyarthritis, aseptic meningitis, myocarditis and conduction block
Leptospirosis	Initially influenza-like or meningitis; second stage can lead to jaundice, renal failure, haemorrhage
Scrub typhus	Influenza-like, may be a vasculitis and rash
Rocky Mountain spotted fever	Blackened eschar at bite, influenza-like, black rash from haemorrhagic vasculitis; renal and other organ failure can follow
Q fever	Fever, rigors, pulmonary consolidation; may develop to endocarditis
Brucellosis	Influenza-like, back pain, may be hepatomegaly and splenomegaly

bacilli are commonly isolated from the blood of septicaemic patients. The most common Gram-negatives are members of the Enterobacteriaceae:

- *Escherichia coli*
- *Klebsiella* spp.
- *Serratia* spp.
- *Pseudomonas aeruginosa*.

Gram-positive bacteria are also commonly isolated, including:

- *Staphylococcus aureus*
- α- and β-haemolytic streptococci
- *Streptococcus pneumoniae*
- *Enterococcus* spp.

In recent years, coagulase-negative staphylococci have been recorded as clinically significant blood culture isolates with increasing frequency. Anaerobic bacteria such as *Bacteroides fragilis* and *Clostridium perfringens* are isolated relatively less frequently. Other species of note include the yeast *Candida albicans* and atypical mycobacteria (from patients infected with human immunodeficiency virus (HIV)). *Haemophilus influenzae* may be isolated from blood cultures, particularly from unvaccinated children. Some patients will have more than one microbial species ('polymicrobial') causing septicaemia.

The microbial species isolated from blood cultures reflect the more severe end of the infectious disease spectrum. There will normally be a mixture of community-acquired and hospital-acquired septicaemias, depending on the case mix of referrals to the hospital in question. The source of organisms invading the patient's bloodstream will usually be:

- a focal source, e.g. a wound or urinary tract infection
- an invasive procedure, e.g. abdominal surgery or cystoscopy

- related to some form of compromised host defences, e.g. administration of glucocorticosteroids or ciclosporin
- no obvious source of infection or precipitating factor (in a significant minority).

Diagnosis

Clinical features The clinical features of septicaemia are various and non-specific, but together they suggest a systemic infective process. The cardinal features include fever (or hypothermia), increased pulse, increased respiratory rate, raised leucocyte count, reduced blood pressure and alterations in clotting function. (Altered temperature, raised pulse and respiratory rate, a probable site of infection and impaired function of one or more organ systems is referred to as the 'sepsis syndrome' and carries a mortality of around 30%.) The patient with severe septicaemia may also be confused, shocked ('septic shock'), in renal failure and have disseminated intravascular coagulation. Hypothermia indicates a relatively poor prognosis. Initially, systemic vascular resistance is reduced, but later it increases, explaining why some patients have 'warm' shock.

Septic shock is most often caused by Gram-negative bacilli such as *E. coli* or *Pseudomonas* sp., but can be caused by Gram-positive bacteria, *H. influenzae*, *Neisseria meningitidis*, other bacteria and a variety of non-bacterial microorganisms. Bacterial cell wall components or other microbial moieties cause the activation of mediator pathways. Fever probably results from release of interleukin-1. Other factors such as tumour necrosis factor contribute to the pathogenesis of multi-system dysfunction. A proportion of patients develop adult respiratory distress syndrome. Renal impairment is multifactorial. There may be cholestatic jaundice.

Laboratory tests A careful history and examination is required unless the primary focus of infection is clearly evident. Blood cultures should always be taken before commencement of antimicrobial chemotherapy. Possible sites of underlying, primary infection should also be cultured. Confirmation of systemic fungal or mycobacterial infection may require special blood culture media. In some less-common systemic infections (e.g. enteric fever), culture of bone marrow may increase the probability of a positive culture. At least two bone marrow samples may increase the probability of a positive culture. At least two blood culture sets are advised; three is optimal, providing these are collected from different venepuncture sites over several hours.

Treatment

A patient with septicaemia cannot wait for the results of definitive, culture-based confirmatory tests before commencing antimicrobial chemotherapy. Presumptive treatment has to be commenced on the basis of the most likely microbial pathogens. Clearly, this will differ according to the clinical setting. However, no single agent is sufficient for all microbial pathogens and in some patients, particularly the immunocompromised, impaired host defences leave little room for indecision. In practice, the initial choice will often have a wider range of antimicrobial activity than is necessary. But that judgement can only be made in retrospect when culture-based data become available. At that point, the agents used should be reduced to the minimum necessary for the causal microorganism. Septicaemia in a patient who has just had abdominal surgery might therefore be treated with ampicillin, gentamicin and metronidazole initially. When the blood culture results confirm the presence of *E. coli*, the ampicillin might be dropped. However, a patient who then became shocked and went into renal failure might be given cefotaxime instead of gentamicin. Patients in septic shock may require intensive care where they can be mechanically ventilated and have their need for fluid replacement and vasopressors carefully monitored.

Prevention

There is no simple means of preventing septicaemia. Its incidence can only be reduced by prevention of the underlying infections and other factors that result in bloodstream invasion by microorganisms. Since septicaemia in hospital patients carries a higher mortality than community-acquired septicaemia, early recognition and treatment of focal infection is important. Care should be taken with all invasive devices and procedures, especially in compromised patients, to avoid the promotion of systemic infection.

Infective endocarditis

Infective endocarditis—infection of the endocardium, usually with systemic consequences—can be caused by almost any species of medically important bacteria, and by other microorganisms. As in septicaemia, relatively few microbial species cause most infections:

- streptococci, particularly the viridans group: most cases
- staphylococci; approximately 25%
- enterococci; approximately 10%
- coagulase-negative staphylococci: prosthetic valve endocarditis
- fungi (mainly *Candida* spp.): in intravenous drug abusers
- *Streptococcus bovis*: endocarditis associated with intestinal polyp, or carcinoma of the colon.

Infection of the endocardium normally occurs in the presence of an abnormal heart valve, i.e. congenital heart disease, rheumatic heart disease or a valvular prosthesis. The abnormal valve causes alterations in the normal pattern of blood flow through the valve orifice, resulting in endothelial damage on the downstream side of the valve. Fibrin and platelets are then deposited on the denuded patch of endothelium to form sterile vegetations. In time, these are colonised by bacteria during transient bacteraemia. Further fibrin and platelet deposition occurs to form more pronounced vegetations. Both *S. aureus* and *S. pneumoniae* can cause endocarditis in the presence of normal heart valves. The vegetation then acts as a source of continuous microbial seeding of the bloodstream. The resulting bacteraemia is thus continual. Larger clumps of microorganisms break off the parent vegetation from time to time, causing the dissemination of septic emboli. If the affected valve is on the left side of the heart, organs with a high blood flow are at high risk of embolic phenomena, i.e. the brain and kidneys. Some of the disseminated lesions are also thought to be the result of deposition of immune complexes.

Diagnosis

Clinical features A patient with infective endocarditis may present with a variety of seemingly non-specific features. Without careful examination, it may be difficult to establish the connection between these features and arrive at the correct diagnosis. It is not surprising that infective endocarditis is one of the commoner causes of PUO. The patient will usually have a fever and will often complain of night sweats and possibly also lethargy and weight loss. A collection of signs may be present on examination of the distal limbs: splinter haemorrhages under the proximal nails, tender nodules in the finger pads (Osler's nodes), haemorrhages on palms and soles (Janeway lesions) and finger clubbing. There may be splenomegaly and in the nervous system, retinal haemorrhages near the optic disc and neurological signs. Most importantly, the majority of patients have a cardiac murmur.

Laboratory tests Urine examination will often reveal proteinuria and microscopic haematuria. If the patient does not have a prosthetic valve, echocardiogram can be used to detect vegetations on heart valves.

A specific laboratory diagnosis is made by taking blood cultures. At least three sets should be collected and unless the patient's condition is rapidly deteriorating antimicrobial chemotherapy should be withheld until those cultures have been collected. Great care should be taken with skin disinfection and no-touch venesection technique to avoid contamination of the cultures with skin organisms that might be interpreted as causal pathogens. The possible diagnosis of infective endocarditis should be clearly indicated to the laboratory so that some of the unusual causes of endocarditis can be excluded by prolonged incubation. It is worth repeating cultures several weeks after commencing antimicrobial chemotherapy to confirm that detectable microorganisms have been eradicated from the bloodstream. In some patients with a clinical presentation strongly indicative of infective endocarditis, no causal pathogen is recovered from blood culture. This is referred to as 'culture-negative endocarditis'. The common causes include prior antibiotic treatment, nutritionally variant streptococci (require special media in the laboratory) and fastidious organisms such as *Coxiella burnetti* or members of the HACEK group (*Haemophilus aphrophilus* and *Actinobacillus, Cardiobacterium, Eikenella, Kingella* spp.). Confirmation of infection with one of these organisms should be discussed with the laboratory.

Treatment

All therapeutic regimens for infective endocarditis aim to eradicate live microorganisms from vegetations. Therapy is therefore given intravenously in high doses for several weeks. Presumptive therapy of infective endocarditis associated with a native valve would normally be directed towards streptococci. High-dose benzylpenicillin is often combined with gentamicin for this purpose. Gentamicin increases the effect of penicillin against enterococci, but at concentrations lower than those required for therapy of Gram-negative septicaemia. It is therefore unnecessary to give a full therapeutic dose of gentamicin in this setting, and if the causal pathogen turns out to be one of the common α-haemolytic streptococci (*S. mitior, S. mutans, S. salivarius* or *S. sanguis*), then high-dose penicillin alone should suffice. If endocarditis affects a previously normal heart valve, staphylococcal or pneumococcal infection should be considered, and an antistaphylococcal penicillin (e.g. flucloxacillin) used as well. Prosthetic valve endocarditis is often caused by coagulase-negative staphylococci. These may be resistant to penicillins and often require the use of vancomycin, which is often useful for endocarditis in patients with penicillin allergy. Candidal endocarditis rarely responds to antifungal therapy alone. Valve surgery is usually required to guarantee eradication of infection. The diagnostic laboratory may test organisms isolated from the blood of patients with infective endocarditis to determine the concentration of antibiotic required to inhibit and to kill the pathogen (i.e. the minimum inhibitory (MIC) and minimum bactericidal (MBC) concentrations).

Prophylaxis

Since patients with valve disease are at increased risk of infective endocarditis, they should be given antibiotic prophylaxis for any medical or dental procedure likely to cause bacteraemia. The agents chosen are given so that peak blood levels occur during the procedure and they should be directed towards the most likely agents of endocarditis, i.e. streptococci in oral and upper gastrointestinal procedures. Enterobacteriaceae very rarely cause endocarditis, and endoscopic investigations of intact mucosal surfaces carry a very low risk of bacteraemia. A standard prophylactic regimen for dental work would be ampicillin given 30 minutes prior to dental surgery, followed by a further dose immediately afterwards. Advice regarding prophylaxis for patients who have had antibiotic therapy in the past month, those with penicillin allergies and those undergoing lengthy operative procedures is best sought from a medical microbiologist or other infectious disease specialist. Nevertheless, the majority of cases of infective endocarditis occur in patients with no identifiable cause of bacteraemia. It is therefore likely that the prophylaxis of infective endocarditis has had little impact on the incidence of the disease.

Syphilis

Syphilis is a treponemal infection with multiple clinical presentations. It is caused by the spiral bacterium *Treponema pallidum* and is transmitted via sexual and transplacental routes. It causes disease in three distinct phases, the first two of which are reviewed in Chapter 10. The first phase is essentially localised whereas the second stage has more generalised symptoms of a spreading maculopapular rash, erosions and folliculitis.

Diagnosis

Clinical features of tertiary syphilis The features of late syphilis are more varied and can make diagnosis difficult. Late (or tertiary) syphilis occurs at least 2 years after secondary syphilis. The dissemination of spirochaetes happens during the secondary stage, so that manifestations of late disease can arise throughout the body. There are three main types of late syphilis:

- benign (also known as gummatous)
- cardiovascular
- neurosyphilis.

In benign tertiary syphilis, granulomas form in the soft tissues, bones or internal organs. These may be confused with malignant disease, with potentially disastrous consequences. Cardiovascular syphilis is less common. The disease attacks the vasa vasorum and has a predilection for the ascending aorta. Aneurysm of the aortic arch may be a late complication. Neurosyphilis is the least common of the three and presents under a number of guises ranging from general paresis, through manic depression to tabes dorsalis. Other neurological complications of syphilitic infection are described. In recent years, it has become clear that HIV-positive patients experience a more rapid progression of syphilis, and neurological consequences, such as necrosing encephalitis, may be devastating.

Laboratory tests A specific laboratory diagnosis is more difficult to obtain than in early syphilis. The Venereal Disease Research Laboratory (VDRL) test may be negative or at best only borderline. The absorbed fluorescent treponemal antibody test (TFA-Abs) can remain positive for many years after infection, whether it has been successfully treated or not. It is unsuitable for the diagnosis of active late syphilis. Up to a third of patients with cardiovascular syphilis may have a negative VDRL result. Finally, although a positive haemagglutination test does not confirm the diagnosis, a negative result does exclude the disease.

Treatment
There have been few reports of treatment failure with two doses of benzathine penicillin for late syphilis. Late neurosyphilis should be treated with procaine penicillin for 2 weeks but in this case the treatment will arrest the development of active disease rather than cure it outright. Patients who have the acquired immunodeficiency syndrome (AIDS) should be given a full 2 weeks of treatment with penicillin intravenously, because treatment failure is much more common.

Lyme disease (Lyme borreliosis)

Lyme disease is a multisystem condition caused by an arthropod-borne infection with the spirochaete *Borrelia burgdorferi*. The spirochaete is transmitted by the bite of a hard-bodied tick of the genus *Ixodes*. The epidemiology of the disease is determined by the distribution and seasonal prevalence of the tick vector, and by human contact with the tick. The normal reservoir of the spirochaete is in small mammals on which the ticks normally feed. Humans are incidental participants in the usual cycle of transmission.

Diagnosis
Clinical features The features of the disease are many and may either progress in series or occur together. They include a spreading, annular erythematous rash (called erythema chronicum migrans), a polyarthritis, cardiological and neurological complications. The rash begins about a fortnight after the tick bite and usually disappears within a matter of weeks. The arthritis is predominantly an arthralgia without significant swelling. In the nervous system, a variety of complications may arise including an 'aseptic' meningitis. The cardiac complications include myocarditis and conduction block.

Laboratory tests Diagnosis is by antibody detection using either serum or cerebrospinal fluid (CSF). There is an early IgM response to infection followed by a rise in IgG. Results need to be interpreted with the help of the clinical features, since positive serology may indicate past infection.

Treatment
The optimal antibiotic treatment of Lyme disease is debatable. Penicillin, tetracycline and third-generation cephalosporins have all been shown to have some effect. However, patients with neuroborreliosis may not improve as a result of antibiotic therapy.

Prevention
Prevention is by avoiding exposure to ticks (long trousers, long sleeves and insect repellent in tick-infested areas) and by swift removal of ticks from the skin if they have embedded.

Leptospirosis

Leptospirosis is a multisystem disease caused by infection with the spirochaete *Leptospira interrogans*. There are several hundred serological varieties of *L. interrogans*, a spirochaete with hooked ends that is able to survive in the proximal tubule of mammalian kidneys and in unpolluted, alkaline surface waters for months. Infection is by skin or mucosal contact with contaminated water. Infected rats or dogs may shed spirochaetes continuously for months. Those at greatest risk include sewer workers, veterinary and farm workers and water sports enthusiasts. Once in the systemic circulation, spirochaetes are disseminated to distant organs where they cause endothelial damage.

Diagnosis
Clinical features The initial infection may resemble influenza or meningitis, with fever, chills, muscle pain, headache and neck stiffness. There may also be back pain and conjunctival injection. After a short asymptomatic interval, there is a second stage of disease, which in some patients leads to jaundice, renal failure and haemorrhage. Some exposed individuals remain asymptomatic.

Laboratory tests *L. interrogans* can be cultured from blood if the blood is collected into a sterile heparinised tube or inoculated into special media at the patient's bedside. The organism can also be cultured from urine during the second week of infection, but the urine must first be made alkaline. Confirmation of growth is by slide agglutination. Most cases are diagnosed clinically or retrospectively using serological methods. In parts of the world where the infection is prevalent, hantavirus infection should also be considered. Nucleic acid amplification tests for detection of leptospiral DNA in blood or other body fluids is now used for diagnosis in some centres.

Treatment

Treatment is with penicillin, but if commenced more than 5 days after the onset of infection (i.e. the first phase), it is unlikely to alter the course of disease. In patients with renal failure, haemodialysis significantly improves the prognosis. Recovery is usually complete when it occurs.

Prevention

Prevention is by avoiding contact with infected animals and contaminated surface waters (sea water is non-hazardous).

Scrub typhus

Scrub typhus is a rickettsiosis caused by an arthropod-borne bacterium called *Orienta tsutsugamushi* (formerly *Rickettsia tsutsugamushi*). It is endemic through south, east and southeast Asia, and northern Australia. It is caused by the obligate intracellular Gram-negative bacillus *O. tsutsugamushi* and is transmitted by the larval stage of trombiculid mites. These mites are found in undergrowth and transitional vegetation (scrub, reclaimed land, jungle and village edge in particular) so rural populations and others passing through (e.g. military personnel) are most at risk of infection.

Diagnosis

Clinical features The infection resembles influenza, with fever, chills and muscle aches. There may also be a macular rash resulting from a general vasculitis. Headache may be severe.

Laboratory tests Laboratory diagnosis depends on serology, since the organism is an obligate intracellular parasite.

Control

Treatment is with tetracycline or chloramphenicol. Chemoprophylaxis has been effective in selected populations (e.g. military personnel).

Rocky Mountain spotted fever

Rocky Mountain spotted fever (RMSF) is a rickettsiosis caused by *Rickettsia rickettsiae*. RMSF is not restricted to the region suggested by its name: it is found throughout North America. The causative organism is an obligate, intracellular Gram-negative bacillus that is transmitted by the bite of a wood tick.

Diagnosis

Clinical features A proportion of patients have a blackened eschar at the site of the tick bite. They develop influenza-like symptoms with severe headache and a black rash caused by the widely disseminated haemorrhagic vasculitis. There may be extensive involvement of the internal organs, and death may result, especially from renal failure

Laboratory tests Laboratory diagnosis is by serology: immunofluorescent antibody test for IgM to detect recent infection or by direct immunofluorescence of skin biopsy. Since the differential diagnosis includes meningococcal infection, blood and CSF culture should also be carried out.

Treatment

Treatment with either a tetracycline or chloramphenicol should be started as early as possible and continued for up to a week after temperature has returned to normal.

Prevention

RMSF can be prevented by avoiding contact with ticks. This entails covering up well during expeditions into wooded areas where the disease is endemic, using insect repellents and removing ticks from the skin after they have attached.

Q fever

Q fever is a febrile illness caused by the rickettsia *Coxiella burnetti*. *C. burnetti* is an obligate, intracellular Gram-negative bacillus that is found in sheep and cattle. Humans are incidental hosts and acquire the infection as a result of contact with infected sheep, cattle and their products. The disease is therefore mainly one of rural populations and livestock workers.

Diagnosis

Clinical features Infection is often via the respiratory route, so that the presenting features may be those of an atypical pneumonia with fever, rigors and pulmonary consolidation. Often this resolves spontaneously but, if the patient has not been treated and has a damaged or prosthetic heart valve, may present at a later date with culture-negative endocarditis.

Laboratory tests Laboratory diagnosis is serological. Immunofluorescent phase two antibody is raised for months after acute infection. Phase one antibody is raised in chronic infection (endocarditis).

Treatment

Treatment is with a tetracycline and may have to be for a prolonged period in cases of endocarditis.

Prevention

Prevention is by avoiding contact with the animal source. In some countries, a vaccine is available to high-risk groups.

Brucellosis

Brucellosis is a systemic infection caused by fastidious Gram-negative bacteria with a principal reservoir in various species of domestic animals. The association between bacterial and animal species is fairly specific: *Brucella melitensis* in goats, *B. abortus* in cattle and *B. suis* in pigs. Brucellas are facultative intracellular parasites and survive in the kidneys, mammary glands and placentas of the host, as well as in soil. Infection is through occupational exposure to animal products or by consumption of dairy products (e.g. goat's milk and cheese).

Diagnosis

Clinical features The disease may take acute or chronic forms. In the acute form, the features are similar to influenza but much more prolonged. There is often a history of back pain, and both hepatomegaly and splenomegaly may be noted. In the chronic form, fea-

tures of disease persist for more than a year and are less clearly defined.

Laboratory tests Diagnosis is by serology using either an enzyme-linked immunosorbent assay (ELISA) or an immunofluorescent antibody test. A small percentage of cases are diagnosed by blood or bone marrow culture in serum-enriched broth.

Treatment

Treatment is with a tetracycline for several weeks. Some authorities add rifampicin, and the tetracycline should be substituted with streptomycin if the patient is female and might be pregnant.

Prevention

Prevention is by vaccination of cattle against Brucellas and by pasteurisation of milk. These measures have led to eradication of brucellosis in some countries.

19.5 Organisms

A checklist of the organisms discussed in this chapter is given in Box 14. Further information is given on the pages indicated.

Box 14 Organisms causing infections that cannot be classed by organ system affected or specialty involved

Bacteria	see page	Fungi	see page
Escherichia coli	248	*Candida* spp.	269
Klebsiella spp.	248		
Enterobacter spp.	248–9	**Viruses**	
Serratia spp.	248	Hantavirus	258
Pseudomonas aeruginosa	249–50		
Staphylococcus aureus	243		
Coagulase-negative staphylococci	243		
Viridans group streptococci (S. *mutans,* S. *mitior, S. salivarius, S. sanguis*)	245		
Enterococcus spp.	245		
Neisseria meningitidis	252–3		
Bacteroides fragilis	252		
Clostridium perfringens	247		
Haemophilus aphrophilus	252		
Actinobacillus sp.	252		
Cardiobacterium sp.	252		
Eikenella sp.	252		
Kingella sp.	252		
Treponema pallidum	255		
Borrelia burgdorferi	256		
Leptospira interrogans	256		
Orienta tsutsugamushi	255		
Rickettsia rickettsiae	255		
Coxiella burnetti	255		
Brucella melitensis	252		
Brucella abortus	252		
Brucella suis	252		

Self-assessment: questions

Multiple choice questions

1. The following conditions can be referred to as 'orphan infections':
   a. Meningitis
   b. Infective endocarditis
   c. Tinea corporis
   d. Late syphilis
   e. Atypical pneumonia

2. In orphan infections:
   a. Invasion of the systemic circulation occurs
   b. A primary focus is usually present
   c. Spread is principally haematogenous
   d. Vasculitis or embolic phenomena may occur
   e. Fever is only caused by endotoxins

3. In the collection of blood cultures:
   a. Blood should be inoculated into three blood culture bottles
   b. Multiple samples should be collected at intervals
   c. The same needle should always be used for collection and culture bottle inoculation.
   d. Less than 5 ml blood per bottle is adequate
   e. Skin disinfection is unnecessary

4. In septicaemia:
   a. *Bacteroides fragilis* is the most common Gram-negative bacterial pathogen
   b. Enterobacteriaceae are common in hospital patients
   c. There is a rising incidence of staphylococcal infection
   d. *Haemophilus influenzae* is more common in children than adults
   e. Coagulase-negative staphylococci isolates are always the result of contamination

5. The origin of septicaemic infection may be:
   a. Soft tissue infection
   b. Deep abdominal abscess
   c. Urinary tract instrumentation
   d. The intestine in a neutropenic patient
   e. Unknown after detailed investigation

6. Infective endocarditis:
   a. Is most commonly caused by enterococci
   b. Causes splinter haemorrhages in the retina
   c. Can cause neurological sequelae
   d. Is a cause of pyrexia of unknown origin (PUO)
   e. Causes heart murmurs in a minority of cases

7. Culture-negative endocarditis can be caused by:
   a. Prior antibiotic treatment
   b. Nutritionally variant streptococci
   c. *Coxiella burnetti*
   d. Non-infective endocarditis
   e. Insufficient blood volume cultured

8. Late syphilis:
   a. Causes granuloma formation
   b. Occurs after an interval of more than 2 years after secondary syphilis
   c. Causes an aortic degeneration known as tabes dorsalis
   d. Is difficult to diagnose by serological methods
   e. Can progress very rapidly in HIV-positive persons

9. The rickettsioses include:
   a. Q fever
   b. Scrub typhus
   c. Rocky Mountain spotted fever
   d. Typhoid
   e. Leptospirosis

10. Lyme borreliosis:
    a. Is associated with exposure to trombiculid mites
    b. Is caused by spirochaetes found in rat or dog kidneys
    c. Results in a rash known as erythema chronicum migrans
    d. Can cause aseptic meningitis
    e. Can be diagnosed by direct immunofluorescence

11. Brucellosis:
    a. Can be transmitted in unpasteurised milk
    b. Primarily affects military personnel
    c. Is difficult to confirm by culture-based methods
    d. Causes back pain in rare cases
    e. Can be effectively treated with tetracycline

Case history questions

History 1

Three young men went on a canoe expedition along a canal network. They broke off their journey early because two of them went down with the 'flu'. About a week later, one of the two started to feel much worse than before and noticed his eyes had turned yellow. He then decided to seek medical help.

1. What bacterial infection might he have?
2. What other serious complication may be present?
3. How would you confirm your suspicions?

History 2

> A 25-year-old woman was admitted to hospital with an intermittent fever, headache, lethargy, and joint, muscle and back pain. She recently visited her extended family, who raise goats in Northern Iran. She was welcomed home with a feast of traditional local dishes. About 2 weeks after her return to Europe, she developed the above symptoms. There were no significant clinical signs on examination other than a fever of 38.0°C.

1. What bacterial infection might she have?
2. How would you confirm the diagnosis?
3. What antibiotics would you choose?
4. How would your choice differ if she were pregnant?

Data interpretation

The following results were obtained from a series of three blood culture sets collected over 24 hours from a patient with a persistent fever and no localising signs of infection:

> *Blood culture 1: Streptococcus bovis*
> penicillin sensitive
> erythromycin sensitive.
> *Blood culture 2: Streptococcus bovis*
> penicillin sensitive
> erythromycin sensitive.
> *Blood culture 3: Streptococcus bovis*
> penicillin sensitive
> erythromycin sensitive.

1. What infection does this result suggest?
2. How would you confirm your suspicions?
3. What precipitating condition should be looked for?
4. If that patient is allergic to penicillin what treatment options remain open?

Objective structured clinical examination (OSCE)

A 54-year-old woman was admitted with a febrile illness and right upper quadrant pain of very recent onset. It was not possible to take a more detailed history but her husband said that she had been healthy until the last few days. On examination she was able to answer a few direct questions but was drowsy. She was tender in the epigastrium and the tenderness extended to the right. There was no evidence of jaundice. Abdominal ultrasound examination showed an echo-dense area consistent with cholelithiasis. Bile obtained under ultrasonic guidance and peripheral venous blood were sent to the laboratory for culture. Specialist advice was sought on the choice of antibiotics. The blood culture was positive after 5 hours of incubation. You are asked the following:

1. Do these features suggest that the patient has gone into septic shock?
2. Is the probable diagnosis septicaemia following cholangitis?
3. Has a non-surgical approach been taken to reduce the risk of major complications by completing treatment of infection before commencing cholecystectomy?
4. Are the presumptive antibiotics advised most likely to have been a combination of intravenous amoxycillin, gentamicin and metronidazole?
5. Is the short time to the blood culture result proof of the severity of disease?

Short notes questions

Write short notes on the following:

1. The sepsis syndrome
2. How rickettsioses can be prevented
3. The consequences of poor blood culture technique

Viva questions

1. Blood cultures have little impact on the immediate management of septicaemia. Discuss.
2. Discuss which spirochaetal disease you think is most difficult to diagnose and why.

Self-assessment: answers

Multiple choice answers

1. a. **False**. Meningitis affects one principal organ system.
   b. **True**. Vegetations seed systemic spread of the infection.
   c. **False**. Tinea affects one principal organ system.
   d. **True**. Can affect multiple organs.
   e. **False**. Pneumonia affects one principal organ system.

2. a. **True**. This is the common feature.
   b. **False**. A primary focus can occasionally be found.
   c. **True**. Invasion of the vascular system is an early stage.
   d. **True**. Particularly in infections of the endocardium.
   e. **False**. Fever can result from release of microbial products by any of the major groups of microorganisms, not only endotoxin (from Gram-negative bacteria).

3. a. **False**. A pair of blood culture bottles should be used: one aerobic and one anaerobic.
   b. **True**. This enables the course of the infection to be assessed and improves the likelihood of detecting some species.
   c. **False**. The same needle can be used for collection and inoculation only if a vacutainer or similar system is used.
   d. **False**. A 5–10 ml blood sample is required per bottle.
   e. **False**. The hands of the venesector and the venesection site should both be carefully disinfected prior to blood culture to avoid contamination with commensal skin organisms.

4. a. **False**. The most common Gram-negative pathogen is *Escherichia coli*.
   b. **True**.
   c. **True**.
   d. **True**.
   e. **False**. Coagulase-negative staphylococci may be significant, especially in patients with intravascular cannulae and in neonates.

5. a. **True**. Often following a wound.
   b. **True**. This is a focal source usually of gut-derived organisms.
   c. **True**. An invasive procedure.
   d. **True**. Immune defences are compromised.
   e. **True**. This is true for a significant minority.

6. a. **False**. Infective endocarditis is most commonly caused by viridans group streptococci such as *S. mutans*.
   b. **False**. Splinter haemorrhages occur in the proximal nailbeds, not the retinal vessels.
   c. **True**. As a consequence of embolism.
   d. **True**. It is a common cause of PUO.
   e. **False**. Murmurs can be heard in most patients with infective endocarditis.

7. a. **True**. This is a common cause.
   b. **True**. These will not grow in standard culture media.
   c. **True**. A fastidious organism that is difficult to culture.
   d. **True**.
   e. **True**. Particularly a problem with the organisms that are harder to culture.

8. a. **True**. This is known as benign syphilis.
   b. **True**. It is at least 2 years and may be substantially more.
   c. **False**. Tabes dorsalis is a form of neurosyphilis.
   d. **True**. Some tests will indicate past infection as well as tertiary syphilis and others can be negative or borderline.
   e. **True**. HIV-positive patients can develop severe neurosyphilis.

9. a. **True**. It is caused by *Coxiella burnetti*.
   b. **True**. It is caused by *Orienta (Rickettsia) tsutsugamushi*.
   c. **True**. It is caused by *Rickettsia rickettsiae*.
   d. **False**. Typhoid is otherwise known as enteric fever and is caused by *Salmonella typhi*.
   e. **False**. Leptospirosis is caused by *Leptospira interrogans*; a spirochaete.

10. a. **False**. The vector of Lyme borreliosis is hard-bodied tick of the genus *Ixodes*.
    b. **False**. The disease is caused by *Borrelia burgdorferi*. The unrelated spirochaete *Leptospira interrogans* is shed via mammalian kidneys.
    c. **True**. A spreading annular erythematous rash.
    d. **True**.
    e. **True**. Direct immunofluorescent stain of skin biopsy taken at the edge of an erythema chronicum migrans lesion can be diagnostic.

11. a. **True**. This includes goat's milk and cheese.
    b. **False**. Brucellosis mainly affects vets, livestock workers and populations that consume unpasteurised dairy products.

c. **True**. Culture requires serum-enriched broth and diagnosis usually is by serology.

d. **False**. Back pain is a surprisingly common feature in acute brucellosis.

e. **True**. Alternatives should be used if the patient is or could be pregnant.

Case history answers

History 1

1. Leptospirosis. In endemic areas, hantavirus infection should be considered as a differential diagnosis.
2. Renal failure, haemorrhage.
3. It might not be too late to attempt isolation of *Leptospira interrogans* from blood (in Fletcher's or similar medium), or from urine after alkalinisation. Otherwise serum should be collected for antigen detection.

History 2

1. Brucellosis. The possibility of goats' milk consumption in an area endemic for brucellosis means the most likely species would be *B. melitensis*.
2. Serology and culture of blood or bone marrow. This case was confirmed by blood culture, although this is achieved in only a minority of cases of brucellosis.
3. A tetracycline, with the possible addition of rifampicin.
4. Tetracycline should not be used. Streptomycin can be used instead, along with the rifampicin. This combination was used for the above patient successfully.

Data interpretation answer

1. This result suggests an infection in the vascular system, most probably infective endocarditis.
2. Careful auscultation may reveal a murmur that was missed at initial examination. In endocarditis murmurs can change. They may also be so subtle as to need confirmation with an echocardiogram.
3. Gastrointestinal pathologies such as polyp or carcinoma are associated with *S. bovis* endocarditis.
4. Erythromycin is not a very satisfactory treatment for endocarditis and a good history of serious adverse reaction to penicillin would make you cautious about using a cephalosporin instead of penicillin. Many would reach for vancomycin, to which this isolate is bound to be sensitive.

OSCE answer

1. Yes. Fever and drowsiness are symptoms and the positive blood cultured was confirmation.
2. Yes. The tenderness is indicative of inflammation of the bile duct and the ultrasound confirmed the presence of gallstones.
3. Yes. Surgery could result in further release of organisms into the systemic system.
4. No. Deteriorating renal function should prompt a choice of antibiotics with Gram-negative activity but not the risk of nephrotoxicity associated with gentamicin.
5. No. While the short incubation time may reflect a high concentration of bacteria in the blood at the time the culture was collected, it is also a function of how quickly the bacteria can grow under laboratory conditions. Numbers of bacteria are not the only measure of severity.

Short notes answers

1. A brief list of clinical features would not be sufficient. A short account of the pathogenesis of the sepsis syndrome should be given. There has been some debate regarding the use of immunomodulators in treatment of the sepsis syndrome. The question requires familiarity with the recent literature.
2. Could be answered in tabular form. Remember the three common rickettsioses covered above: scrub typhus, RMSF and Q fever. All can be prevented by reducing exposure; the first two by vector-related methods (clothing, repellents and behaviour). In Q fever, the disease is transmitted by another route requiring different precautions. A vaccine is available in some countries. (Laboratory workers are also at risk if they handle live rickettsiae.)
3. Requires a little imagination! Probably best to go through the procedure in chronological sequence, thinking about contamination, missed diagnosis, needle-stick injury (and even added discomfort to the patient).

Viva answers

1. You should discuss the importance of initiating antimicrobial therapy *immediately*, using a multiagent regimen based on the clinical features and local conditions. Blood for culture should be taken before therapy is started and this will influence later modification of the presumptive regimen. You should also mention that infections

can be polymicrobial and can be with organisms that are difficult to culture.

2. Base your answer on syphilis (*Treponema pallidum*), Lyme disease (*Borrelia burgdorferi*) and leptospirosis (*Leptospira interrogans*). List the methods available for each in the laboratory and the contribution of

clinical features, geographical location and history to diagnosis. If syphilis is confined to tertiary syphilis (spirochaetes can be demonstrated in the early stage) then this probably has the most problematic laboratory results and the least defining clinical features.

20 Emerging infections

Overview

The growing number of emerging infections has brought a new challenge to the microbiology and treatment of infectious diseases. As the global population expands into new and diverse microbial habitats, people are being exposed to never-before-encountered diseases. Previously known infections may re-emerge by exploiting changes in behaviour and in distribution of the human population. An initial lack of professional expertise or diagnostic laboratory support can lead to significant underdiagnosis of emerging infections and an underestimate of the scale of the problem. Molecular epidemiology, information technology and regional surveillance networks all form a part of the response to emerging infections. Caution should be exercised in pronouncing the eradication of a given infectious disease.

20.1 Emerging and re-emerging infections

Learning objectives

You should:
- be aware of the reasons for the emergence of new infectious diseases
- know the major examples.

In the late 20th century there was optimism that infectious diseases were in decline, at least in developed countries. The announcement that smallpox had been eradicated seemed to confirm that view. This led to a growing indifference towards public and environmental health measures in developing countries, some of which regarded the rise of non-communicable diseases as a measure of developed nation status. A laissez-faire and sometimes frankly complacent attitude to infectious diseases led to the gradual relaxation of public health infrastructure in many parts of the world during the 1970s. The outbreak of Legionnaires' disease in Philadelphia, USA probably marks the turning point, though it was not until the arrival of a previously unknown acquired immune compromise syndrome (AIDS) in homosexual men in North America that the tide of complacency began to turn. Since the late 1970s, a long list of new infections and infectious agents has been compiled. Inevitably, these conditions are at first underdiagnosed. Until clinical and diagnostic expertise has built up, the epidemiology cannot be elucidated.

Notable examples of new infections are given in Table 36.

20.2 Epidemiology

Learning objectives

You should:
- be aware of the infections that are new to humans
- know of the existence of diseases with an unknown infective agent
- be aware of the role of new strains, new toxins and drug resistance in giving rise to new or re-established infections.

Emerging infectious diseases have been defined as including new infections and those infections that already existed but which have undergone a rapid increase in incidence or geographical distribution. The process implied by the word 'emerging' includes:

- movement into a new population
- establishment/dissemination within that population.

Table 36 Selected emerging infectious diseases and their infective cause in approximate chronological order of discovery

Infective agent	Disease
Rotavirus	Major cause of infantile diarrhoea worldwide
Parvovirus B19	Fifth disease, aplastic crisis in chronic haemolytic anaemia
Cryptosporidium parvum	Acute enterocolitis
Ebola virus	Ebola haemorrhagic fever
Legionella pneumophila	Legionnaires' disease
Hantavirus	Haemorrhagic fever with renal syndrome (HFRS)
Campylobacter sp.	Enteritis
Staphylococcus aureus	Toxic shock syndrome
Escherichia coli O157:H7	Haemorrhagic colitis, haemolytic uraemic syndrome
Borrelia burgdorferi	Lyme disease
Human immunodeficiency virus (HIV)	Acquired immunodeficiency syndrome (AIDS)
Helicobacter pylori	Gastric ulcers
Human herpesvirus-6 (HHV-6)	Roseola subitum
Ehrlichia chaffeensis	Human ehrlichiosis
Hepatitis C	Parenterally transmitted non-A, non-B hepatitis
Vibrio cholerae O139	Epidemic cholera
Bartonella (= *Rochalimaea*) *benselae*	Cat-scratch disease, bacillary angiomatosis

There are several features that emerging infections share other than newness, changing incidence or range. Most test the limits of diagnostic laboratory technology, particularly if the infective agent has not previously been encountered in the setting of human disease (e.g. human immunodeficiency virus (HIV) or *Rochalimaea henselae*). But new or altered strains of known infective agents can pose a similar technological challenge if they gain the ability to produce a previously unknown toxin (e.g. *Staphylococcus aureus* in toxic shock syndrome and *Escherichia coli* in haemolytic uraemic syndrome). The problem of emerging infections has increased since the group includes those recently described diseases of presumed infective aetiology whose infective agent has yet to be discovered. The recognition of and progress in understanding major emerging infections such as AIDS have demonstrated how quickly the scientific and medical community can respond to the challenge and have also spurred on critical developments in laboratory medicine. Another group of emerging infections include those caused by previously known infective agents that have acquired significant new antimicrobial resistance mechanisms. While antibiotic resistance per se does not necessarily qualify an infective agent for emerging infection status, the expression of novel resistance factors can significantly alter the presentation of disease or change its epidemiology so that its decline is reversed (e.g. pulmonary tuberculosis in locations with a significant proportion of multidrug-resistant strains). Finally, there are exotic new diseases that appear where the human population has altered its conventional interaction with other animal species (e.g. new variant Creutzfeldt–Jakob disease in western Europe). Strictly speaking, as *Helicobacter pylori* gastritis probably existed long before the causal agent was identified, this infection cannot be properly described as 'emerging'.

Influenza, by comparison, though clearly the cause of epidemics more than a century ago, produces new epidemics as a result of antigenic drift and shift. It is these new influenza events that give the infection its 'emerging' status.

20.3 Ecology

Learning objectives

You should:

- know the factors that assist microbial mobility among populations
- be aware of the ecological reservoirs for infectious agents
- know the role that human manipulation has played in creating new or more virulent pathogens.

The epidemiology of emerging infections highlights the importance of the interaction between humans and their biological environment. Infections that are communicable either directly or indirectly between humans will respond to changes in population distribution, density or behaviour as their causal infective agent gains a selective advantage through the specific features of those changing conditions. Microbial mobility or traffic is a key concept in understanding the complex ecology of emerging infections. Factors that increase the probability of microbial traffic include:

- environmental: climate, agriculture, forestry practice, water supply and natural flow
- human demography and behaviour: urbanisation, war, commerce, tourism, substance abuse, sexual activity

- technological and industrial development: mechanisation, food processing
- microbial adaptation: gene transfer, phenotypic phase variation.

The increasing volume of rapid international travel has contributed to the efficient spread of infectious disease on a global scale. Urbanisation provides increased opportunities for infections that spread easily in overcrowded habitation, such as meningitis and tuberculosis. As the cities sprawl and encroach on the rural environment, so the human population has come into contact with animal and insect vectors of infective agents that they have not previously encountered and to which they may have no effective immunity. The complex ecology of vector-borne and zoonotic infection was appreciated by early parasitologists and tropical medicine specialists. Clearly the domesticated animal population is an important reservoir for human infection, and wild animals probably represent another reservoir of potential human pathogens. Only recently have we begun to understand the wider significance of the inanimate environment to other infectious diseases: events that occur within the mediating environment and modulate the quantity and quality of interactions we have with the microorganisms that live there. These include factors such as phase variation in bacteria and the stress-starvation response, both of which may significantly alter the virulence of a given bacterial strain.

Ecological issues affecting the interaction between human and other species do not only operate on a grand scale. They also function at a cellular and molecular level. This multilevel understanding of ecological interaction between humans and infective agents is referred to as 'biocomplexity' and has been applied with considerable success to certain community-acquired bacterial infections, starting with cholera. It is likely that application of non-linear mathematic techniques will assist the development of predictive models for emerging infection since the characteristics of epidemic spread of some infections have already been analysed using the mathematics of complexity. Universality and scaling are features of complex non-linear systems such as epidemics of emerging infections, which will allow a more mechanistic understanding of the ecology of emerging infection in future. In the meantime, we are restricted by the limits of medical technology to a descriptive approach, which suggests that our best efforts have only met with modest success.

The most sinister recent development in the ecology of emerging infection is the consequence of deliberate human manipulation of infective agents. When human experimentation leads to a more virulent novel strain of infective agent, or to a new agent altogether, the product

of these experiments must be carefully contained. Inadequate laboratory disposal methods or inadvertent release into the surrounding environment can have tragic consequences (e.g. the Sverdlovsk anthrax incident). Deliberate release of infectious agents (such as *Bacillus anthracis*) with enhanced or atypical infectivity, for military or terrorist purposes illustrates how a knowledge of the ecology of infections can be twisted and abused for sinister ends.

20.4 Diagnosis

Learning objectives

You should:

- be aware of the use of genetic and typing technology in identifying and surveying infections
- be aware of internet sources of information on newer infections.

By definition, emerging infections are diseases in which infectious disease physicians, microbiologists and public health specialists have limited expertise. Until clinical and diagnostic experience has built up, diagnoses may be missed or significantly delayed, particularly in clinical settings where workload is high and laboratory support poor. It is not practicable to maintain the high-end technology (such as broad-band polymerase chain reaction (PCR) and other molecular diagnostic techniques used for syndromes with presumed infective aetiology) in more than a handful of reference centres. The optimal diagnostic approach at the face-to-face bedside level appears to be a low threshold of suspicion in cases of undiagnosed infection. Persistence may be necessary in establishing the identity of the causal agent or a non-infective explanation in diseases of presumed infective aetiology. Use of the whole range of conventional diagnostic laboratory technology including histopathology, haematology, biochemistry and immunology will help to delineate the pathology of the condition even if it proves impossible to put a name to it. Thorough diagnostic imaging may lead to the discovery of occult loci of focal infection or the involvement of additional organ systems. The internet, worldwide web and other emerging technologies are a useful source of up-to-date information on the diagnosis of emerging infections. Nucleic acid amplification technology (PCR) has become increasingly important in the laboratory diagnosis of emerging infections caused by non-culturable microorganisms. Newer bacterial subtyping methods, which when combined can give a high degree of discrimination between strains of a given species, are being used by sentinel public health laboratories for surveillance of key community-acquired infections. DNA macrorestriction (pulsed field gel electrophoresis) is now used extensively by food hygiene laboratories for subtyping food-borne pathogens and the results are exchanged via the internet in a system called PulseNet. A standard Southern blotting protocol based on insertion sequence IS 6110 has been used internationally to track the spread of *Mycobacterium tuberculosis*. A more recent technique called spoligotyping is now being used to characterise the same species.

20.5 Treatment and global response

Learning objectives

You should:

- be aware of new treatment modalities
- know about the central collection of data and means of accessing information.

Treatment

Once a specific emerging infection has been successfully diagnosed, the attending physician may feel that the bigger part of the challenge has been completed. In some cases this is true. However, the majority of emerging infections remain difficult to treat and in some cases no specific treatment is yet available. The longer lead time to specific aetiological diagnosis can hamper the beneficial effects of antimicrobial therapy. Clearly, in the case of diseases such as AIDS, major advances have been made in effective antiretroviral therapy. Bacterial infections such as *Campylobacter* enteritis and *H. pylori* gastritis can be treated with specific agents from a range of antibacterial agents already available. But specific antiviral treatment for some of the emerging viral infections (e.g. hantavirus pulmonary syndrome) is not available.

Global response to emerging infections

The scale of the emerging infectious diseases problem has provoked a worldwide response, beginning with a collaboration between several leading centres in North America, western Europe and further afield. In less than a decade, an international network of interested professionals has grown. Organisations such as the World Health Organization (WHO), the Centers for Disease Control and prevention (DC; Atlanta, USA), various national public health laboratories and other reference centres exchange information that supplements WHO

and national notifiable disease data. Information gathering requires specific case definitions, backed by accurate diagnostic laboratory results. Only when the data are able to discriminate between strains or subtypes of an infective agent that cause different disease outcomes can they be used to guide disease control interventions, as happened when hepatitis C virus was identified as the commonest cause of non-A non-B viral hepatitis, and when capsular type b *H. influenzae* was recognised as the commonest cause of invasive *H. influenzae* infection. Information gathering is difficult to sustain unless the interest of the supplier is kept alive by a matching feedback of useful information. The internet and worldwide web have provided an effective means of sharing information, analyses and insights rapidly. Internet bulletin board systems (e.g. ProMED) and on-line journals (e.g. EID (Emerging Infectious Diseases)) are an important component of the global response to the emerging infection challenge. However, it is inevitable that there will be further emerging infection incidents, some catastrophic, in future years. Another essential aspect of the global response is the regional collaborative network that functions both as a collective early warning system and as a means of accessing specialist assistance when local resources are insufficient for the task. Locally, regionally and internationally, the capacity to respond rapidly to an outbreak requires close professional collaboration, a high level of laboratory infrastructure with additional capacity for unplanned contingencies, and public health leadership. Currently, these factors exist in combination in only a few major reference centres. Until the growing complexity of infectious diseases is matched by a better framework for communicable disease surveillance and control, the front-line physician will remain vulnerable to unforeseen emerging infections.

20.6 Specific emerging infections

Learning objectives

You should:

- know the characteristics of the current emerging infections
- know the factors contributing to their occurrence
- know the basis of their management.

Influenza

Influenza follows a pattern of seasonal peaks on which are superimposed periodic epidemics and pandemics. Seasonal epidemics are the result of subtle changes in surface antigens: antigenic drift. Major epidemics and pandemics are caused by genetic recombination events involving avian influenza virus. Pig–duck proximity is thought to have been an important source. The H5N1 epidemic in Hong Kong was brought under control quickly as a result of effective surveillance and prompt public health intervention.

New variant Creutzfeldt–Jakob disease

New variant Creutzfeldt–Jakob disease is a fatal neuro-degenerative disease epidemiologically linked to the European bovine spongiform encephalopathy epidemic. While the origins of the outbreak remain controversial, changes in livestock rearing practice and in particular the supply of rendered bovine material in animal feed are generally thought to have contributed to the genesis of the bovine infection. The majority of human cases so far have been diagnosed in the UK, where the cattle epidemic was largest.

Acquired immunodeficiency syndrome

AIDS was first recognised in the 1980s. It is now thought to have arisen earlier in central Africa, where there may have been initial transfer of HIV from another primate species. It is likely that initial interspecies transmission went unnoticed as long as it resulted in sporadic cases in relatively isolated rural communities. It has been suggested that the AIDS pandemic might have been contained if a better health infrastructure had been present in central Africa. However, HIV has demonstrated abilities that exploit aspects of sexual behaviour, intravenous drug abuse, the presence of other infections such as tuberculosis and travel patterns to the point where AIDS has affected the entire world population.

Resistant Staphylococcus aureus

Strains of *Staphylococcus aureus* resistant to the oxazolyl penicillins (MRSA) were thought of as hospital pathogens until recently, when they began to appear more frequently in community-acquired infections. This development significantly reduces the choice of antibiotics available for treatment of staphylococcal infections. The appearance of *S. aureus* strains with reduced sensitivity to vancomycin (VISA) presents a threat of further reduction in key therapeutic options. Nursing home and extended care facilities have become an important reservoir of MRSA that bridges the gap between hospital and community.

Tuberculosis

Tuberculosis was in decline in most developed countries in the early 1980s. Since then, several countries have shown a reversal of this decline and in some locations there has been a significant rise in pulmonary tuberculosis. A part of this trend has been attributed to AIDS. But other factors, most notably the occurrence of multidrug resistance, have played an important part in the re-emergence of tuberculosis.

Lyme disease

Lyme disease has become a noted infection in parts of North America and western Europe where infection with *Borrelia burgdorferi* results from the bite of an *Ixodid* (hard-bodied) tick. In the eastern United States, Lyme disease is a problem in communities near areas of reforestation where deer ticks are the vector and forest deer the principal host for *B. burgdorferi*.

Enterohaemorrhagic Escherichia coli

Haemorrhagic colitis and haemolytic uraemic syndrome are caused by verotoxin-bearing strains of *E. coli*, in particular *E. coli* O157:H7. Sporadic cases and occasional outbreaks have been associated with butchering and meat processing practices that contaminate raw meat with toxin bearing strains. Minced and other beef products have been an important food vehicle for verotoxin-positive *E. coli* and thus a source of human infection.

20.7 Further reading

Bonn D 2001 Biocomplexity: look at the whole, not the parts. Lancet 357: 288

Emerging Infectious Diseases on-line journal: http://www.cdc.gov/ncidod/eid/index.htm

Garrett L 1995 The coming plague: infectious diseases in a world out of balance. Virago, London

Garrett L 2000 Betrayal of trust: the collapse of global public health. Hyperion, New York

Morse SS 1995 Factors in the emergence of infectious diseases. Emerging Infectious Diseases 1: 8–10

Satcher D 1995 Emerging infections: getting ahead of the curve. Emerging Infectious Diseases 1: 1–7

Self-assessment: questions

Multiple choice questions

1. The following conditions can properly be referred to as 'emerging infections':
   a. Meningococcal meningitis
   b. Hantavirus pulmonary syndrome
   c. MRSA
   d. VISA infection
   e. Pneumococcal pneumonia

2. In emerging infections, the infection is:
   a. New to the population
   b. Of increasing incidence
   c. Of increasing geographical range
   d. Of increased severity
   e. Of increased duration

3. The following bacterial agents of infection were first described during the 1980s and 1990s:
   a. Ebola virus
   b. Human immunodeficiency virus 1
   c. *Escherichia coli*
   d. Hepatitis B
   e. *Bartonella henselae*

4. The following factors contribute to the risk of emerging infections:
   a. Rainforest clearance
   b. Reforestation
   c. International travel
   d. Local travel
   e. Novel food technology

5. Of the following, the three most important components of the response to emerging infections are:
   a. Improved antibiotic susceptibility testing methods
   b. Prospective surveillance of specific infectious agents
   c. Networked information dissemination
   d. Capacity for rapid outbreak response
   e. Local expertise with a wide range of new infective agents

Objective structured clinical examination (OSCE)

After admission of a 23-year-old woman with clinical features of encephalitis and acute respiratory distress, it is discovered from discussions with other residents and staff that there have been three other young adults with a similar clinical presentation admitted during the last week. The necessary diagnostic tests and immediate supportive measures are arranged. After review by an intensivist, she is moved to the intensive care unit. You are asked to consider this in regard to what might be going on in the community.

1. Do you think that the initial non-specific tests are of little epidemiological value?
2. Do you think that the rumours from other patients are not important?
3. Should the public health physician only be notified once a notifiable disease has been properly diagnosed?
4. Once the obvious infective diagnoses have been excluded, do you think that the microbiology laboratory will have anything else to offer?
5. Even if a case cluster can be confirmed, do you think it is likely to excite wider professional interest?

Viva questions

1. What is the relevance of domestic animals to emerging infectious diseases?
2. What features of infection would make you suspect a biological weapon attack?
3. How does the diagnostic laboratory contribute to emerging infection surveillance?

Self-assessment: answers

Multiple choice answers

1. a. **False**. This has a long history.
   b. **True**. Hantavirus also causes haemorrhagic fever.
   c. **False**. This is a form of the bacterium *Staphylococcus aureus* (methicillin-resistant *S. aureus*), not an infection per se.
   d. **True**. Intermediate vancomycin susceptibility *S. aureus* infections are only recently described.
   e. **False**. This has a long history.

2. a. **True**. Emerging infections include those that move into a new population.
   b. **True**. A rapid increase in incidence can allow an existing infection to be considered as emerging.
   c. **True**. Changing human behaviour, such as travel, can contribute.
   d. **False**. Not in the original description.
   e. **False**. Not in the original description.

3. a. **False**. It was first observed in 1976.
   b. **True**. Identified in the early 1980s.
   c. **False**. But the O157:H7 strain was first recognised in 1982.
   d. **False**. Hepatitis C is a recent discovery.
   e. **True**. The cause of cat-scratch disease was recognised in 1992.

4. a. **True**. This allows microbial and human traffic to and from an area with new insect and animal vectors.
   b. **True**. Zoonotic infections such as Lyme disease increase.
   c. **True**. This allows individuals to come into contact with (and transmit) diseases for which they have no natural immunity.
   d. **True**. Local travel between city and rural communities or vice versa may contribute to the traffic of microorganisms in various ways.
   e. **True**. This can bring new microorganisms into the human foodchain and in fact has led to the emergence of haemorrhagic colitis.

5. a. **False**.
   b. **True**.
   c. **True**. Allows both a collective early warning system and rapid access to specialist advice.
   d. **True**. This provides a laboratory infrastructure and a planned response with specialist support.
   e. **False**. Impractical for all but the largest reference centres.

OSCE answer

1. No. All laboratory tests that produce an out-of-range result may contribute to a case definition.
2. Yes. Other patients that have been admitted earlier are likely to have completed a more comprehensive diagnostic workup. Some hospitals are using software to accelerate diagnosis of unusual syndromes by comparing a new patient's dataset with those of other patients with similar presentations.
3. No. Public health measures such as disease control or environmental health interventions need to be introduced as quickly as possible to arrest an outbreak of acute, communicable disease. The earlier the authorities have the information, no matter how incomplete, the better prepared they will be when action is required.
4. Yes. At the very least, serum and any tissue specimens should be stored by the laboratory for future analysis. Some reference laboratories may be able to use molecular methods based on broad band polymerase chain reaction or small subunit RNA to identify a presumed infective agent, even in the absence of specific clues. A specific aetiological diagnosis can be established in a proportion of cases by serological tests since some patients may be late seroconverters.
5. Yes. There are several international projects underway that target syndromes of presumed infective aetiology. Your cluster may be the one that adds the missing detail. If not, it may still provide the world with a new infective agent to worry about.

Viva answers

1. Domestic animals act as a reservoir for zoonotic infections and add a further step in the ecology of infections that require a vector. Integrated pig–duck farming may have contributed to recent influenza outbreaks in East Asia. Domestication of new species could introduce new pathogens to the human food chain or to livestock handlers. Changes in food production practice have led to the emergence of haemorrhagic colitis and possibly to new variant Creutzfeldt–Jakob disease.
2. A biological weapon (BW) attack should be suspected if the infective agent is on the known BW list, is very unusual in that epidemiological setting (e.g. pulmonary plague in a developed country, anthrax in an urban setting) or has an unusual

clinical presentation (whole body vesiculopustular rash as in smallpox). The list of possible features is very long. Probably the single most important consideration is to expect the unexpected. Remember that a higher level of biocontainment will be required than might at first seem necessary. Leave speculation about who is to blame to the police. Leave heroics to the security forces and film actors.

3. The diagnostic laboratory is often the first line of hard data collection for surveillance of emerging infections. Laboratory case descriptions are becoming increasingly important in monitoring the emergence and spread of infection as public health authorities move towards evidence-based practice. Specific pathogen data are needed before disease control or environmental health measures can be effectively targetted. Trends must be examined to assess the impact of those measures. Subtyping of infective agents improves the specificity of surveillance and targetting of interventions. Molecular epidemiology is being used with increasing confidence for surveillance purposes, and as part of the laboratory's contribution to outbreak response. The larger reference laboratories with an interest in specific emerging infections often provide confirmatory diagnostic methods that are not available commercially.

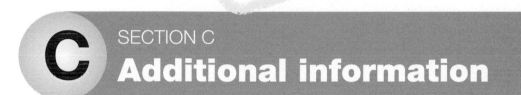

SECTION C
Additional information

21 Bacteriology

Overview

This chapter is concerned with the more common bacterial causes of infection. Bacteria are grouped according to their major classes. Their biology, ecology, mechanisms of disease, identification, therapy and typing are reviewed.

Learning objectives

You should:

- know the principal groups of bacteria
- know the infections they cause
- know key laboratory tests used to detect and identify them
- know antibiotics used to treat their infections.

21.1 Gram-positive bacteria

Cocci

Staphylococci

The staphylococci are a group of Gram-positive cocci that tend to form clusters. Although 14 species are known to cause human infections, the vast majority of infections are caused by *Staphylococcus aureus, Staphylococcus epidermidis* and *Staphylococcus saprophyticus*. Of these, the single most important species is *S. aureus*.

Characteristics

Staphylococci grow easily under aerobic conditions on blood and other non-selective agars. They are catalase positive, and almost all *S. aureus* strains are also coagulase positive. Confirmation of the rare coagulase-negative strains can be made by detection of protein A or DNAase. *S. saprophyticus* can be distinguished from *S. epidermidis* by its resistance to the antibiotic novobiocin. Another useful property of *S. aureus* is its ability to ferment mannitol.

Staphylococci are found on the skin and mucosal surfaces of humans and other animals. *S. aureus* has a predilection for the anterior nares, the groins and perineum. *S. epidermidis* tends to be spread more widely over the skin surface. Around 25% of adults have nasal colonisation with *S. aureus*, and the number is higher in patients with diabetes or renal failure. Some strains produce a polysaccharide capsule that may help them to resist phagocytosis. *S. epidermidis* can produce a matrix of extracellular polysaccharide (slime) that assists in adhesion to plastic medical devices. Around 100% of patients with chronic skin disease are colonised by *S. aureus*.

Staphylococcus aureus

S. aureus, the most pathogenic of staphylococci, produces a variety of enzymes and toxins that are thought to contribute to the development of disease. The exact role of many of these is not yet known, but the important factors include catalase (inactivates hydrogen peroxide), coagulase, leukocidin and the toxins TSST (toxic shock syndrome toxin), enterotoxin and exfoliatin.

S. aureus produces invasive and toxin diseases. The invasive diseases include:

- superficial pustule or boil
- surgical wound infection
- abscesses of deep soft tissue, brain or lung
- osteomyelitis
- septicaemia.

The toxin diseases depend on the action of *S. aureus* toxins and are:

- toxic shock syndrome
- scalded skin syndrome
- food poisoning.

Toxic shock syndrome is a condition that was originally seen in women using hyperabsorbent tampons. It includes fever, hypovolaemia, vomiting and other multisystem features. It has also been recognised in male patients and in patients with pre-existing invasive staphylococcal infection. These toxins belong to the family of molecules known as superantigens.

Staphylococcus epidermidis

S. epidermidis is an important bacterial pathogen in compromised hospital patients, particularly premature neonates and patients with invasive medical devices such as intravascular cannulas. It produces extracellular polysaccharide that enables it to stick to plastic devices. Infection may be difficult to eradicate without first removing the device.

Staphylococcus saprophyticus

S. saprophyticus only appears to cause infection in the urinary tract, almost exclusively in adult women, in which it accounts for around 10% of cases of cystitis.

Control

Staphylococci can be treated with a variety of antibiotics. Unfortunately, acquired resistance has reduced the choice available, particularly in hospital practice. Less than 10% of *S. aureus* from hospital patients are sensitive to penicillin. The remainder produce β-lactamases, and must be treated with a β-lactamase-resistant isoxazolyl penicillin (e.g. flucloxacillin, dicloxacillin). A proportion of these strains have also acquired resistance to this group of antibiotics ('methicillin resistance', known as MRSA) and must be treated with a non-β-lactam agent such as vancomycin. Methicillin resistance is caused by alterations in a penicillin-binding protein PBP_2.

In view of the frequency of hospital-acquired infections with *S. aureus*, it is often necessary to perform typing studies on strains isolated from several patients to establish whether or not an outbreak has occurred. Phage typing, or one of the newer molecular techniques (e.g. pulsed field gel electrophoresis (PFGE)) help to determine just how indistinguishable staphylococcal strains from different sources are. The earlier typing systems are limited by a high proportion of untypable strains, making the system more suitable for excluding a common source than for confirming one.

Streptococci

The streptococci are a group of Gram-positive cocci that have a tendency to form chains. There are several genera of streptococci, classified according to their salient features, which include:

- the type of haemolysis produced on blood agar
- the optimal condition for growth
- susceptibility to inhibitor compounds.

Beta-haemolytic streptococci

The β-haemolytic streptococci are a group of Gram-positive, chain-forming cocci that produce haemolysins, which cause a zone of clearing around bacterial colonies growing on blood agar. The effect is best seen on sheep blood agar. This group of streptococci is further subdivided according to the polysaccharide antigen present in the bacterial cell wall. This is detected by latex agglutination (Table 37). Important groups encountered in medical practice are A, B, C, D, F and G, although others are isolated from time to time.

Group A. The one species in this group *S. pyogenes* is an important cause of human disease. Conditions caused are:

- invasive: impetigo, pharyngitis, lymphangitis, necrotising fasciitis, septicaemia
- toxic: streptococcal toxic shock syndrome, scarlet fever
- postinfective: rheumatic fever, glomerulonephritis, Sydenham's chorea.

A recent increase in streptococcal pyrogenic exotoxin-bearing strains has accompanied increasing reports of invasive group A streptococcal disease in developed countries. The majority of group A streptococci are penicillin sensitive, although increased minimum inhibitory concentration (MIC) is recognised with increasing frequency. Resistance to the macrolides (e.g. erythromycin), a useful alternative for penicillin-sensitive patients, is much more common. Typing of clinical isolates is not commonly practised and relies on differences in M and T antigens. The M antigen is antiphagocytic and, therefore a virulence factor. DNA macrorestriction analysis (PFGE) is a more recent option for molecular typing.

Group B. These streptococci are present in the indigenous vaginal flora of healthy adult women.

Table 37 Streptococci grouped by polysaccharide antigen

Group	Species	Diseases
A	*S. pyogenes*	Impetigo, pharyngitis, lymphangitis, septicaemia, necrotising fasciitis, toxic shock syndrome, rheumatic fever, scarlet fever, rheumatic heart disease, glomerulonephritis, Sydenham's chorea
B	*S. agalactiae*	Neonatal septicaemia, meningitis
C	*S. equi, S. equisimilis, S. zooepidemicus, S. equinus*	Pharyngitis, septicaemia
D	*S. bovis*	Septicaemia, endocarditis
F	*S. anginosus/ milleri*	Abscess, endocarditis, septicaemia
G	*S. anginosus*	Pharyngitis, endocarditis

However, they may cause septicaemia and meningitis in newborn infants, particularly following prematurely ruptured membranes. The species is susceptible to penicillin and ampicillin.

Groups C and G. These β-haemolytic streptococci are found in the oropharynx of healthy subjects and may rarely contribute to pharyngitis. However, they do not cause the severe invasive, toxic or postinfective disease associated with group A streptococci. Some strains of group C streptococci have occasionally been known to cause fatal septicaemia.

Group D. In this group, *S. bovis*, a penicillin-susceptible species, is associated with colonic carcinoma. It is occasionally isolated from patients with bacteraemia. The enterococci (see below) are closely related to this group but are bile salt tolerant.

Group F. These streptococci are part of a group of streptococci that some microbiologists know as *S. milleri*. This group is found on human mucosal surfaces and can cause invasive disease involving deep soft tissues, including bacterial liver abscess. This streptococcus is sometimes recognised in the laboratory by its characteristic caramel odour.

Viridans group streptococci

The viridans streptococci are α-haemolytic, i.e. they cause green discoloration of a thin ring of blood agar around each colony through the action of an α-haemolysin. The group includes a number of commensal species present in the oropharyngeal flora, each with slightly different preferred sites: *S. mitior*, *S. mitis*, *S. mutans* and *S. salivarius*. Production of the sticky substance dextran by *S. mutans* contributes to the formation of dental caries. The other biomedical significance of these species is that bacteraemia resulting from dental procedures (scaling, tooth extraction) will disseminate these species into the bloodstream. In patients with damaged natural heart valves or prosthetic valves, infective endocarditis may result. These species are usually penicillin susceptible, but some strains may be tolerant, i.e. while being inhibited by penicillin, they require much higher concentrations to ensure a bactericidal effect.

Streptococcus pneumoniae ('pneumococcus')

S. pneumoniae is a Gram-positive diplococcus that appears α-haemolytic on blood agar. Mature colonies can have a depressed centre caused by autolysis, resulting in the so-called 'draughtsman' appearance. The cocci are slightly elongated along their long axis and may possess a polysaccharide capsule. *S. pneumoniae* is susceptible to optochin (ethyl hydrocuprein), a specific antibacterial compound. They are also susceptible to lysis in the presence of bile salts; a feature that is sometimes used to make a presumptive identification in the laboratory. The capsular polysaccharide, of which there

are over 80 types known, is a major virulence factor since it interferes with phagocytosis. *S. pneumoniae* is found in the oro- and nasopharyngeal flora of healthy individuals. The organism is transmitted via the respiratory route in droplet nuclei and can cause a variety of life-threatening diseases including pneumonia and meningitis. Asplenic patients are at risk of pneumococcal peritonitis. *S. pneumoniae* can also cause infection in the structures adjacent to the upper respiratory tract, resulting in acute sinusitis and otitis media.

Penicillin is the treatment for severe pneumococcal infections, but there have been recent reports of increasing penicillin MIC in clinical isolates. These moderately resistant strains may be missed in the diagnostic laboratory unless specific tests for these strains are carried out. Erythromycin is often used as an alternative treatment in patients with penicillin allergy (though not suitable for meningitis), but resistance is common in some centres. Alternatives include chloramphenicol and the third-generation cephalosporins.

Epidemiological studies are usually based on the capsular typing using specific antisera. Only a few capsular types predominate in a particular area. This information is used to help in the manufacture of the polyvalent pneumococcal vaccine.

Enterococci

The enterococci are a group of bacteria closely related to group D streptococci. They have group D polysaccharide and are bile tolerant, which enables them to grow in the gastrointestinal tract where they are present as minority members of the indigenous flora. They can therefore be grown on MacConkey agar. The most common member of the genus is *Enterococcus faecalis*, which is a cause of urinary tract and hospital-acquired infections. The other species encountered in hospital practice is *Enterococcus faecium*. Both species are intrinsically resistant to penicillin but can usually be treated with ampicillin. Nitrofurantoin or trimethoprim is usually satisfactory for enterococcal urinary tract infection. There are increasing reports of ampicillin-resistant *E. faecium*, and gentamicin- and vancomycin-resistant *E. faecalis*.

Anaerobic streptococci

Some streptococcal species are unable to tolerate even low concentrations of oxygen and are therefore obligate anaerobes. These include peptococcus and peptostreptococcus: species found in the enteric and vaginal flora. Full identification of these species is often not completed in the diagnostic laboratory since it may add substantial delays to the release of laboratory reports.

These species are isolated from polymicrobial collections such as abscesses in the brain, abdomen and pelvic organs. Both species are usually sensitive to penicillin and metronidazole.

Bacilli

The Gram-positive bacilli (rod-shaped) include five major groups of organism:

- aerobic spore-formers
- aerobic non-spore-formers
- irregular staining non-spore-formers
- branching bacilli
- anaerobic species.

Aerobic spore-forming bacilli

Bacillus cereus

Bacillus cereus is a spore-forming Gram-positive bacillus that grows easily on blood agar under aerobic conditions. It forms rough, spreading colonies with root-like projections and is haemolytic. *B. cereus* is widely spread throughout the environment and is also present as a commensal member of the intestinal flora.

Two important enterotoxins are known: one emetic and the other diarrhoeagenic. The species is responsible for food poisoning, and the emetic form is commonly seen after consumption of Chinese fried rice. Culture of single stool specimens for *B. cereus* is rarely helpful, unless quantitative methods are used as part of a larger epidemiological study.

Bacillus anthracis

Bacillus anthracis is a spore-forming Gram-positive bacillus that grows on blood agar with a characteristic non-haemolytic 'medusa-head' colony. The species is found in the environment, particularly in association with domestic animals.

B. anthracis is responsible for a rare ulcerating skin infection and for a rapidly fatal pulmonary infection transmitted by inhalation of spores. For this reason, diagnostic specimens and bacterial isolates from patients with suspected anthrax must be handled by laboratory staff under a high level of biocontainment to prevent laboratory-acquired infection. *B. anthracis* is susceptible to penicillin.

Aerobic non-spore-forming bacilli

The aerobic non-spore formers include *Listeria* and *Erysipelothrix*. Both of these species are found in the environment and in the intestinal tract of a variety of species.

Listeria spp.

The genus *Listeria* includes *L. monocytogenes* and *L. ivanovii*: the two species responsible for human infection. Listeria grows on blood agar and produces small grey/blue colonies with a narrow zone of β-haemolysis. The genus is catalase positive, a feature useful in differ-

entiating it from streptococci. Listeria also has a characteristic tumbling motility when incubated in broth at 22°C. Listeria can grow at low temperatures and can be selected in the laboratory by cold enrichment.

It is still not clear exactly how listeria causes disease in humans, but disease takes a variety of forms from a mild, influenza-like condition to neonatal meningitis, septicaemia and stillbirth (extreme variant is granulomatosis infantiseptica). Infants, the immunocompromised and elderly people are at particular risk of infection. There has been debate over how the disease is transmitted. Epidemics have been associated with consumption of soft cheeses, other dairy products and processed meats. Endemic disease may also be associated with a variety of foods, particularly those stored at low temperature after cooking for consumption at a later date.

Erysipelothrix rhusiopathiae

Erysipelothrix rhusiopathiae is another non-spore-forming Gram-positive bacillus that grows on blood agar under aerobic conditions. There is no haemolysis and the bacillus is catalase negative, distinguishing it from *Listeria* spp. *Erysipelothrix* sp. is widely dispersed in the environment and is particularly common in the intestines of pigs and some fish.

E. rhusiopathiae causes a superficial skin infection known as erysipeloid, in which the skin becomes indurated and bluish in colour. Cases of endocarditis have been reported.

E. rhusiopathiae is resistant to vancomycin and the aminoglycosides and should be treated with penicillin.

Irregularly staining non-spore-forming bacilli

Coryneform bacteria

The coryneform bacteria are irregularly staining Gram-positive bacilli belonging to the genus *Corynebacterium*. They tend to line up in irregular patterns on Gram stain, known as 'Chinese letter' or 'picket fence' formation. The most important member of the genus is *C. diphtheriae*, the cause of diphtheria. This species is an aerobic Gram-positive rod that grows on blood agar but, because of the presence of a luxuriant regional flora, requires the use of selective media such as tellurite agar. Growing on tellurite medium, *C. diphtheriae* has characteristic features that help in identification and also in differentiation of biovars into *gravis*, *intermedius* and *mitis* types. Staining of individual colonies of *C. diphtheriae* with methylene blue shows up prominent metachromatic granules.

Pathogenic members of the species produce a toxin that causes formation of an inflammatory exudate in the oropharynx of the infected patient. Systemic dissemination of the toxin results in cardiac and neurotoxicity. Expression of the toxin depends on the presence of a bacteriophage: β-phage.

The main reservoir of *C. diphtheriae* appears to be asymptomatic and convalescent carriers, and during epidemics β-phage-negative strains can be isolated. Bacteriological diagnosis of diphtheria depends on both isolation of the organism and then demonstration of the toxin either by animal test or by in vitro assay.

There are other corynebacteria (e.g. *C. ulcerans*, an important veterinary pathogen) that cause pharyngitis without more severe consequences. Other corynebacteria such as *C. jeikeium* have been associated with infections in immunocompromised patients.

Branching bacilli

Nocardia spp.
The most important branching Gram-positive bacilli are the nocardioform bacteria. These are bacteria that form slow-growing wrinkled colonies. Some have mycelia and sporulate, thus bearing a superficial resemblance to fungi. However, these species have no defined nucleus or intracellular organelles. They are prokaryotes and are bacteria because their cell walls contain muramic acid. The most common species encountered is *Nocardia*. Nocardias are moderately acid fast and can be demonstrated in a modified Ziehl–Neelsen stain. They require a prolonged period of incubation before the typical 'breadcrumb' colonies can be recognised. *N. asteroides* can cause focal, cavitating pulmonary infection, which may be mistaken for pulmonary tuberculosis. Infection by these organisms is associated with renal transplantation and other types of compromised defence. *Nocardia* species are usually susceptible to sulphonamide antibiotics and some cephalosporins.

Actinomyces spp.
Another group of branching Gram-positive bacilli are the actinomycetes, the commonest of which is *Actinomyces israelii*. These bacteria are not acid fast but grow on blood agar quite slowly, the colonies initially producing fine, spidery projections. Many strains grow better under anaerobic conditions, though they may not necessarily be true obligate anaerobes.

Actinomycetes are present in soil and are only opportunist pathogens, but they can cause a range of invasive infections, including cervicofacial, thoracic, abdominal and pelvic actinomycosis. *A. israelii* causes inflammatory exudate and fibrosis, and it has the ability to spread across tissue planes, causing confusion with malignant disease from time to time. In chronic disease, sinus tracks may form and purulent exudate with flecks of

tangled bacteria ('sulphur granules') may be discharged.

Actinomycetes are usually susceptible to penicillin. Detailed identification and typing has to be carried out by reference laboratories and may require gas–liquid chromatography.

Anaerobic bacilli

Clostridium perfringens
Clostridium perfringens is a spore-forming Gram-positive bacillus that grows preferentially under anaerobic conditions to form spreading grey colonies. Spores are rarely formed under conditions of optimal growth. A variety of exotoxins are formed including a lecithinase.

C. perfringens causes a progressive necrosis of striated muscle, either following contamination of a traumatic wound or in the presence of impaired circulation; a condition known as 'gas gangrene' or clostridial myonecrosis (there are other members of the genus that can cause gas gangrene, e.g. *C. noyvii* and *C. septicum*).

Some strains of *C. perfringens* produce an enterotoxin that can cause food poisoning, typically with abdominal pain and diarrhoea after a 12-hour incubation period. In rare instances, a more severe intestinal disease, necrotic enteritis, can follow ingestion of *C. perfringens*. *C. perfringens* is present in the intestinal flora of humans and other animals and is widespread in the environment, particularly where human sewage or animal manure has been distributed.

The organisms are susceptible to penicillin and metronidazole. Serological typing of *C. perfringens* is sometimes performed by reference laboratories as part of the investigation of food-borne outbreaks.

Clostridium tetani
Clostridium tetani is a Gram-positive bacterium with terminal spores that give the bacillus a drum-stick appearance. The species is highly anaerobic but can be grown on blood agar, on which it forms flat, irregular edged, spreading colonies. Though present in similar habitats to *C. perfringens*, *C. tetani* is difficult to isolate in clinical practice.

C. tetani produces a potent neurotoxin, tetanospasmin, that binds to presynaptic inhibitory neurones. Deep inoculation into a traumatic wound, no matter how small, can cause tetanus, a disease almost entirely caused by the action of bacterial toxin.

C. tetani is susceptible to penicillin and metronidazole.

Clostridium botulinum
Clostridium botulinum is a spore-forming Gram-positive bacillus that will only grow on blood agar in a strictly anaerobic environment.

C. botulinum produces a potent neurotoxin that acts on the bulbar cranial nerves and motor neurones to produce a flaccid paralysis of respiratory and facial muscles. The organism is widespread in the environment and is present in the enteric flora of domestic animals. The spores of *C. botulinum* are relatively heat resistant, so that neurotoxic food poisoning can result from ingestion of the bacterium. Foodstuffs implicated are home bottled or canned items, such as honey. Outbreaks have involved duck pâté and yoghurt.

Clostridium difficile

Clostridium difficile is an anaerobic, spore-forming Gram-positive bacillus commonly found in the enteric flora of a variety of animal species, including humans. *C. difficile* grows on blood agar and can be isolated from specimens contaminated with other species if heat shock or alcohol pretreatment is used.

This species is responsible for antibiotic-associated diarrhoea and pseudomembranous colitis, preceded by overgrowth caused by the elimination of antibiotic-sensitive bacteria as a result of antimicrobial chemotherapy.

While resistant to many of the β-lactam antibiotics, *C. difficile* is sensitive to vancomycin, metronidazole and bacitracin. Molecular typing has been used to demonstrate patient-to-patient spread in a hospital setting.

21.2 Gram-negative bacteria

Enteric bacilli

The proper name for this group of bacteria is the Enterobacteriaceae, though they are sometimes colloquially known as 'coliforms'. These are a group of Gram-negative bacilli that ferment glucose, are oxidase negative, grow both aerobically and anaerobically (facultative anaerobes) and are commonly found in the intestinal flora. All these species will grow quickly on blood agar and will grow in the presence of bile salts.

The enteric Gram-negative bacilli all have a lipopolysaccharide (endotoxin) in the cell wall that bears the type-specific polysaccharide O chain. Some species are motile as a result of the action of flagella. Some species have an antiphagocytic capsule and some produce important exotoxins.

Members of this group are amongst the most common bacterial species encountered in hospital practice, while many are also important causes of infectious disease in community practice. The enteric Gram-negative bacilli are present in the intestinal contents of many other animal species and are widely distributed in the inanimate environment, particularly where sewage or manure has been.

Escherichia coli

E. coli is the most commonly isolated member of the Enterobacteriaceae and is an indole-positive lactose fermenter. Some specific serotypes of *E. coli* have pathogenicity factors that assist adherence to mucosal cells, invasion into underlying tissues, or cause alterations in mucosal function.

E. coli can cause enteric infection, urinary tract infection, septicaemia and endotoxic shock, and a variety of hospital-acquired infections (Table 38).

Many clinical isolates have plasmid-borne antibiotic-resistance factors, such as β-lactamases, making it difficult to predict antimicrobial susceptibility. Comparison of clinical isolates is usually done on the strength of phenotypic characteristics, but genetic typing methods may be required in specific settings.

Klebsiella–Enterobacter–Serratia group

The K–E–S group contains three metabolically active genera that are particularly important as a cause of hospital-acquired infections.

Klebsiella is a lactose-fermenting genus that often produces very mucoid colonies on solid media.

Serratia spp. may produce colonies that are naturally pigmented red.

They may cause community-acquired urinary tract infection, severe Gram-negative pneumonia and other infections. *Klebsiella* spp. are easily spread in hospitals on the hands of staff.

Many isolates are resistant to ampicillin (almost 100% klebsiellas), and this group has seen an increased incidence of resistance to extended-spectrum cephalosporins (e.g. cefotaxime, ceftriaxone and ceftazidime) and to aminoglycosides in recent years. Typing of klebsiellas is with type-specific antisera or by molecular methods.

Salmonella spp.

The genus *Salmonella* is probably the most complex of the Enterobacteriaceae. It is currently in the process of

Table 38 *Escherichia coli* variants and enteric disease

Short form	Full name	Disease
ETEC	Enterotoxigenic *E. coli*	Traveller's diarrhoea
EPEC	Enteropathogenic *E. coli*	Diarrhoea in infants
EIEC	Enteroinvasive *E. coli*	Diarrhoea, specific serotypes
EHEC	Enterohaemorrhagic *E. coli*	Haemorrhagic colitis (haemolytic uraemic syndrome)

being rearranged on the basis of recent molecular taxonomic work. Salmonellae are non-lactose fermenters, urease negative and with the exception of *S. typhi* are hydrogen sulphide producers. They are motile and possess O saccharide antigens and H flagellar antigens. *S. typhi* also has an antiphagocytic Vi antigen. There are three type species, *S. typhi*, *S. choleraesuis* and *S. enteritidis*, of which the last has the greatest number of serotypes (over 2000). These are arranged into groups according to the presence of certain O antigens detected with agglutinating antisera, and into types according to their H antigens. The full description is not usually given on clinical laboratory report forms, and many laboratories only carry a limited range of typing antisera. Typing is by serological methods and bacteriophage studies initially. Molecular methods are being used increasingly in the investigation of salmonella infection outbreaks.

The salmonellas are responsible for enteric fever (caused by *S. typhi* or *S. paratyphi*), gastroenteritis and septicaemia. While the only reservoir for *S. typhi* is humans, with convalescent carriage or subclinical disease, the other salmonellas are often found in association with other animals, in which they may be a cause of disease. The association between *S. enteritidis* and poultry is probably responsible for the role of poultry products as the single most commonly implicated foodstuff in food-borne salmonellosis.

Shigellae spp.

The shigellae are a group of non-motile Gram-negative bacteria, closely related to *E. coli*. There are four species, *S. sonnei*, *S. boydii*, *S flexneri* and *S. dysenteriae*, of which *S. sonnei* is the most commonly isolated and the cause of the mildest intestinal disease. Only a small number of bacilli are required for intestinal infection, and the strains causing the most severe forms of infection produce toxins, such as verotoxin. Shigella infection is usually limited to the large intestine. Severe disease may cause invasion of the intestinal wall, but distant spread within the body is rare.

The invasive nature of severe shigella infection means that antibiotics may have to be prescribed, but resistance to all the commonly used agents is common. Typing of strains other than *S. sonnei* is done initially with antisera.

The Proteae

The Proteae include three genera, *Proteus*, *Morganella* and *Providencia*, of which *Proteus* is the most commonly encountered. *Proteus* spp. are non-lactose-fermenting Gram-negative bacilli that are strongly urease positive and motile. Some members of this group spread in a wavelike growth over solid media (called 'swarming'). Those strains that swarm can be typed by Dienes' phenomenon, which is the formation of a line of demarcation between non-identical isolates from different sources.

Proteus spp. are responsible for urinary tract infections and have a particular association with nephrolithiasis and long-term indwelling urinary catheters. Septicaemia, endotoxic shock and a variety of hospital-acquired infections can also be caused by members of the Proteae.

P. mirabilis, the most common *Proteus* sp., is usually sensitive to ampicillin and cephalosporins. *P. vulgaris* is ampicillin resistant.

Yersinia spp.

There are three important members of this group of Gram-negative bacilli: *Yersinia enterocolitica*, *Y. pseudotuberculosis* and *Y. pestis*. The yersinias are only rarely isolated from clinical specimens but can grown on conventional solid media. They have a characteristic Gram-stain appearance, with prominent staining at each end of the bacillus.

Y. enterocolitica and *Y. pseudotuberculosis* cause enteric infection in children (mesenteric adenitis) and adults. They may also cause septicaemia following blood transfusion. *Y. pestis* is the cause of bubonic, septicaemic and pneumonic plague.

Environmental Gram-negative bacilli

There are a number of medically important Gram-negative environmental genera, such as *Pseudomonas*, *Burkholderia*, *Acinetobacter* and *Stenotrophomonas*. Most of these bacteria do not ferment glucose and some are strongly oxidase positive. Their widely differing metabolism and wide temperature range allow them to survive and grow in various locations in the inanimate environment. Some species utilise decaying organic material as an energy source. These species may be isolated from soil, water and many locations in the hospital environment. This and their ability to accumulate multiple antibiotic-resistance factors, has led this group of bacteria to become a common cause of hospital-acquired infection.

Pseudomonas spp.

The *Pseudomonas* spp. include *P. aeruginosa*, *P. fluorescens* and a number of related motile, oxidase-positive Gram-negative bacilli. *P. aeruginosa* produces a blue–green pigment called pyocyanin and forms irregular colonies on solid media. These often have a musty, grape-like smell.

P. aeruginosa causes a wide variety of hospital-acquired infections from catheter-associated urinary tract infection to chronic osteomyelitis. It is a common cause of nosocomial pneumonia, burn and wound infection. Mucoid variants are an important cause of chronic pulmonary infection in patients with cystic fibrosis.

P. aeruginosa is often resistant to extended spectrum β-lactam agents and aminoglycosides. Antimicrobial agents commonly used to treat pseudomonas infections include piperacillin, the 4-aminoquinolones and the carbapenems.

Typing studies on *Pseudomonas* isolates are required when a hospital outbreak is suspected. These utilise the antibacterial activity of pyocines: substances produced by a given *P. aeruginosa* strain that are inhibitory to other strains.

Burkholderia spp.

The *Burkholderia* genus includes a number of bacteria formerly known as members of the genus *Pseudomonas*, of which *B. pseudomallei* and *B. cepacia* are medically important.

B. pseudomallei is an oxidase-positive Gram-negative non-fermenter that produces dry, wrinkled colonies on blood agar after several days. *B. cepacia* is slow growing on conventional solid media and susceptibility testing is difficult.

B. pseudomallei is found in soil and surface water and is the cause of melioidosis, a potentially fatal granulomatous disease that affects the lungs and soft tissues and is endemic to southeast Asia and northern Australia. The organism has to be handled carefully in the diagnostic laboratory to prevent occupationally acquired infection by inhalation. *B. pseudomallei* is usually susceptible to ceftazidime, co-trimoxazole and doxycycline and meropenem.

B. cepacia is an environmental Gram-negative bacillus that can act as an opportunist pathogen and has been associated with pulmonary disease in cystic fibrosis.

Stenotrophomonas maltophilia

Stenotrophomonas maltophilia is another Gram-negative species that used to be classified as a member of the *Pseudomonas* genus. It is oxidase negative, or very weakly positive, and produces yellow pigmented colonies. It also is found in the inanimate environment and in the human intestine.

S. maltophilia has been recognised increasingly as an opportunist pathogen of compromised patients such as leukaemics. It is often resistant to conventional antipseudomonal agents and is always resistant to the carbapenems: treatment with these agents is liable to select *S. maltophilia*.

Acinetobacter spp.

Acinetobacter is a genus of small Gram-negative coccobacilli that are oxidase negative and that can grow on MacConkey agar. All members of the genus are non-motile non-fermenters, but their ability to utilise carbohydrates by other metabolic pathways varies with species.

These species are widely dispersed in the hospital environment and often cause hospital-acquired infection, particularly in compromised patients and high-dependency wards, such as intensive care units. The most common member of the genus encountered in clinical practice is *A. baumannii* (formerly *A. calcoaceticus* var *anitratus*), which often possesses multiple antibiotic resistance. The less frequently seen *A. lwoffii* is less antibiotic resistant. Epidemiological studies using molecular methods such as polymerase chain reaction (PCR) typing of *Acinetobacter* spp. may be required to investigate hospital outbreaks.

Curved and spiral species

Vibrio spp.

The vibrios are a group of oxidase-positive, glucose-fermenting curved Gram-negative bacilli that are motile and have a preference for alkaline environments. There are over 30 species, of which the most important to medicine are *V. cholerae*, *V. vulnificus* and *V. parahaemolyticus*.

Isolation of vibrios in the diagnostic laboratory is usually performed by growth on TCBS (thiosulphate, citrate, bile salt) or an equivalent selective agar. Further selection can be achieved by enrichment of vibrios in alkaline peptone water prior to inoculation of solid media. *V. cholerae* produces yellow colonies on TCBS. *V. vulnificus* and *V. parahaemolyticus* produce yellow colonies. Vibrios are found in aquatic environments contaminated by human sewage and can be found in shellfish. Infection results from consumption of contaminated seawater or seafood.

V. cholerae is the organism responsible for cholera, a potentially life-threatening watery diarrhoea. *V. cholerae* has around 60 O antigen types. The single most important is type O1, which causes the most severe disease. This single type is subdivided into serotypes Inaba, Ogawa and Hikojima. Further subdivision of all three types can be made into the classical and the El Tor biovars.

Many *Vibrio* species as well as type O1 *V. cholerae* can produce watery diarrhoea. *V. cholerae* causes the most severe diarrhoeal disease because of the action of a toxin that binds to ganglioside receptors on the intestinal mucosa, stimulating production of cyclic AMP and blocking resorption of sodium and water from the small intestine. Pandemics of cholera occur around once per decade. The last pandemic was caused by the El Tor biotype, which spread to South America. The classic biotype is currently spreading from an initial focus in south Asia (Bengal strain). The classic biotype causes more aggressive disease but does not survive in the environment as easily as the El Tor biotype.

The mainstay of management is fluid and electrolyte replacement, but treatment with tetracycline or co-trimoxazole can shorten the duration of diarrhoea and volume of fluid lost.

V. vulnificus can cause more invasive disease, sometimes resulting in a septicaemia with high mortality rate, especially in patients with liver disease.

Campylobacter spp.
The Campylobacters are a group of microaerophilic, capnophilic curved Gram-negative bacilli. The most commonly encountered member of the genus is *C. jejuni*, which is probably the most common bacterial cause of diarrhoea. Isolation of the species in the laboratory requires microaerophilic conditions (10% CO_2 and 90% N_2), selective agar (such as Preston or Skirrow's medium) and incubation at 42°C. These measures prevent the growth of commensal enteric bacteria. Other campylobacters such as *C. fetus*, *C. coli* and *C. lari* can be distinguished from *C. jejuni* by results of susceptibility testing with cephalothin and nalidixic acid, and by hippurate hydrolysis.

The campylobacters are an important cause of intestinal disease in domestic animals such as cattle and poultry, which may act as a primary source of infection. In humans infection typically causes a short-lived, bloody diarrhoea. Systemic spread may occur at extremes of age, and cases of arthritis and meningitis have been reported.

C. jejuni is usually sensitive to erythromycin, but diarrhoea in adults and older children does not usually require antibiotic therapy.

Helicobacter pylori
Formerly known as *Campylobacter pylori*, this bacterium has been recognised as a factor in the pathogenesis of peptic ulcer disease. *H. pylori* is a urease-positive, curved Gram-negative bacillus that can be grown under microaerophilic conditions on modified blood agar. The primary source is not known at the time of writing.

Ingestion of *H. pylori* has been shown to produce gastritis, and eradication of the organisms by antibiotic therapy has reduced the recurrence rate of gastric ulceration. There is some evidence to suggest that *H. pylori* may be a contributor to the development of certain intragastric malignancies.

Some strains are resistant to metronidazole.

Fastidious bacilli
Several genera of Gram-negative bacilli are difficult to culture under laboratory conditions because of specific growth factor or atmospheric requirements. However, provision of those growth requirements in supplemented media or modification of the gaseous environment used for incubation enables isolation of these genera from clinical specimens. The occurrence of these genera is under-reported since many diagnostic laboratories lack the incubators or do not stock the media required to isolate them. Moreover, their fastidious nature guarantees that a proportion of potential isolates will not be recovered, even in optimal laboratory conditions.

Haemophilus spp.
Haemophilus is a genus of small Gram-negative coccobacilli that require growth factors present in blood to grow on solid media. Important members of the genus include *H. influenzae*, *H. aegyptius*, *H. ducreyi* and *H. parainfluenzae*, which can be distinguished in part by their differing requirement for X (haemin) and V (NAD) factors (Table 39). *H. influenzae* can be typed by its capsule type and by biochemical characteristics.

Haemophilus spp. are found on mucosal surfaces in the upper respiratory tract and genital tract. *H. influenzae* is the most common human pathogen and causes invasive disease such as meningitis, cellulitis, epiglottitis and septicaemia in young children, and lower respiratory tract infection in adults. The majority of invasive infections are caused by strains possessing a polysaccharide capsule type b (composed of ribose). Non-capsulated strains can cause invasive disease, particularly in patients with lymphoid malignancies.

H. aegyptius is closely related to certain biotypes of *H. influenzae*. This species is responsible for conjunctivitis, and the life-threatening condition known as Brazilian purpuric fever.

H. ducreyi is the species that causes the sexually transmitted genital infection chancroid.

H. parainfluenzae is less often associated with symptomatic infection and is a common commensal species in the upper respiratory tract.

Haemophilus spp. are penicillin resistant, and an increasing proportion of *H. influenzae* strains show resistance to ampicillin that is mediated by a β-lactamase, and/or resistance to chloramphenicol. Invasive *H. influenzae* disease has decreased in communities where one of the new conjugated PRP (capsular type b substance) vaccines has been introduced.

Table 39 *Haemophilus* spp. and growth factor requirements

Species	Factor X	Factor V
H. influenzae	+	+
H. parainfluenzae		+
H. aegyptius	+	+
H. ducreyi	+	−
H. aphrophilus	+/−	−

HACEK group

'HACEK' is an acronym for *Haemophilus aphrophilus*, *Actinobacillus actinomycetemcomitans*, *Cardiobacterium hominis*, *Eikenella corrodens* and *Kingella kingae*. These are all Gram-negative bacilli that grow slowly and require CO_2 for growth. They are found among the commensal flora of the oropharyngeal or genital mucosae and are a rare cause of infective endocarditis on abnormal heart valves.

Pasteurella spp.

Pasteurella is a genus of small, oxidase-positive Gram-negative bacilli of which the most important member is *P. multocida*. This species can be found in the oral cavities of cats, dogs and other animals and is recognised as a cause of infection following animal bites. The species is usually sensitive to penicillin.

Brucella spp.

The more commonly encountered members of this genus are *B. melitensis*, *B. abortus* and *B. suis*. These are oxidase-positive Gram-negative bacilli that require serum supplemented media for growth.

These species cause brucellosis: a zoonotic infection resulting from ingestion, inoculation or inhalation of bacteria in animal products (these include milk, placenta, meat and animal body fluids). Brucellae can cause granulomas, particularly in musculoskeletal, lymphoreticular and central nervous tissues.

Doxycycline, streptomycin or rifampicin are effective against members of the genus in vivo.

Legionellaceae

The Legionellaceae are a group of fastidious aerobic Gram-negative bacilli found in a wide variety of aquatic environments, both natural and artificial. It is thought that they may survive in close association with free-living amoebae. Legionellas are difficult to culture and require special media (BCYEa: buffered charcoal, yeast extract, α-ketoglutarate). Confirmation is by direct immunofluorescent antibody stain. The same reagent or silver stain can be used on direct smears from clinical specimens for rapid diagnosis.

There are many members of the genus, but over two thirds of human infections are caused by *L. pneumophila* serotype 1. The most common infection is a pneumonia, usually bilateral with little if any sputum and with non-pulmonary features including confusion, diarrhoea and myalgia. A self-limiting febrile condition known as Pontiac fever is also associated with respiratory exposure to Legionella.

The genus is susceptible to erythromycin and rifampicin. Typing is by serological methods or plasmid studies.

Anaerobic Gram-negative bacilli

The anaerobic Gram-negative bacilli are fastidious anaerobes; they do not tolerate exposure to oxygen. They include *Bacteroides*, *Prevotella* and *Fusobacterium* spp., all of which are associated with abscess formation, deep soft tissue infection and polymicrobial infections at various sites in the body from the brain to the pelvic organs and muscular fascia. Infection by these species usually occurs after contamination of traumatised, ischaemic or necrotic tissues with material from the mouth or intestines.

Bacteroides spp. are most commonly isolated, and *B. fragilis* is the single most common species. *B. fragilis* is a bile-tolerant, anaerobic Gram-negative bacillus, normally found in the commensal flora of the lower intestine. The species is resistant to penicillin.

Prevotella is a genus that includes all the species formerly known as the pigmented Bacteroides group (e.g. *B. melaninogenicus*, now *P. melaninogenica*). These are highly anaerobic, slow-growing species, with pigmentation that may only be apparent after weeks of incubation. They are found in the upper gastrointestinal tract and, along with *Fusobacterium necrophorum* (an anaerobic Gram-negative bacillus with tapered ends), they are the more common anaerobic species in pulmonary infection following aspiration into the lungs. These species are usually penicillin sensitive.

All the anaerobic Gram-negative bacilli are sensitive to metronidazole and most are sensitive to clindamycin.

Gram-negative cocci

The Gram-negative cocci most commonly seen in medical practice belong to two genera: *Neisseria* and *Moraxella*. *Neisseria* includes *N. gonorrhoeae*, *N. meningitidis* and several commensal species such as *N. lactamica*. *Moraxella catarrhalis* is the most common member of the genus *Moraxella*.

Neisseria spp.

The Neisseriaceae are Gram-negative cocci that often occur in pairs (therefore they are called diplococci), have fastidious growth requirements and prefer a humid, CO_2-rich environment. They are found on human mucosal surfaces, adhering by pili. *N. meningitidis* has a polysaccharide capsule that provides resistance to phagocytosis. Presumptive identification is by Gram stain of the appropriate specimen. Colonies are oxidase positive. Identification of species is confirmed by a sugar utilisation test or immunological means (Table 40).

N. gonorrhoeae is the cause of variety of sexually transmitted infections of the urinogenital tract and other body orifices and of septicaemia and neonatal infec-

Table 40 Biochemical reactions of the Neisseriaceae

Species	Sugar utilisation				DNAase
	Glucose	Maltose	Lactose	Sucrose	
N. gonorrhoeae	+	−	−	−	−
N. meningitidis	+	+	−	−	−
N. lactamica	+	+	+	−	−
M. catarrhalis	−	−	−	−	+

tions. Specimens from external body surfaces require selective media (such as vancomycin, colistin, trimethoprim, amphotericin agar) to suppress the growth of commensal species. Identification must be confirmed for medico-legal reasons, by either sugar utilisation or co-agglutination test. Penicillin resistance, caused either by β-lactamase production or by altered penicillin-binding proteins, tetracycline resistance and even quinolone resistance are seen with increasing frequency. Current recommendation for treatment of gonococcal infections in localities with high rates of resistance is ceftriaxone. Laboratory typing can be done by analysis of metabolic substrate requirements (auxotyping). One particular type—the AHU auxotype (arginine, hypoxanthine, uracil)—has a strong association with disseminated gonococcal infection in adult women.

N. meningitidis is the other clinically important member of the genus and is responsible for bacterial meningitis and septicaemia, which occur most often in preschool children and institutionalised young adults. There are several capsular serotypes, of which A, B and C are the most common. Type A is often responsible for epidemic disease, while type B is the cause of much endemic disease. N. meningitidis can be grown on chocolate agar in a humid CO_2 incubator. Penicillin resistance is, fortunately, uncommon but some β-lactamase producers have been noted in recent years. Epidemiological typing is by serogrouping with antisera to capsular polysaccharide and serotyping according to outer membrane protein type.

Moraxella **spp.**

The most common member of the genus encountered clinically is M. catarrhalis (formerly known as *Neisseria catarrhalis*) and then *Branhamella catarrhalis*. M. catarrhalis is a Gram-negative coccus that is relatively asaccharolytic, DNAase positive and usually β-lactamase positive.

The species is found in the oropharyngeal flora, particularly in children and older adults and was for many years thought to be non-pathogenic. In recent years it has become clear that the species can be a cause of infection in structures adjacent to the upper respiratory tract (e.g. causing otitis media and sinusitis) and may be an opportunist pathogen in the lower respiratory tract,

causing exacerbations of chronic bronchitis. It may also cause bacteraemia in the immunosuppressed.

M. catarrhalis is usually penicillin resistant because of its β-lactamase.

21.3 Mycobacteria

The mycobacteria are slow-growing acid-fast bacilli. They have a cell wall structure that differs from Gram-negative and Gram-positive species in several respects. The mycobacterial cell wall does not rely for its integrity on peptidoglycan. Instead, it has mycolic acid and waxes, which make it resistant to conventional stains. The mycobacterial cell wall requires either heat or a prolonged staining period with concentrated dye before stain permeates the organism. Staining with concentrated carbol fuchsin that resists decolorisation with acid–alcohol, as in the Ziehl–Neelsen stain, explains the acid-fast property of this group of bacteria.

Mycobacteria can be grown on specialised media such as Lowenstein–Jensen or Middlebrook agar. Lowenstein–Jensen medium contains inspissated egg, starch and malachite green, while Middlebrook contains defined chemicals, albumin, biotin and catalase. Growth is best in the presence of added CO_2 and results in colonies with variable size, shape and colour, features that can help in identification (Table 41). Other characteristics used to identify mycobacteria include optimal temperature range, niacin accumulation, catalase and hydrolysis of the detergent Tween. *Mycobacterium leprae*, the cause of leprosy, cannot be cultivated on artificial media and has only been grown in armadillos and suckling mice. The slow growth of mycobacteria has led to improved methods of isolation, including detection of $^{14}CO_2$ produced from ^{14}C-palmitic acid in the broth used in an automated radiometric (BACTEC) detection system. Slow rates of growth also cause problems for determination of antibiotic susceptibility, which can require further lengthy delays.

Mycobacterium tuberculosis

M. tuberculosis is the single most important human pathogen in the group. This species is responsible for

Table 41 Identification of mycobacteria

Species	Growth at (°C) 37	Growth at (°C) 30	Growth	Pigmented	Niacin
M. tuberculosis	+	−	Slow	−	+
M. bovis	+	−	Slow	−	−
M. avium and M. intracellulare	+	−	Slow	−	−
M. kansasii	+	−	Slow	+	−
M. fortuitum	+	−	Fast	−	−
M. chelonae	+	−	Fast	−	−
M. ulcerans	−	+	Slow	−	−
M. marinum	−	+	Slow	−	−

pulmonary tuberculosis, tuberculous meningitis and a variety of extrapulmonary tuberculous infections. The principal reservoir is in the human population, in post-primary recrudescent disease. There are increasing reports of *M. tuberculosis* infection, partly as a result of disease secondary to infection with the human immunodeficiency virus (HIV). There are also increasing rates of resistance to commonly used antimycobacterial agents such as streptomycin, rifampicin and isoniazid. Subtyping can now be performed with a variety of molecular methods, and these methods are being used with increasing frequency as an adjunct for infection control interventions in future. The related species *M. bovis* is also found in cattle and may cause mycobacterial infection in cattle-rearing communities.

Mycobacterium avium and *M. intracellulare*

The second most commonly isolated causes of human mycobacterial infection are now *M. avium* and *M. intracellulare*. These species are non-pigmented mycobacteria found in the inanimate environment. They are a common cause of both pulmonary and extrapulmonary infection in patients with HIV infection and are defusing illnesses for the acquired immunodeficiency syndrome (AIDS). However, they have also been known to cause infection in immunocompetent individuals.

Mycobacterium kansasii

M. kansasii is a mycobacterial species that produces pigment on exposure to light and is a cause of cavitating pulmonary infection in patients with AIDS and in other patients.

Mycobacterium ulcerans and *M. marinum*

M. ulcerans and *M. marinum* are both species that have a lower optimal temperature range than *M. tuberculosis* and cause infection primarily affecting the skin and soft tissues.

Mycobacterium fortuitum–chelonae complex

The *M. fortuitum*–*M. chelonae* complex includes species that grow very rapidly for mycobacteria and can be isolated on conventional media such as MacConkey agar (without crystal violet). These species tend to cause skin and soft tissue infection with a tendency to abscess formation.

21.4 Bacteria not grown in the laboratory

Several groups of bacteria are not normally identified by culture in the routine diagnostic laboratory, either because they require specialist culture techniques (e.g. cell culture) or because they cannot be grown at all. The standard approach to diagnosis of infections caused by non-cultivatable bacteria is to use immunological methods, including direct immunofluorescence and antibody detection in patient serum. More recently, nucleic acid probes have been employed successfully to detect the presence of these organisms in clinical specimens. The main bacteria included in this grouping are the mycoplasmas, chlamydias, rickettsias and spirochaetes.

Mycoplasmas

The mycoplasmas are a group of small bacteria with limited metabolic capabilities and no rigid cell wall. They grow slowly on special agar media and are occasionally isolated as minute colonies on chocolate agar. The lack of cell wall prevents staining with the Gram stain and renders β-lactam antibiotics ineffective. Under the plate microscope, mycoplasma colonies pit the agar, giving a 'fried egg' appearance. The slow growth, requirement for special media and difficulty obtaining specimens in the case of respiratory infection mean that many laboratories do not attempt mycoplasma culture. Infections are diagnosed either by serological methods retrospectively or by a rapid DNA probe or PCR.

The most important species is *Mycoplasma pneumoniae*, which causes atypical pneumonia, upper respiratory infections and central nervous system complications, including Guillain–Barré syndrome. *M. hominis* and *Ureaplasma urealyticum* (a related genus that hydrolyses urea) are two other species found in the respiratory and genitourinary tracts; their role in human disease has been debated extensively. Both are thought to cause sexually transmitted disease, including non-gonococcal urethritis in males and infections of the pelvic organs in females.

Most isolates are sensitive to erythromycin and tetracycline, but resistance to both agents has been reported.

Chlamydias

The chlamydias are a group of small Gram-negative bacteria that require an intracellular environment for growth. The infective form of the organism is the elementary body (EB), which after penetration of the host cell transforms into a perinuclear cytoplasmic inclusion body that can be stained with Giemsa, iodine or group-specific immunofluorescent antibody. Chlamydias can be cultured using shell vials similar to those used for virology.

There are three medically important species: *C. trachomatis, C. psittaci* and *C. pneumoniae* (Table 42).

The most commonly encountered species is *C. trachomatis*, which causes eye disease (trachoma and inclusion conjunctivitis), urethritis and cervicitis, and lymphogranuloma venereum. While culture remains a reference centre gold standard, most clinical laboratories rely on a direct immunofluorescent stain for rapid diagnosis of *C. trachomatis*.

C. psittaci, the cause of psittacosis (an uncommon respiratory infection acquired from contact with psittacine birds such as parrots), is normally diagnosed by serological methods.

C. pneumoniae is a recently recognised member of the genus with features distinctive from the other two species. It is known to cause an atypical pneumonia. Although culture is possible, serological methods are used for diagnosed.

Chlamydial infection is treated with tetracycline.

Rickettsiae and coxiellae

The rickettsiae are a group of obligate intracellular Gram-negative bacteria with a preference for vascular endothelium.

Rickettsial diseases are associated with a petechial (vasculitic rash) and multisystem disease. They are usually transmitted by arthropods (Table 43). The three groups of diseases are typhus, scrub typhus and spotted fever.

Coxiella is a related genus that causes acute disease (atypical pneumonia) and chronic disease (infective endocarditis) following contact with infected cattle. Organisms in this group can be isolated from laboratory animals but are highly infective. Diagnostic laboratories, therefore, rely on immunofluorescent stain of skin biopsy or serological tests on serum.

Spirochaetes

The spirochaetes are spiral-shape bacilli that, with few exceptions, cannot be cultivated in the laboratory. They include three important genera: *Treponema, Borrelia* and *Leptospira*. Spirochaetal infections are often multiphasic, with distinct pathology at successive stages of infection. Transmission of several species is via arthropods, the ecology of which is an important determinant of human infection. Spirochaetes are usually sensitive to the penicillins.

Treponema spp.

There is one species of importance in the genus, *Treponema pallidum*, a spirochaete responsible for distinctive early and late manifestations. Its most common subspecies, *T. pallidum* ssp. *pallidum*, is the cause of syphilis. Syphilis has early and late stages, with chancre, disseminated disease, gummata, neurological, cardiovascular, osseous and congenital complications. Other subspecies

Table 43 Rickettsiae and coxiellae

Species	Arthropod vector	Disease
R. prowazeki	Pediculus humanus	Louse-borne typhus
R. typhi	Xenopsylla cheopis	Murine typhus
Orienta tsutsugamushi	Leptotrombidium mites	Scrub typhus
R. rickettsiae	Dermacentor andersoni	Rocky mountain spotted fever
C. burnetti	–	Q fever

Table 42 The chlamydias

Species	EB shape	Sulphonamide sensitivity	Iodine staining	Infections
C. trachomatis	Round	Sensitive	+	Trachoma, conjunctivitis, genital and neonatal infections
C. psittaci	Round	Resistant	–	Psittacosis
C. pneumoniae	Oval	Resistant	–	Pneumonia

(spp. *pertenue, endemicum* and *carateum*) are responsible for endemic non-venereal variations of treponemal disease in the tropics (Table 44).

Treponemes cannot be cultivated in the laboratory. Diagnosis is by microscopic and serological methods.

Treatment is with penicillin, against which no acquired resistance has been documented.

Borreliae

The borreliae are a genus of spiral bacilli that include *B. burgdorferi* and *B. recurrentis*. *B. recurrentis* causes louse- and tick-borne relapsing fever. *B. burgdorferi* causes Lyme disease, a multiphase condition with skin rash (erythema chronicum migrans), arthritis and neurological complications that is transmitted by hard-bodied ticks.

B. recurrentis is diagnosed by microscopy of a blood film, while *B. burgdorferi* infection is diagnosed by serological methods.

Leptospira interrogans

The one disease-causing species in the genus *Leptospira* is *L. interrogans*. This species has several serovars (e.g. serovar *icterohaemorrhagiae*) that cause differing patterns of disease. Disease is multiphasic: an initial infective stage giving way to an immune stage later on.

The spirochaetes are very small and difficult to detect in a blood film. The organism can be cultivated in reference laboratories equipped with the necessary semisolid agar and skilled in handling these organisms. However, diagnosis depends more often on agglutination of live non-pathogenic leptospiras by patient serum. DNA probes have been used for diagnosis.

Table 44 Endemic non-venereal treponemal infections

T. pallidum subspecies	Disease	Location
pertenue	Yaws	Tropical Asia, Africa, Americas
endemicum	Endemic syphilis	Asia, Africa, Middle East
carateum	Pinta	South and Central America

22 Viruses

Overview

This chapter deals with the major groups of viruses, the infections they cause, and how they are diagnosed and treated. Information on infection is presented by microorganism, rather than by disease or syndrome. The chapter is meant as an alternative entry into information presented in previous chapters and as a supplementary learning resource.

Learning objectives

You should:

- know the principal groups of viruses
- know the infections they cause
- know key laboratory tests used to detect and identify them
- know the antiviral agents used to treat their infections.

22.1 DNA viruses

Adenoviridae

The adenoviruses are a group of naked, icosahedral viruses with double-stranded linear DNA. They are found in tonsils, adenoids and stools of humans and are often found in healthy people. There are many serotypes: 1–37, 40 and 41. After penetration of the host cell, adenoviruses are transported to the nucleus where they replicate. Infection can cause cell lysis.

The clinical consequences of adenovirus infection include conjunctivitis, diarrhoea and a variety of infections of the respiratory tract (common cold, pharyngitis, and pneumonia).

Hepadnaviridae

The hepatitis B virus is a member of the hepadnaviridae. It is an enveloped virus with double-stranded DNA that is found in humans. Transmission is via blood, tissues and body secretions. Important antigens of this virus are the surface, core and e antigens and DNA polymerase.

The hepatitis B virus has a tropism for hepatocytes and causes acute lytic infection, chronic infection and transformation, leading eventually to hepatocellular carcinoma.

The virus cannot be grown in tissue culture. Diagnosis is by serological techniques that detect viral antigens or the corresponding antibody response. The surface antigen is used as the most important marker of antigenaemia, but e antigen is regarded as a more effective indicator of infectivity. Anti-core antibodies are the first to be detected after the antigenaemia begins to decline.

There is no really effective therapy. Prevention is by immunoprophylaxis with a recombinant surface antigen (subunit) vaccine, and postexposure administration of hyperimmune globulin.

Herpesviridae

The herpesviruses are a group of enveloped, icosahedral viruses with double-stranded linear DNA. The group includes herpes simplex virus I and II, varicella-zoster virus, cytomegalovirus, Epstein–Barr virus and human herpesvirus 6. These are viruses of humans, and several members of the group (herpes simplex, varicella-zoster) are capable of persisting for prolonged periods at privileged sites in the body (latency). Members of this group have tropism for different human cell types.

Herpes simplex viruses I and II are spread by contact between oral and genital tracts. Infections at both sites, keratitis, encephalitis and neonatal infections can all be caused by herpes simplex. They can be treated with nucleoside analogues, e.g. aciclovir.

Epstein–Barr virus causes infectious mononucleosis.

Cytomegalovirus can cause both a mononucleosis-type disease and congenital infection. It can also cause pneumonia and retinitis in the immunocompromised patient. Cytomegalovirus infections can be treated with ganciclovir or foscarnet.

Varicella-zoster virus causes chickenpox and shingles. A live attenuated virus vaccine is now available in some countries.

Human herpesvirus 6 is the cause of a common exanthematous disease, exanthem subitum ('roseola').

Parvoviridae

Parvovirus B19 is a small, naked icosahedral virus with a single strand of linear DNA. It is the only virus incapable of transforming host cells. Parvovirus B19 undergoes replication in the nucleus of erythropoietic cells, causing a relatively minor infection known as erythema infectiosum, fifth disease or 'slapped cheek' syndrome after the rash it causes in young children. In patients with thalassaemia or sickle cell disease, parvovirus B19 infection may cause severe anaemia. During pregnancy, it can cause severe fetal infection resulting in stillbirth or hydrops fetalis.

Diagnostic tests are not widely available since the virus is difficult to grow in cell culture. DNA probes and polymerase chain reaction (PCR) have been used. Specific IgM antibody detection has been used to diagnose recent infection.

Papovaviridae

The papovaviruses are a group of small, icosahedral viruses with double-stranded circular DNA. The most important member is the human papillomavirus (HPV) of which there are 60 serotypes. The virus cannot be cultivated and has species specificity: types known to be human pathogens are only found in humans. Transmission is by inoculation into breaks in the epidermal surface, in either the skin or mucosal surfaces. Infection of the basal layer of the skin leads to cell proliferation and the characteristic papillomas or warts. Oncogenic transformation occurs in a small minority of infections, particularly those associated with certain serotypes, resulting in intraepithelial neoplasia and carcinoma. The majority of cervical carcinomas have detectable human papillomavirus DNA.

Treatment of papillomata is by removal with surgery, laser destruction or freezing. There is no specific antiviral therapy or vaccine.

Poxviridae

The poxviruses are the largest viruses known. They have no envelope and linear, double-stranded DNA. Poxviruses are present in humans and animals. The group includes variola (smallpox), vaccinia, orf and molluscum contagiosum. Members of the group have a large genome and are the only DNA viruses where replication occurs in the host cell cytoplasm.

Variola virus is of historical importance now that smallpox has been eradicated. It remains a potential threat only in the context of biological terrorism. However, the pox viruses are potentially useful in the construction of recombinant vaccines. Pox are viral skin lesions that begin as vesicles, turning to sterile pustules before crusting over.

Molluscum contagiosum is a viral infection restricted to the skin, where direct inoculation of the virus results in small umbilicated nodules.

Orf, or contagious pustular dermatitis, is an infection of animal workers, who develop a single nodular lesion, usually on the hand.

Diagnosis of these infections is usually clinical, but electron microscopy of material from the lesions may be helpful in certain cases.

22.2 RNA viruses

Arenaviridae

The arenaviruses are enveloped viruses with single-stranded RNA. The group includes Lassa, Junin and Machupo viruses, which are commonly restricted to small mammals.

Infection in humans causes fever, haemorrhage and shock. In Lassa fever, there may also be pharyngitis and hepatitis.

Ribavirin has been used for treatment. Patients with active arenavirus infection are highly contagious and require special isolation precautions.

Bunyaviridae

The bunyaviruses are a group of enveloped, single-stranded RNA viruses with helical symmetry. There are a number of human pathogens in the group, including Hantavirus, a cause of haemorrhagic fever and renal failure. Hantavirus is found in small mammals and transmitted by inhalation or inoculation.

Ribavirin has some beneficial effect when given early in the course of infection.

Caliciviridae

Caliciviruses are non-enveloped, icosahedral viruses with single-stranded linear RNA. Norwalk agent and related viruses are probable members of this group of resilient viruses found in the human gastrointestinal tract. Despite their resistance to heat, acid and ether, they cannot be grown in cell culture.

Together with the other caliciviruses, they are spread by the faecal–oral route and cause gastroenteritis. The incubation period is only several hours.

Diagnosis is by immuno- or conventional electron microscopy, or by enzyme immunoassay.

Coronaviridae

The coronaviruses are enveloped viruses with single-stranded RNA and helical symmetry. Electron microscopy shows a ring or corona of club-shaped projections surrounding the virus particle. Transmission is via the respiratory route, resulting in infection of the upper (and rarely lower) respiratory tract.

Laboratory diagnosis is by serological methods where required.

Filoviridae

The filoviruses included Marburg and Ebola; two viruses named after the places where they first caused outbreaks of human infection. These are enveloped viruses with single-stranded linear RNA that can form filamentous, curved forms in tissue culture and human infections.

Filoviruses are found in humans and other primates, from which human infection is normally acquired. Infection is highly contagious. The primary reservoir is not known. The disease they cause is a haemorrhagic fever with a high case-fatality rate.

Diagnosis is by isolation of the virus or by immunofluorescence, conducted in special reference laboratories because of the potential health risk to laboratory staff.

There is no specific treatment or effective vaccine.

Orthomyxoviridae

The orthomyxoviruses are a group of enveloped, single-stranded RNA viruses, which includes influenza virus types A, B and C. These viruses are found in humans and other animals. Influenza viruses cause endemic and epidemic influenza, most epidemics being attributed to type A. The viral envelope has two important proteins: a haemagglutinin and neuraminidase. The haemagglutinin mediates attachment to receptors on the surface of respiratory tract epithelial cells. Major changes in these antigens are referred to as antigenic shift. Minor changes are called antigenic drift. It is antigenic shift that is responsible for the new epidemic strains that periodically (every 8–10 years) cause influenza pandemics. The virus is transmitted in droplets to the upper respiratory tract where primary infection occurs. Multiplication in ciliated epithelial cells impairs ciliary function. Cytotoxic and immunological damage results in desquamation of respiratory epithelium and secondary bacterial infection. Apart from influenza, these viruses rarely cause pneumonia and Reye's syndrome.

Laboratory diagnosis is by virus isolation from the nose or throat swabs.

Amantidine has been found to have some beneficial effect for both early treatment or prevention of influenza. However, prevention relies on a killed virus vaccine composed of current strains.

Paramyxoviridae

The paramyxoviruses are a group of enveloped viruses with single-stranded RNA and helical symmetry. The group includes parainfluenza 1–4, mumps, measles and respiratory syncytial viruses. Members of the group possess haemagglutinin and neuraminidase. Unlike members of the orthomyxoviridae, these agents show no significant spread or direct contact.

Infections caused include mumps, measles and a variety of respiratory syndromes.

Mumps Mumps begins as a primary infection in the respiratory tract followed by viraemia and spread to glandular tissues, including the salivary glands, pancreas, testes and ovaries. Glandular epithelia swell and desquamate. Some patients develop an aseptic meningitis.

Laboratory diagnosis is by viral isolation from blood, cerebrospinal fluid or urine or by serodiagnosis.

There is no effective antiviral agent, but the live attenuated mumps vaccine has been highly successful.

Measles Measles virus also causes a primary infection in the respiratory tract followed by viraemia and spread to distant sites including lymphoid tissues and lymphocytes. Measles infection, therefore, results in a compromised immune system. In patients with prior immune compromise, usually because of malnutrition in poorer countries, measles may be progressive and more often results in secondary bacterial infection or encephalitis. A slowly progressive brain syndrome known as subacute sclerosing panencephalitis occurs as a late sequel in a very small proportion of measles infections.

Diagnosis is by virus isolation from oropharyngeal secretions or urine, or by serological tests (e.g. complement fixation or haemagglutination inhibition).

Respiratory syncytial virus Respiratory syncytial virus is so-called because of its tendency to cause cell fusion in cell cultures. It causes bronchiolitis and pneumonia in infants. Immunity does not appear to be protective after infection and an effective vaccine has yet to be developed.

Laboratory diagnosis is by rapid immunofluorescent test, cell culture or by PCR. Early treatment with ribavirin has been effective in some studies.

Parainfluenza virus The parainfluenza viruses are responsible for croup, bronchitis and some cases of viral pneumonia in young children.

Picornaviridae

The picornaviruses are small, icosahedral viruses with single-stranded linear RNA and no envelope. The group includes polioviruses 1–3, coxsackieviruses A and B, echoviruses, enteroviruses and rhinoviruses. Members of this group cause a variety of clinical syndromes from aseptic meningitis and encephalitis to gastroenteritis, pleurodynia and the common cold. Spread is by faecal–oral or respiratory routes. The picornaviruses are relatively resistant to disinfectants. With the exception of the rhinoviruses, there is much overlap in the syndromes caused by each of the viruses in the group.

Diagnosis is by culture of virus from throat swab, stools or body fluids. There is no effective antiviral treatment.

Poliovirus Poliovirus causes mild infection in young children from poorly developed countries. A small proportion develop infection of the central nervous system, usually a self-limiting aseptic meningitis. In countries with better sewage disposal and higher standards of personal hygiene, infection occurs later in life and has a higher risk of paralytic disease. Paralysis is caused by viral infection of the anterior horn cells. Prevention is by administration of either a killed virus vaccine or a live attenuated virus. The live virus is given as three separate doses, separated by several months to allow types 1–3, respectively, the opportunity to establish local infection. Reversion to the pathogenic wild type very rarely occurs.

Coxsackievirus Coxsackieviruses are divided into groups A and B according to their differing neuropathic effects on newborn mice. There is some overlap in the conditions they cause, which include pleurodynia; hand, foot and mouth disease; and herpangina. Serodiagnostic tests are unreliable indicators of recent infection.

Rhinovirus Rhinoviruses account for most cases of the common cold. There are around 100 serotypes and they all have a lower temperature optimum than most other viral pathogens of humans, which may explain their preference for the epithelium of the nasopharynx. Rhinoviruses cause little epithelial damage and leave little immune protection against further infection. There is no effective vaccine.

Reoviridae

The most important reovirus is rotavirus: a non-enveloped, icosahedral single-stranded RNA virus with a characteristic double-shelled outer capsid. There are three serogroups, and group one contains four serotypes. Spread is by the faecal–oral route and the virus is found in human and animal gastrointestinal tracts.

Rotavirus is the most frequent cause of diarrhoea in infants and also causes outbreaks in homes for the elderly. Infection is primarily in the small intestine where villous blunting occurs. There is delayed gastric emptying and a reduction in brush border enzymes resulting, respectively, in vomiting and malabsorption. Infection with rotavirus results in long-term immunity.

Diagnosis is by electron microscopy, antigen detection by latex agglutination or enzyme immunoassay.

There is no effective antiviral treatment or vaccine.

Retroviridae

Retroviruses are a group of viruses that only came to attention as a result of the human immunodeficiency virus (HIV) pandemic. They are enveloped viruses with a double copy of single-stranded RNA. The group includes the human T cell leukaemia viruses (HTLV) I and II, and HIV 1 and 2. These viruses are found in tissues, blood and body fluids of humans. Transmission is via blood, tissues and body fluids either through inoculation or by sexual contact. Vertical transmission may also occur.

HTLV I and II are oncoviruses that integrate their genome into the host cell genome, which results in indefinite virus production without cell lysis, leading to conditions such as adult T cell or hairy cell leukemia.

HIV 1 and 2 integrate into host cell DNA and persist for a long and variable period, after which cytolysis begins.

Members of the retrovirus group possess the enzyme reverse transcriptase, which allows the virus to make a double-stranded DNA copy using viral RNA as a template. HIV is known to attach to CD4 lymphocytes (T helper cells) using an envelope glycoprotein (gp120). Fusion with the cell membrane is assisted by another glycoprotein (gp41). Infected CD4 cells then form syncytia with other lymphocytes. The cell-mediated immune system is thus progressively impaired, leading to increasing risk of infection with opportunistic pathogens. Infection of astrocytes and glial cells in the brain, and fibroblasts throughout the body, occurs via other mechanisms. The three main conditions caused by HIV infection are the acquired immunodeficiency syndrome (AIDS), polyglandular lymphadenopathy (PGL) and the AIDS-related complex (ARC). Laboratory diagnosis is by enzyme immunoassay for antibody response to specific viral components or by Western blot. p24 antigenaemia and PCR also have a role in the evaluation of specific patient groups. The reverse transcriptase inhibitor azidothymidine (AZT) was the first drug to slow down the progression of immune compromise and to reduce the risk of vertical transmission from an HIV-infected pregnant mother to her unborn child. However, AZT is expensive, causes significant side effects and resistant strains of virus are common. Newer reverse transcriptase inhibitors, inhibitors of HIV protease and alternative chemotherapeutic agents have become available and are used in complex multidrug regimens (highly active antiretroviral therapy, HAART). All these drugs have problems with side effects and with the development of drug resistance. Side effects and the complex dosing schedule lead to problems with compliance. There is no prospect of widely available, curative chemotherapy or an effective vaccine for HIV in the immediate future. Prevention depends on protection of blood and organ donation and avoidance of risky patterns of sexual behaviour and intravenous drug use.

Rhabdoviridae

The most important rhabdovirus is the rabies virus; an enveloped bullet-shaped virus with a single strand of linear RNA. Rabies virus is found in domestic and wild animals, particularly in Asia. Infection occurs as a result of inoculation by animal bite and occasionally through inhalation. The virus travels from muscle via the neuromuscular junction and axons to the central nervous system where it replicates, forming eosinophilic inclusion bodies (Negri bodies) in the cytoplasm of nerve cells. Rabies virus also reaches the salivary glands of infected animals.

Infection causes a universally fatal encephalitis and respiratory paralysis, unless postexposure prophylaxis with killed cell vaccine and hyperimmune globulin is given. This therapy relies on the lengthy incubation period of the infection (weeks to 1 year). There is no effective antiviral agent. Those at high risk of rabies infection can also benefit from pre-exposure vaccination with human diploid cell vaccine.

Togaviridae

The togaviruses are a group of enveloped, icosahedral single-stranded RNA viruses, which include rubella virus and arboviruses groups A and B.

Several togaviruses are transmitted from other animals by the bite of a mosquito. These arboviruses include the agents of Western equine encephalitis, Eastern equine encephalitis and Venezuelan equine encephalitis; all diseases encountered in the Americas. These viruses have a tropism for central nervous tissues, but the majority of infections are subclinical. The most severe infections are usually in infants.

Diagnosis is by inoculation into mouse brains or nucleic acid amplification.

Prevention is by vaccination of horses and specialist laboratory workers.

Rubellavirus Rubellavirus causes a mild, self-limiting exanthematous disease in children and adults. There may be a transient arthritis in some adult patients. The primary event is viral infection of the respiratory tract, followed by viraemia and dissemination to lymphoid tissues, skin and internal organs. Its greatest importance is as a cause of an intrauterine infection that results in interference with organogenesis during the first trimester of pregnancy. The severity of congenital malformation depends on how early in pregnancy the maternal infection occurred. Viral shedding continues after birth. There is a significantly reduced risk of fetal malformation following inadvertent vaccination of pregnant woman.

Diagnosis is by serological methods, and many centres screen pregnant women for rubella immune status. Haemagglutination inhibition, immunofluorescent and enzyme immunoassay techniques are used. Recent infection can be detected using an IgM-specific assay.

Prevention is by vaccination of children, or adolescent females, and hospital workers with a live attenuated rubella virus.

23 Parasitology

Overview

This chapter deals with the major groups of parasites, the infections they cause, and how they are diagnosed and treated. Information on infection is presented by microorganism, rather than by disease or syndrome. The chapter is meant as an alternative entry into information presented in previous chapters and as a supplementary learning resource.

Learning objectives

You should:

- know the principal groups of medically important parasites
- know the infections they cause
- be aware of the key laboratory tests used to detect and identify them
- know the antibiotics used to treat their infections.

23.1 Life cycles

Readers who are interested in details of specific parasite life cycles should refer to a medical parasitology textbook. Only the infective and diagnostic stages are mentioned in the account below.

23.2 Protozoa

Plasmodium

The plasmodia are sporozoan protozoa. There are four main species of medical importance: *Plasmodium falciparum*, *P. vivax*, *P. malariae* and *P. ovale*. The sporozoite stage of the parasite is transmitted to humans by the bite of a female anophelene mosquito, resulting in malaria. *P. falciparum* infections account for the majority of fatal infections.

Diagnosis is by observing different stages of the parasite's life cycle in smears made from peripheral blood (thin or thick films, stained with Giemsa, Wright's or similar stain). Parasite forms that can be observed, depending on the species and stage of infection, are trophozoites (ring form), schizonts and gametocytes. Newer diagnostic methods include acridine orange/buffy coat and gene amplification by the polymerase chain reaction (PCR).

Treatment of acute infection is with chloroquine unless resistance is suspected, in which case quinine, mefloquine or an alternative may be required. Primaquine must be used in *P. vivax* or *P. ovale* infections to prevent late relapse.

Community-wide prevention is by vector control methods such as draining mosquito breeding sites or spraying with residual insecticides. Personal prevention is by avoiding contact with the mosquito vector (bed nets, clothing and insect repellent) and by chemoprophylaxis, which is becoming increasingly complex because of increasing levels of resistance to currently used agents.

Babesia spp.

Babesia spp. are sporozoan parasites transmitted by the bite of ticks. The parasite causes babesiosis: a febrile disease in which there may be hepatosplenomegaly. Infection is more severe and more likely to endanger life in splenectomised patients.

The diagnostic stage of the parasite can be seen as tiny ring forms or Maltese crosses in erythrocytes in Giemsa-stained peripheral blood smears.

Patients do not respond to conventional antimalarial treatment but may benefit from a combination of quinine and clindamycin.

Toxoplasma gondii

Toxoplasma gondii is a sporozoan parasite belonging to the Coccidia. Toxoplasmosis is transmitted by ingestion of raw or poorly cooked meat containing sporulated oocysts. Infection may also be acquired by hand-to-mouth transmission following disposal of contaminated cat litter, since cats can act as a primary host for the parasite. Transplacental transmission may occur resulting in congenital disease.

Many infections are asymptomatic, but clinically apparent infection can range from mild to fulminant disease. The immunocompromised are at particular risk of severe disease.

Diagnosis is by demonstration of a rising titre or specific IgM antibody in serum.

Treatment is with pyrimethamine in combination with other agents. Spiramycin is used for treatment of toxoplasmosis diagnosed during pregnancy. Prevention is by thorough cooking of meat and safe disposal of cat litter.

Cryptosporidium sp.

Cryptosporidium sp. is a sporozoan parasite belonging to the Coccidia. Cryptosporidiosis is an intestinal infection caused by ingestion of sporulated oocysts. The entire life cycle is in the gastrointestinal tract of humans and the usual primary host, young calves or lambs. Immunocompromised patients are at increased risk of severe disease. In patients with the acquired immunodeficiency syndrome (AIDS), the diarrhoea of cryptosporidiosis may resemble cholera.

Diagnosis is by microscopy of diarrhoeal stool. The cysts can be stained by a modified acid-fast method.

There is no effective antimicrobial treatment and prevention is by thorough filtration of drinking water. Cysts are resistant to the usual level of chlorine added to potable water.

Microsporidium spp.

Microsporidium spp. are intracellular sporozoan parasites with an unusual coiled organelle, the polar filament, that injects sporoplasm into an intestinal mucosal cell. Microsporidia cause enteritis, particularly in immunocompromised patients.

Diagnosis is difficult and requires electron microscopy. There is no known effective treatment.

Cyclospora spp.

Cyclospora is a newly recognised genus of coccidian parasite responsible for diarrhoea in international travellers, particularly those visiting Central America and East Asia.

Diagnosis is by microscopy of diarrhoea stool.

There is no effective antimicrobial treatment at present.

Isospora belli

Isospora belli is a sporozoan parasite belonging to the Coccidia that causes diarrhoea or malabsorption following ingestion of oocysts.

Diagnosis is by microscopy of stool or duodenal aspirate.

Treatment with pyrimethamine/sulfadiazine or trimethoprim/sulfamethoxazole combinations may be effective.

Entamoeba spp.

The genus *Entamoeba* includes *E. histolytica*, *E. hartmanii* and *E. coli*, which are members of the Rhizopoda (amoe-bae). Certain strains of *E. histolytica* are pathogenic for humans and cause amoebic dysentery and soft tissue abscesses (e.g. in liver) after ingestion of amoebic cysts.

Definitive diagnosis is by recognition of motile amoebae (trophozoites) containing erythrocytes in the patient's stool or biopsy material. Microscopic detection of amoebic cysts of correct size and appearance in faecal specimens is suggestive but not conclusive evidence. These must be differentiated from the cysts of the non-pathogenic *Escherichia coli*. Serological tests are used to help to confirm invasive *Entamoeba* infection in the absence of diarrhoea.

Treatment is with metronidazole and diloxanide.

Prevention is by safe disposal of human faeces.

Naegleria spp.

Naeglerias are free-living amoebae (Rhizopoda) capable of causing a severe, life-threatening meningoencephalitis. Diagnosis is by microscopy of fresh, uncentrifuged cerebrospinal fluid (CSF) at room temperature. There is no universally effective antimicrobial agent, but amphotericin has been said to help in a few cases.

Acanthamoeba sp.

Acanthamoeba sp. is a free-living amoeba (Rhizopoda) known to cause meningitis in the immunosuppressed and keratitis in contact lens wearers or following minor corneal trauma.

Diagnosis is by microscopic detection of cysts and trophozoites in biopsy material, or by growing cysts from clinical specimens on a lawn of bacteria.

Treatment of keratitis is with propamidine, but the response is often poor.

Ciliates

Balantidium coli is the only ciliate to cause infection in the human gastrointestinal tract. Infection of the caecum and ileum follows ingestion of cysts and results in bloody diarrhoea.

Diagnosis is by recognition of trophozoites in biopsy material or stool preparation.

Treatment is with metronidazole.

Pneumocystis carinii

Pneumocystis carinii is a protozoan parasite of uncertain designation (some authorities propose that the species is more closely related to the fungi). *P. carinii* causes interstitial pneumonia in immunocompromised patients, including those with AIDS, in those on high doses of glucocorticoids and in premature infants.

Diagnosis is by silver methenamine or immunofluorescent stain of bronchial biopsy or bronchoalveolar lavage material.

Treatment is with co-trimoxazole or pentamidine. Prevention in patients with human immunodeficiency virus (HIV) infection is with continuous co-trimoxazole treatment.

Flagellates

Trichomonas **spp.**

The trichomonads are a genus of flagellate with an undulating membrane running along one side of the cell. They inhabit the human gastrointestinal and genitourinary tract. Only *Trichomonas vaginalis* causes disease in humans: vaginitis and urethritis. No cyst stage has been identified. Infection is by direct transfer either during sexual intercourse or in some cases by indirect contact. Asymptomatic infection is common.

Diagnosis is by microscopic detection of trophozoites in vaginal secretions.

Treatment is with metronidazole.

Giardia lamblia

Giardia lamblia is a flagellate protozoan that causes diarrhoea and malabsorption following ingestion of the cyst stage. The leaf-shaped trophozoite grows on the duodenal mucosa.

G. lamblia trophozoites can sometimes be detected by microscopy of diarrhoea stool. Normally, diagnosis is by detection of the cyst stage in stools, or less often by detection of the trophozoite in duodenal aspirate or biopsy material.

Treatment is with metronidazole or tinidazole.

Leishmania **spp.**

The *Leishmania* spp. are a complex group of flagellated protozoa that cause cutaneous, mucocutaneous and visceral leishmaniasis (kala–azar) following transmission of the promastigote stage by the bite of a sandfly (Table 45).

Diagnosis is by bone marrow tap or splenic biopsy and recognition of the non-flagellated, amastigote stage in phagocytic cells.

Treatment is with pentavalent antimonial compounds.

Prevention is by vector control and avoiding contact with sandflies.

Trypanosoma **spp.**

The genus *Trypanosoma* includes the haemoflagellates *T. brucei* and *T. cruzi* and causes, respectively, African sleeping sickness and Chagas disease (Table 46). Metacyclic epimastigotes of *T. brucei* var *gambiense* or *rhodesiense* are transmitted by the bite of the tsetse fly *Glossina* sp. Metacyclic epimastigotes of *T. cruzi* are transmitted in the faeces of reduviid or cone-nosed bugs following a blood meal.

Diagnosis of African trypanosomiasis is by microscopic detection of trypomastigotes in blood, bone marrow or lymph node biopsy material. Treatment is with suramin and melarsoprol, both of which are highly toxic.

Diagnosis of *T. cruzi* infection is by serological methods, and treatment with nifurtimox is still under investigation.

Prevention is by vector control.

23.3 Helminths (worms)

The helminths include:

- nematodes: roundworms that can be intestinal, blood and tissue parasites
- Flatworms (platyhelminths)
  —cestodes (tapeworms): ribbon-like segmented worms; intestinal and multiorgan parasites
  —trematodes: leaf-like flukes; intestinal, liver, lungs or blood parasites.

Table 45 Leishmanial infections

Leishmaniasis	Species	Location
Visceral	*L. donovani, L. infantum, L. chagasi*	Old, New Worlds
Cutaneous	*L. tropica, L. major, L. aethiopica*	Old World
Mucocutaneous	*L. mexicana, L. brasiliensis* complexes	New World

Table 46 Trypanosome infections

Location	Disease	Progression	Epidemiology	Trypanosome	Vector
West Africa riverside, woodland	Sleeping sickness	Subclinical or slow	Endemic	*T. brucei* var *gambiense* group	*Glossina palpalis*
East Africa savanna	Sleeping sickness	Rapid	Episodic	*T. brucei* var *rhodesiense* group	*Glossina morsitans*
South America	Cardiomegaly megaoesophagus/ colon	Slow	Endemic	*T. cruzi*	Reduviid bug

Nematodes

Enterobius vermicularis

Enterobius vermicularis is a nematode or roundworm that causes perianal itching. The organism is commonly known as pinworm or threadworm and is transmitted by hand-to-mouth transfer of eggs.

The diagnosis is made when the adult worms are seen at the anal margin or on the stools, or by microscopic detection of eggs on a Sellotape swab preparation.

Treatment is with mebendazole and should be given to all family members.

Prevention is by high standards of personal hygiene, particularly among young children.

Trichuris trichiura

Trichuris trichiura is a nematode (roundworm), often called whipworm. Trichuris is spread by eggs transmitted via the faecal–oral route. Infection causes diarrhoea, abdominal pain and may even lead to rectal prolapse.

Diagnosis is by recognition of the characteristic eggs in stool preparations for microscopy.

Treatment is with metronidazole and prevention is by hygienic disposal of faeces.

Toxocara spp.

Toxocara canis and *T. cati* are nematodes (roundworms). Transmission of eggs from moist soil contaminated by cat or dog faeces can lead to visceral larva migrans or endophthalmitis.

Definitive diagnosis is difficult since a high proportion of seropositive individuals have had asymptomatic infection previously.

Treatment with thiabendazole may be beneficial.

Prevention is by deworming cats and dogs and by covering sandpits used by young children when the pits are not in use.

Hookworms

Hookworms are intestinal nematodes (roundworms). The two most important species are *Ancylostoma duodenale* and *Necator americanus*. These species used to be distributed in the Old World and New World respectively, but there is now considerable overlap in their distributions. Infection follows penetration of the skin of the lower limb by filarial larvae. The adult worm inhabits the intestine consuming blood from the intestinal mucosa and releasing eggs into the intestinal lumen.

Diagnosis is by recognition of the eggs in faeces.

Treatment is with mebendazole.

Prevention is by hygienic disposal of faeces and mass treatment of communities where the infection is endemic.

Strongyloides stercoralis

Strongyloides stercoralis is a nematode (roundworm) that causes a range of conditions (diarrhoea, bronchitis, eosinophilia) known under the general heading of strongyloidiasis. Infection follows penetration of the skin by filariform larvae from the soil. Three routes of transmission have been documented: direct in temperate climates, indirect in tropical conditions and autoinfection.

Diagnosis is by detection of the rhabditiform larvae in stool specimens.

Treatment is with thiabendazole.

Prevention is by hygienic disposal of faeces.

Trichinella spiralis

Trichinella spiralis is a nematode (roundworm) that causes parasite dissemination to striated muscle following consumption of meat containing the larval stage of the parasite.

Diagnosis is by serology or muscle biopsy.

Mebendazole has been beneficial in some cases.

Prevention is by thorough cooking of meat from omnivores and carnivores and by sterilisation of pig feed.

Ascaris lumbricoides

Ascaris lumbricoides is a nematode (roundworm) that causes intestinal infection following ingestion of embryonated eggs in faecally contaminated food. There is some debate about the public health importance of ascariasis, but obstruction of the intestine and associated hollow organs can be caused by *A. lumbricoides*. Infection may also have an adverse effect on nutrition.

Diagnosis is by detection of the eggs in faeces.

Treatment is with piperazine, which relaxes the adult worm, allowing its expulsion from the intestine.

Wuchereria and Brugia spp.

Wuchereria bancrofti, *Brugia malayi* and *B. timori* are tissue nematodes transmitted as microfilaria by various species of mosquito. The microfilariae migrate to the lower limbs where the adult stage causes blockage of lymphatics, resulting in lymphangitis and elephantiasis.

Diagnosis is by detection of microfilariae on microscopy of a blood smear.

Treatment is with diethylcarbamazine or ivermectin.

Prevention is by avoiding contact with the mosquito vector or by mass treatment of communities where infection is endemic.

Onchocerca volvulus

Onchocerca volvulus is the tissue nematode responsible for onchocerciasis, otherwise known as river blindness. Infection results from transmission of microfilariae by the blackfly *Simulium* sp.

Diagnosis is by microscopy of preparations of biopsy material from skin snips over the subcutaneous nodules caused by the infection.

Treatment is with ivermectin.

Prevention is by vector control measures and by periodic mass treatment programmes.

Loa loa

Loa loa is the infection caused by a tissue nematode transmitted by *Chrysops* flies in parts of equatorial Africa. Infection results in various conditions, including Calabar swellings of the limbs and migration of the adult worm across the conjunctiva.

Diagnosis is by detection of microfilariae in peripheral blood smears.

Treatment is with repeated courses of diethylcarbamazine.

Dracunculus medinensis

Dracunculus medinensis is a tissue nematode that causes dracontiasis: a condition in which the adult worm settles in a subcutaneous location and forms a painful swelling which bursts on contact with water, releasing larvae. Infection is by drinking water containing a later larval stage.

Diagnosis is clinical.

Treatment is with metronidazole and careful removal of the adult worm.

Prevention is by protection of potable water supplies.

Cestodes

Taenia spp.

Taenia spp. are cestodes or tapeworms. The genus includes *T. saginata* (beef tapeworm) and *T. solium*. Both species cause tapeworm infection of the gastrointestinal tract after ingestion of the cysticerci (larval stage) in poorly cooked infected meat. *T. solium*, the pork tapeworm, can also cause disseminated disease (cysticercosis) when the first-stage larva penetrates the gastrointestinal wall and spreads to distant sites including the skin, muscles and brain.

Diagnosis is by detection of eggs in faeces or proglottids (mature segments of tapeworm) passed per rectum.

Treatment is with niclosamide, which causes release and expulsion of the tapeworm.

Prevention is by meat inspection, stopping pigs consuming raw sewage and adequate cooking of pork and beef.

Diphyllobothrium latum

Diphyllobothrium latum is a tapeworm associated with consumption of raw or poorly cooked freshwater fish. The adult is the longest tapeworm species found in humans. Infection is by ingestion of the plerocercoid (larval stage). Infection can result in macrocytic anaemia.

Diagnosis is by detection of eggs on stool microscopy or proglottids passed per rectum.

Treatment is with niclosamide.

Prevention is by cooking freshwater fish and avoiding sewage contamination of fishing lakes and rivers.

Echinococcus granulosus

Echinococcus granulosus is the minute tapeworm responsible for hydatid disease. Dogs and wild canines are the primary host for the tapeworm, and infection results from hand-to-mouth transmission of eggs from their faeces. Penetration of the gastrointestinal wall leads to formation of cysts, which may grow to a large size. The commonest sites are the lungs and liver, but the abdomen, pelvis and brain are sometimes involved.

Diagnosis is by serological tests such as enzyme-linked immunosorbent assay (ELISA) and may require confirmation by detection of the arc 5 antigen.

Treatment is by careful surgical removal of cysts and treatment with albendazole.

Prevention requires routine deworming of dogs in endemic areas.

Trematodes

Fasciola hepatica

Fasciola hepatica is a tissue trematode (fluke) that causes infection of the liver following consumption of watercress or contact with grass containing the cercarial stage of the fluke.

Diagnosis is by identification of the operculated eggs in faeces or bile.

Treatment is with dichlorophenol.

Prevention is by treatment of domestic animals, particularly sheep, and growing watercress away from pasture land.

Clonorchis sinensis

Clonorchis sinensis is also known as the oriental liver fluke: this trematode causes infection of the hepatobiliary system following consumption of raw or undercooked fish containing parasitic metacercariae.

Diagnosis is by detection of the operculated eggs in faeces.

Treatment is with praziquantel.

Prevention is by thorough cooking of fish.

Paragonimus westermanii

Paragonimus westermanii is also known as the lung fluke; this tissue trematode causes pulmonary infection following consumption of cercariae in raw or partly cooked crabs and crayfish in east Asia.

Diagnosis is by detection of eggs in sputum.

Treatment is with praziquantel.

Prevention is by avoiding consumption of raw crustaceans.

Schistosoma

The genus *Schistosoma* includes *S. mansoni*, *S. japonicum* and *S. haematobium*, the three main pathogenic species in humans (Table 47). Infection results from penetration of intact skin by cercariae during contact with contaminated water. Disease (schistosomiasis) manifestations depend on the species, the time after exposure and a variety of host factors. In chronological sequence, dermatitis, fever and fibro-obstructive disorders can be expected. The adult worms inhabit the venous plexus of affected organs and release eggs into the tissues, promoting a fibrous reaction. Eggs are released in the faeces or urine, depending on the species.

Diagnosis is by microscopic detection of eggs in clinical specimens.

Treatment is with praziquantel.

Prevention is by hygienic disposal of urine and faeces, control of the snails that act as intermediate hosts, and by mass treatment campaigns.

Table 47 Infection with *Schistosoma* spp.

Species	Location	Site of disease	Specimen
S. mansoni	Africa, South America	Colon, liver	Stool, rectal biopsy
S. japonicum	East Asia	Liver, colon	Stool, rectal biopsy
S. haematobium	Africa, Middle East	Urinary tract	Urine

24 Mycology

Overview

This chapter deals with the major groups of fungi, the infections they cause, and how they are diagnosed and treated. Information on infection is presented by microorganism, rather than by disease or syndrome. The chapter is meant as an alternative entry into information presented in previous chapters and as a supplementary learning resource.

Learning objectives

You should:

- know the principal groups of fungi
- know the infections they cause
- be aware of the key laboratory tests used to detect and identify them
- know the antibiotics used to treat their infections.

Aspergillus spp.

Aspergillus fumigatus is a filamentous fungus that causes opportunist lung infections in immunocompromised patients, allergic bronchopulmonary disease and fungal balls (mycetoma) in patients with pre-existing pulmonary cavities.

Diagnosis of invasive pulmonary disease is by microscopy of biopsy material and in allergic disease by serological methods.

Treatment of invasive disease is with amphotericin. Mycetomas may require surgical removal.

Another member of the genus, *A. niger*, is responsible for superficial infection of the external auditory meatus.

Candida spp.

Candida are single-celled, budding fungi or yeasts, present as a minority member of the indigenous flora of the gastrointestinal tract in some people. They cause a variety of opportunist infections and are important as a cause of infection in the immunocompromised patient. The commonest clinically important species is *Candida albicans*.

Diagnosis is by microscopy in clinical specimens and culture on Sabouraud or similar agar.

Treatment of candidiasis is with a variety of antifungal agents including nystatin, miconazole, fluconazole, amphotericin and flucytosine, depending on the site and severity of infection.

Cryptococcus neoformans

Cryptococcus neoformans is a single-celled fungus, or yeast, that causes meningitis and occasionally focal lesions, mainly in immunocompromised patients. In cerebrospinal fluid specimens, the yeast is capsulated and can be seen at microscopy using India ink.

Treatment is with fluconazole or amphotericin.

Dermatophytes

Dermatophytes are filamentous fungi with a preference for epithelial body surfaces. They are responsible for fungal skin infections. This group includes *Trichophyton*, *Epidermophyton* and *Microsporum* spp.

Treatment is with a topical antifungal agent. Persistent infections may require on oral agent.

Epidermophyton floccosum

Epidermophyton floccosum is a filamentous fungus in the dermatophyte group that causes skin infection. It can be differentiated from other dermatophytes by the microscopic appearance of a lactophenol cotton blue preparation.

Microsporum spp.

These filamentous fungi are responsible for a variety of superficial mycotic infections.

Fusarium spp.

Fusarium spp. are filamentous fungi associated with keratitis and a variety of opportunist infections in immunocompromised patients.

Trichophyton spp.

Trichophyton is a genus of filamentous fungi that causes common skin infections. Important species include *T. rubrum* and *T. mentagrophytes*.

Histoplasma capsulatum

Histoplasma capsulatum is a dimorphic fungus since it can grow in both yeast and mycelial forms. It causes systemic fungal infection and is most commonly found where there are large amounts of bird or bat droppings. Immunocompromised patients are more susceptible to severe infection.

Treatment is with amphotericin.

Mucor spp.

Mucor spp. are filamentous, sporing fungi or moulds, responsible for severe, life-threatening infections (e.g. rhinocerebral mucormycosis) in immunocompromised patients. These infections have a poor prognosis despite aggressive surgical and antifungal therapy.

Pityrosporum spp.

Pityrosporum ovale is the yeast form of a dermatophytic fungus responsible for pityriasis. *Pityrosporum orbiculare* has also been associated with seborrhoeic dermatitis and may be present as indigenous flora of the normal skin.

Sporothrix schenckii

Sporothrix schenckii is a dimorphic, soil-living fungus responsible for infections of the skin, lymphatic vessels and other sites.

Specific diagnosis is often by silver stain of biopsy material.

Treatment is with oral itraconazole.

25 Entomology

Overview

This chapter deals with the major groups of medically important arthropods, the infections they act as vectors for, and their recognition and control. The chapter is meant as a supplementary learning resource.

Learning objectives

You should:

- know the principal groups of medically important arthropods
- know the infections they act as vectors for
- know the key features used in their recognition
- know the methods used in their control.

Mosquitoes

Mosquitoes are small, winged, biting insects; the females require a blood meal before their eggs can complete their development. The most important types of mosquito are the anophelene and culicine varieties. Anophelene mosquitoes are responsible for transmission of malaria, some arbovirus infections and filarial disease. Culicine mosquitoes transmit arbovirus and filarial infections but not malaria. The adult mosquito can be identified by its resting angle (the proboscis, thorax and abdomen of anophelenes form a straight line, while culicines are bent), its palps and the arrangement of wing scales. Important disease vectors include *Anopheles gambiae* (malaria in Africa), *Culex tritaeniorhyncus* (Japanese encephalitis in East Asia), *Aedes aegypti* (dengue and yellow fever) and *Mansonia* spp. (filarial disease in southeast Asia).

Many mosquito species have developed biological or behavioural resistance to previously effective insecticides. Vector control, therefore, depends heavily on eradication of breeding sites. Personal measures to avoid contact with disease-carrying mosquitoes have become more important.

Sandflies

Sandflies are very small, winged, biting insects with a limited range. They are responsible for transmission of leishmaniasis, sandfly fever and bartonellosis. The genus *Lutzomyia* is important in South America. *Phlebotomus* spp. are the dominant sandfly vectors elsewhere. Sandflies have been successfully controlled by spraying housing with a residual insecticide such as DDT (dichlorodiphenyltrichloroethane).

Tsetse flies

Tsetse flies are relatively large biting insects capable of rapid flight. They feed on mammalian blood and transmit the trypanosomes responsible for African sleeping sickness. Two main groups are important as vectors of human disease: *Glossina morsitans* and *Glossina palpalis*. The *G. morsitans* group is found in the savanna of west, central and east Africa and transmits *Trypanosoma brucei* var *rhodesiense*. The *G. palpalis* group is found in riverside forests in west Africa and transmits *T. brucei* var *gambiense*.

Control methods include destruction of game animals, clearance of preferred bush habitats, aerial spraying with insecticides such as DDT or permethrin and insect trapping.

Blackflies

The genus *Simulium* (blackfly) comprises small biting insects that are found by fast flowing streams in west Africa and parts of Central America. Blackflies transmit *Onchocerca volvulus*, the cause of river blindness.

Vector control is being attempted in some endemic areas by aerial spraying with pyrethroid or organophosphorus insecticides.

Fleas

Fleas are wingless insects with a worldwide distribution. Both males and females require mammalian blood. The flea family is important in the transmission of several diseases: plague (tropical rat flea, *Xenopsylla cheopis*), murine typhus and tularaemia. In addition, one member of the family, *Tunga penetrans*, is able to penetrate human skin and causes a lesion known as jiggers.

The most common reason for implementing measures to control fleas is during an outbreak of bubonic plague. The use of insecticide to eradicate fleas should precede rat extermination to avoid rat fleas seeking human hosts.

Lice

Lice are insects with a wingless thorax and prominent graspers that require a blood meal to survive. Lice infestation is with *Pediculus humanus* (human body louse) or *Pthiris pubis* (the pubic or crab louse) and causes local irritation. Lice are important as vectors of relapsing fever, epidemic typhus and trench fever.

Control is by topical application of insecticide and the destruction of infested clothing.

Reduviid bugs

Some species of reduviid or cone-nosed bugs feed on human blood, biting at night. Their chief medical significance is as vectors of *Trypanosoma cruzi*: the cause of Chagas disease.

Vector control is by improving conditions to eradicate breeding sites and by the use of residual insecticides.

Sarcoptes

The itch mite *Sarcoptes scabei* produces an intensely itchy lesion by burrowing into the skin. The condition is known as scabies.

Diagnosis is by microscopy of a mite removed from its burrow with a sterile needle after covering the burrow with oil.

Treatment is with lindane or benzene hexachloride. Family contacts may require treatment at the same time, and clothing and bedding should be thoroughly cleaned.

Ticks

Ticks are arachnids and belong to two main groups: argasid (soft-bodied) and ixodid (hard-bodied) ticks. Argasid ticks are important as vectors of tick-borne relapsing fever (caused by *Borrelia duttoni*). Ixodid ticks are involved in the transmission of tick-borne typhus (e.g. Congo–Crimea haemorrhagic fever) and Lyme disease. Removal of ticks is achieved mechanically or with grease or chloroform.

Acid-fast stain

Multiple-step stain for acid-fast bacteria such as mycobacteria and *Nocardia* sp. The most commonly used stains of this type include Ziehl–Neelsen (concentrated carbol fuchsin, heated, followed by acid–alcohol and a counterstain) and auramine–phenol.

Agar

Term used to refer to a type of solid growth medium for bacteria or fungi that contains agar solidifying agent. Examples include blood (contains intact erythrocytes) agar, chocolate (haemolysed blood) agar, CLED (cysteine lactose electrolyte-deficient) agar, MacConkey (lactose, pH indicator and bile salt) agar, sorbitol–MacConkey, XLD (xylose lysine decarboxylase) agar, DCA (deoxycholate citrate) agar, and VCAT (vancomycin colistin amphotericin trimethoprim) agar.

Agglutination

Fine clumping caused by a reaction between a test organism and agglutinating antisera. Antisera can be carried on inert particles such as latex, erythrocytes or staphylococci to enhance the visible agglutination reaction.

Anaerobic cabinet

An airtight incubator from which oxygen has been expelled and in which obligate anaerobic bacteria can be grown.

Anaerobic gas jar

A portable alternative to the anaerobic cabinet, suitable for a smaller number of agar plates. The gaseous contents must be replaced each time the jar is resealed.

Antibiotic susceptibility test

Antibiotic susceptibility of a pathogen tested in the laboratory by a variety of methods. In the disk diffusion method, a lawn of test organism is spread evenly on the surface of an agar plate, and then antibiotic-containing disks are placed on top. After incubation, susceptibility is indicated by a zone of growth inhibition, whereas resistance corresponds to a reduced, absence of, inhibition zone. A variation on this method used a control species with known susceptibilities on the same agar plate for comparison. A more accurate but cumbersome method is the minimum inhibitory concentration (MIC), which requires the growth of the organism in a series of progressively dilute antibiotic solutions. The MIC is the lowest concentration that inhibits microbial growth.

Antibody detection

Antibody detection methods include complement fixation test, haemagglutination assay, indirect fluorescent antibody test (IFAT) and enzyme-linked immunosorbent assay (ELISA). Serodiagnosis by IgG detection usually requires paired serum specimens with an interval of 7–10 days, during which a fourfold increase in titre would be a minimum threshold for positive results. However, single positive IgM assays can provide evidence of recent infection.

Antigen detection

A variety of methods including direct fluorescent antibody (DFA) test and enzyme-linked immunosorbent assay (ELISA). The detection of significant levels of microbial antigen in sterile tissues or body fluid is probably indicative of infection, but positive results on specimens from body surface sites may require careful interpretation.

Bench-top tests

Simple, rapidly performed laboratory tests that help towards a presumptive diagnosis but which rarely provide the definitive answer.

Beta(β)-lactamase test

Test for the enzyme responsible for resistance to penicillin or cephalosporin antibiotics by lysing the β-lactam ring. Commonly used screening versions of the test employ a chromogenic cephalosporin (nitrocefin) or paper strips impregnated with penicillin and a pH indicator.

Blood culture

Used to detect bacteria or fungi in the systemic circulation (bacteraemia). Performed by sampling peripheral blood using a no-touch or aseptic venipuncture method. At least 10 ml blood should be withdrawn and dispensed into two blood culture bottles, one for aerobic and one for anaerobic culture. Multiple sets of bottles should be inoculated at intervals for patients with suspected infective endocarditis. Blood culture bottles are incubated in the laboratory and examined regularly either by eye or by using an automated device. When microbial growth is suspected, the contents of the bottle are Gram stained and subcultured onto solid media.

Capsule stain

Single-step negative stain to detect the presence of bacterial or fungal capsules (usually polysaccharide).

Catalase test
A bench-top test that uses hydrogen peroxide to demonstrate the presence of catalase in certain bacteria—used to distinguish streptococci (negative result) from staphylococci (positive result).

Catheter specimen of urine
Urine specimen obtained from a patient with indwelling urinary catheter. Bacteriuria is common in these patients and, in the absence of pyuria, may not reflect true urinary tract infection, since urinary catheters are prone to microbial colonisation.

Cell culture
Term referring to use of cell monolayer for cultivation of obligate intracellular pathogens, such as viruses and chlamydias.

Clone
Genetically identical individuals or cells. In DNA cloning, a particular gene is isolated and multiplied to allow its use or identification. A clonal immune response is the proliferation of lymphocytes with a particular specificity in response to an antigen; the lymphocytes then produce monoclonal (identical) antibody molecules.

Coagglutination
An agglutination test method in which staphylococci are used as carrier particles for the test antibody, the Fc fragment of which adheres to protein A bound to the staphylococcal cell surface. Used to detect bacterial antigen as a rapid diagnostic method in meningitis and used to confirm the identity of *Neisseria gonorrhoeae*.

Coagulase test
A test that employs rabbit plasma as a substrate for the coagulase produced by *Staphylococcus aureus*. The definitive test is the tube coagulase test performed in a test tube, and the rapid, bench-top test is the slide coagulase test—for clumping factor.

Colony-forming units (cfu)
The number of colonies of bacteria or fungi that grow on the surface of solid media corresponds to the number of colony-forming units (cfu) present in the inoculum. This number is approximately equal to the number of cells present only if the species is not prone to cluster or clump.

Complement fixation test (CFT)
An antibody detection test used for serodiagnosis of various infections. The CFT relies on a reaction between sought-for complement-fixing antibody and sensitised erythrocytes to produce a visible endpoint, on which the titre is based.

C-reactive protein (CRP)
A protein produced as part of the acute-phase reaction that happens to react with pneumococcal C substance. Elevated levels are found during any acute systemic inflammatory response, but very high levels can be found during severe *Streptococcus pneumoniae* infection.

Culture
A term referring to the growth of microorganisms under artificial conditions, or the results of microbial growth on artificial culture media.

Differential count
The relative percentage of different leucocyte cell lines in peripheral blood or other fluid examined. Applied to cerebrospinal fluid, it is used to assist the differentiation between viral and bacterial meningitis.

DNA sequencing
Identifying an organism by analysing its DNA base sequence. Rapid, automated DNA sequencing is now used widely in diagnostic microbiology laboratories to identify a variety of viruses, mycobacteria and various other microorganisms. Sequencing at the 16S ribosomal DNA locus is an important method of identifying otherwise difficult to identify bacterial species.

Enzyme-linked immunosorbent assay (ELISA)
An antibody or antigen detection system that uses antibody linked to an enzyme to produce a colour reaction indicating a positive result. Widely used for serodiagnosis of different infectious diseases.

Erythrocyte sedimentation rate (ESR)
The speed at which a column of red blood cells settles. This can be used as a non-specific indicator of systemic disease. Not specific to infectious diseases.

Fatty acid analysis
Cell wall fatty acids from bacterial isolates analysed by gas liquid chromatography of their methyl ester products (fatty acid methyl esters, or FAME). The pattern of peak retention times generated by this type of analysis is often characteristic of a given bacterial species. These data can be used to confirm the identity of bacteria that are otherwise difficult to identify.

Fluorescent treponemal antigen (FTA)
A specific test for the serodiagnosis of syphilis. It becomes positive during the secondary stage of disease and may remain positive for many years after treatment. The test uses treponemes bound to glass microscope slides to bind sought-for antibody, to which anti-human fluorescent antibody is bound. Used to confirm a specific diagnosis but does not necessarily indicate active or current infection.

Gram stain
A multiple step stain that is widely used to demonstrate the fundamental cell wall structure and the shape of bacteria. An initial staining with methyl violet is followed

by the addition of iodine as a mordant, decolorisation with alcohol or acetone, and counterstaining with dilute carbol fuchsin. Gram-positive bacteria have a thick peptidoglycan layer in their cell wall and retain methyl violet despite decolorisation: they stain dark blue-purple. Gram-negative bacteria do not retain methyl violet because they have only a thin peptidoglycan layer and take up the colour of the counterstain: pink. The shape of bacteria that have been Gram stained is also used in their classification, e.g. streptococci (chain-forming, spherical bacteria), bacilli (sausage-shaped).

Haemagglutination assay
Antibody detection assay relying on agglutination of erythrocytes for the visible endpoint, followed by calculation of titre.

Haemolytic; β(beta)-, α(alpha)-
Alteration of blood agar surrounding a bacterial colony. This change is used to classify streptococci into α-haemolytic (e.g. the viridans group), β-haemolytic (e.g. *Streptococcus pyogenes*) and non-haemolytic (e.g. *Streptococcus faecalis*). The α-haemolytic streptococci discolour the surrounding agar green, while β-haemolytic streptococci clear the red cells from the agar. Other bacterial species can cause haemolysis on blood agar.

Helper cell count
Count of T helper cells (i.e. T lymphocytes bearing the CD4 cell surface antigen). This is used to support a diagnosis and to monitor disease progression in the acquired immunodeficiency syndrome (AIDS).

Helper/suppressor cell ratio
The ratio of T helper to T suppressor lymphocytes. This is used to support a diagnosis of AIDS or human immunodeficiency virus (HIV) infection.

Identification: preliminary, definitive
The process of giving a name to a microorganism recovered in the diagnostic laboratory. Preliminary identification is often partial and provisional, in the interests of speed, whereas definitive identification requires the completion of all relevant identification tests. This may involve delays of days to weeks for slow-growing organisms that require laboratory manipulation. Identification of microbial pathogens is used to arrive at a specific aetiological diagnosis, guide antimicrobial chemotherapy and sometimes to assist in epidemiological investigations.

Immunofluorescence: direct, indirect (IFAT)
A method of detecting either antibody or antigen. Direct and indirect methods are used. A positive result depends on the detection of recognisable microorganisms under an ultraviolet microscope. Applications include detection of *Legionella pneumophila*, *Pneumocystis carinii* and antibodies to *Entamoeba histolytica*.

Incubation
The provision of a suitable temperature and gaseous atmosphere for the cultivation of microorganisms on or in artificial media. Commonly used gaseous conditions include aerobic (room air), anaerobic (from which oxygen has been eliminated), capnophilic (for organisms that require a higher than usual CO_2 concentration). The most commonly used temperature is 37°C, but other temperatures are used for specific purposes.

Inoculation
The application of live microorganisms to an environment supportive of microbial growth. The term is usually used in the diagnostic laboratory to refer to inoculation of artificial growth media (see *Agar, Media*).

Lactose fermenter
A term usually used to refer to bacterial species that belong to the Enterobacteriaceae that are capable of fermenting lactose.

Latex agglutination test
A form of agglutination reaction that uses latex particles as a carrier for the agglutinating antibody used in the test. Uses include grouping of β-haemolytic streptococci.

Media
A term used to refer to the artificial media employed to provide the appropriate solid, liquid or cellular environment for the growth of microbial pathogens. Solid media usually contain agar as a solidifying agent and often have a liquid equivalent that lacks agar. These media can be either selective or non-selective depending on the range of growth substrates and inhibitory compounds they contain. Non-selective media are usually used to grow fastidious microorganisms from normally sterile sites, while selective media are used to isolate potential pathogens from non-sterile sites. See *Cell culture* for more information.

Microscopy
Use of various types of microscope in diagnostic microbiology. This is an important part of diagnosis since microorganisms cannot, by definition, be seen without the assistance of a magnifying device. Light (brightfield) microscopy is the most widely used technique, usually with a stain to improve contrast and provide information on microbial structure. Other types of light microscopy include darkfield, phase contrast, ultraviolet and confocal laser microscopy. The much higher magnification electron microscope (either scanning or transmission) is required to see the structure of viral particles and the ultrastructure of other microorganisms.

Midstream urine (MSU)
Specimen of urine passed for laboratory examination after discarding the first few drops of the urine stream

(to reduce contamination with urethral commensals) and before completion of micturition. An MSU should only be collected after careful cleansing of the external genitalia and cannot be collected from babies or from patients with an indwelling urinary catheter.

Minimum bactericidal concentration (MBC)

Similar to the minimum inhibitory concentration (MIC, see below), but it is the lowest concentration at which no growth occurs on subculture of an inoculum at varying antibiotic dilutions. A large difference between MBC and MIC may be caused by antibiotic tolerance, which can result in treatment failure.

Minimum inhibitory concentration (MIC)

A method of determining *Antibiotic susceptibility* that uses a serial dilution of antibiotic as a growth medium for the test species. The lowest concentration at which growth occurs is referred to as the MIC. Used to confirm disk diffusion test results, particularly where borderline results may adversely affect clinical outcome. Methods include broth macrodilution, broth microdilution and plate incorporation.

Molecular epidemiology

A catchphrase used to describe the application of molecular microbial typing methods to the investigation of possible outbreaks or epidemics. A rapidly growing list of methods is available using mainly molecular genetic techniques.

Monoclonal antibody

Specific antibody produced using the mouse hybridoma technique. Monoclonal antibodies (mAbs) are widely used in serodiagnosis of infectious diseases.

Nagler plate

Egg yolk-containing agar, half of which is covered with clostridial antitoxin. Lecithinase-producing *Clostridia* spp. (e.g. *C. perfringens*) cause changes in the underlying agar that are inhibited by antitoxin. It is used to identify *C. perfringens*.

Neutrophil count

Count of neutrophil polymorphonuclear cells. Used in diagnosis of meningitis (count in cerebrospinal fluid) and urinary tract infection (count in midstream urine specimen, usually as total leucocyte count).

Oligonucleotide probe

A reagent of known nucleotide sequence used to detect uncultivatable microorganisms or the genetic determinants of pathogenicity (e.g. toxins).

Oxidase test

Rapid, bench-top test to detect the presence of cytochrome oxidase. Used in the presumptive identification of some bacteria, including *Pseudomonas* spp. and *Neisseria* spp.

Phage typing

The application of a recognised set of bacteriophages with specificity for particular strains of the bacterial species in question. The commonest species to be typed with bacteriophages is *Staphylococcus aureus*. The results of phage typing can be used for epidemiological studies.

Plasmid typing

Distinguishing apparently phenotypically identical bacterial species by extracting any plasmid DNA present in each strain and separating it into its constituent bands by gel electrophoresis. Strains of a given species with more than one band in common are very likely to have originated from the same progenitor and are referred to as indistinguishable. Plasmid typing is widely used in the investigation of outbreaks.

Polymerase chain reaction (PCR)

A method of rapid DNA amplification. When combined with a gene probe for a known/sought-for nucleotide sequence (called a 'primer'), PCR provides a very sensitive means of detecting non-cultivatable microorganisms. PCR is used in many areas of clinical microbiology.

Pulsed field gel electrophoresis (PFGE)

A highly discriminating method of molecular typing bacteria for epidemiological purposes. It employs infrequent cutting restriction endonuclease enzymes to cut bacterial DNA into large fragments that can be separated in an agarose gel with a pulsed field electric current. This method can be applied to a wide range of bacterial pathogens responsible for hospital- and community-acquired infections.

Pyocine typing

Inhibitory substances (pyocines) produced by *Pseudomonas aeruginosa* that act on other strains of the same species. If a collection of known pyocine types are tested against an unknown clinical isolate, its pyocine type can be determined. Pyocine typing of *P. aeruginosa* has been used to investigate possible outbreaks of nosocomial infection caused by this organism.

Radial haemolysis

A serological test in which serum is placed in wells in a gel containing sensitised erythrocytes. Presence of haemolytic antibodies results in clearing of the gel. The test is used to assess the rubella immune status of pregnant women.

Rapid diagnostic tests

Tests that provide results fast enough to influence immediate clinical management. The results of diagnostic investigations that rely on growth of live organisms may not be available for days, or in some cases even weeks. Rapid diagnostic tests do not as a rule rely on cultivation of microorganisms. In practice, a result must be available no more than 30–60 minutes after specimen collection to be of use in immediate clinical decisions.

Report

The verbal or written communication from the diagnostic laboratory that contains the result of laboratory investigations. When the diagnostic process is lengthy, a preliminary report may be issued containing provisional information of immediate value to the physician managing the patient. A definitive report may follow. The preliminary and definitive reports may correspond to the respective stages of identification of a causal pathogen.

Request form

The request form is the principal means of communicating relevant clinical information to the diagnostic laboratory with the clinical specimen. Since the request form is a communication between medical staff, it should be completed by the physician who requests the investigation and not by nursing or other paramedical staff. Many laboratories use the request form as a laboratory worksheet and may even return a part of the form as the *Report*.

Ribotyping

A molecular typing method for epidemiological investigation of bacterial infections. In this method, DNA from bacterial isolates is cut into fragments using restriction endonuclease enzymes. The DNA fragments are separated on a nitrocellulose membrane, which is then probed with a labelled nucleic acid probe designed to bind to the 16s ribosomal operon. The method has been automated, allowing rapid completion of the process, storage of data in digital form and transmission to distant sites for comparison of strains detected in outbreak investigations.

Salmonella serotyping

Identification of salmonella serovars by serology. The large number of salmonella serovars means that a full identification of *Salmonella* spp. isolated from clinical specimens requires a serological method. The one usually employed is agglutination with a panel of antisera. Preliminary screening of suspected colonies is done with polyvalent antisera to the O and H antigens, and to the Vi antigen (for *S. typhi*). A panel of O and H antisera are then used to narrow the possible options to common groups, following the Kaufmann–White scheme. Slide agglutination reactions require confirmation by a tube agglutination method. Only large teaching centres and reference laboratories carry the full range of antisera required to identify all salmonella serovars. Most hospital laboratories can only provide a provisional identification, and even then this is 24 hours or more after submission of the specimen.

Serology

The application of antibody- and antigen-detection methods for the diagnosis of infectious diseases. These methods are usually applied to infections caused by microorganisms that are difficult or impossible to cultivate in the laboratory.

Silver stain

A very sensitive staining process that deposits silver salts in microorganisms. Used to detect the presence of *Pneumocystis carinii* in bronchial lavage fluid and fungal hyphae in tissues.

Slide agglutination test

Agglutination reaction performed on a glass slide, rather than in a test tube or microtitre tray (see *Agglutination* above).

Spore stain

A modified version of the Ziehl–Neelsen acid-fast stain used to drive stain into the thick-walled spores present in some bacteria. It is used to assist in their identification.

Stool microscopy

The examination of faeces (before or after concentration techniques). This is usually restricted to the detection of enteric parasites, where the microscopic appearance can be used to identify the infection.

Streptococcal grouping

Identification of the group to which β-haemolytic streptococci belong. This is achieved by detecting the group-specific capsular polysaccharide. Commonly used methods include a rapid latex agglutination technique.

Substrate utilisation test

Biochemical tests used to help to identify bacteria or fungi that usually rely on utilisation of a specific substrate to produce an easily identifiable colour reaction. These tests can be performed in single containers, or in a commercially available gallery of multiple tests.

Swabs

Fine cotton or alginate tipped swabs widely used to obtain clinical specimens for diagnostic microbiology. The standard cotton swab is dry and does not allow prolonged survival of fastidious bacterial species. These require either specialised swabs (e.g. *Neisseria gonorrhoeae*, charcoal swab; *Bordetella pertussis*, alginate swab) or a special transport medium (e.g. *Chlamydia trachomatis*). If the specimen is purulent exudate, it is better to send a large quantity in a suitable container than a small amount on a dry cotton swab.

Therapeutic drug monitoring

Assessment of serum levels of drugs to ensure that adequate concentrates are reached and that toxic levels are avoided. Some antibiotics are toxic at easily attained concentrations and must have their serum level monitored during therapy. These can be measured either by a bioassay method or by rapid automated methods.

Thick film

A thick film of blood on a microscope slide. Diagnosis of malaria is best done by examination of a stained thick film in which the cells have been lysed. This method is considerably more sensitive than the *Thin film* method (see below).

Thin film

A thin film of peripheral blood on a microscope slide. Diagnosis of malaria is often confirmed by microscopic examination of a thin smear of peripheral blood that has been Giemsa stained. The microscopist looks for intraerythrocytic ring forms, schizonts and gametocytes to confirm a diagnosis and identify the species of *Plasmodium* responsible for infection. The method is not as sensitive as *Thick film* examination (see above) and should always be repeated at least once per patient, because parasitaemia may be intermittent.

Transport medium

A solution used to preserve viable microorganisms during transfer from the patient to the diagnostic laboratory. Most often used for viruses, chlamydias and fastidious bacteria such as *Neisseria gonorrhoeae*.

Venereal Disease Reference Laboratory (VDRL) test

A non-specific serological test for infection with *Treponema pallidum*. Biological false-positive reactions occur with influenza, leprosy and infectious mononucleosis, but the VDRL test is a useful early indicator of active infection.

Western blot

An immunological method that uses a nitrocellulose strip containing microbial antigens separated by electrophoresis to detect the presence of antibodies in serum specimens. The method is used to confirm the presence of antibodies to a range of viral antigens in patients with HIV-related disease.

Ziehl–Neelsen stain

A stain that employs concentrated carbol fuchsin (heated to drive in the stain), acid, alcohol and a counterstain to demonstrate acid-fast bacteria such as *Mycobacterium tuberculosis* and *Nocardia asteroides*. A modified version can be used to stain bacterial spores.

27 Antimicrobial agents

Aciclovir

A purine nucleoside analogue (acycloguanosine) with activity residing in its phosphorylated metabolite. The enzymes required to produce this metabolite are not present in human cells other than those infected with virus. Viral thymidine kinase, therefore, activates the compound, resulting in high potency against herpes simplex virus (HSV) and varicella-zoster virus and low toxicity. Resistant HSV has been described. Uses include treatment of HSV keratitis, encephalitis and genital tract lesions.

Amantidine

A compound with inhibitory activity against influenza type A virus. It is used for treatment and prevention during outbreaks of type A influenza. Resistance has been documented among influenza type A strains.

Aminoglycosides

A group of potent antibacterial aminosugar–aminocyclitol compounds. The group includes gentamicin, amikacin, tobramycin, streptomycin and others. These have good activity against many Gram-negative bacteria, particularly the Enterobacteriaceae and *Pseudomonas* spp., less useful activity against Gram-positive bacteria, and no useful action against obligate anaerobes. Antibacterial activity is significantly reduced in the presence of a low pH, anaerobic environment or a high concentration of divalent cations (e.g. Ca^{2+}). There is little useful uptake from the gastrointestinal tract and all agents in the group are prone to cause auditory and renal toxicity. Aminoglycoside antibiotics are therefore administered parenterally, and the peak and trough serum concentrations are measured regularly. Uses include the treatment of Gram-negative septicaemia and as supplementary agents in chemotherapy of tuberculosis and some Gram-positive infections.

Amphotericin

A polyene antifungal agent with a complex ring structure. Amphotericin has a spectrum of activity that includes many yeast, filamentous and dimorphic fungal species. It is insoluble in water and has to be given as a suspension in deoxycholate or a liposomal preparation by intravenous infusion. The bile salt suspension has a high rate of toxic effects including fever and thrombophlebitis. Its principal use is in treating systematic fungal infection, sometimes in conjunction with other antifungal agents.

Ampicillin

A member of the penicillin group of β-lactam antibiotics. Ampicillin is more active against many Gram-negative bacteria and less susceptible to gastric acid than phenoxymethyl penicillin. Its widespread use as an oral penicillin, particularly in treating upper respiratory and urinary tract infections, has led to the development of resistance to this and related compounds, most significantly by the spread of plasmids and transposons carrying a group of antibiotic-inactivating enzymes, the β-lactamases.

Antimonials, pentavalent

Pentavalent antimonial compounds interfere with parasite glucose metabolism and are used to treat leishmaniasis, although they are relatively toxic to humans.

Arsenicals

Arsenical agents were amongst the first antimicrobial agents to be used but are highly toxic and are therefore rarely used now. One exception is melarsoprol which is used to treat African trypanosomiasis. The action is on glucose metabolism.

Beta (β)-lactam agents

A group of antibiotics derived from moulds with antibacterial activity that depends on interference with cross-linkage of peptidoglycan in the bacterial cell wall. Interference with this process leads to a loss of the affected bacterial cell's structural integrity and consequently to cell death. The group includes the penicillins, cephalosporins, monobactams and carbapenems (see below). These antibiotics have considerable between-compound variation in the range of species against which they can act. Resistance is now common, especially amongst bacteria from hospital patients, either because of the presence of enzymes that rupture the β-lactam ring (β-lactamases) or because of changes in the cell wall permeability. True toxic effects are rare with these agents, but allergic reactions are relatively common and can be fatal. Members of this group have been used to treat most types of bacterial infection, though a β-lactam antibiotic is not always the best or only choice available.

Carbapenems

A group of β-lactam-type antibacterial agents with a penem structure that includes meropenem and imipenem. The prototype compound imipenem is inactivated by renal tubular dipeptidase and is therefore provided in fixed combination with a dipeptidase inhibitor, cilastatin. Meropenem is not inactivated by dipeptidase and achieves better levels in the cerebrospinal fluid. This group of agents has useful activity against bacterial intracellular pathogens.

Cefotaxime

One of the cephalosporin antibiotics (a β-lactam), often referred to as a 'third-generation cephalosporin'. Cefotaxime has potent activity against many Gram-negative bacteria, though much poorer activity against Gram-positive organisms than the earlier cephalosporins. It is resistant to some of the β-lactamase antibiotic-inactivating enzymes, but novel β-lactamases have now been described in Enterobacteriaceae that are capable of inactivating cefotaxime. These new resistance enzymes have become common in centres where there is heavy use of third-generation cephalosporins. Cefotaxime also reaches therapeutically useful levels in the cerebrospinal fluid, which has made it an acceptable choice for treatment of some intracranial infections.

Cefoxitin

Another cephalosporin. It differs from other third-generation agents (see *Cefotaxime* above) in having relatively greater activity against anaerobic bacteria. However, cefoxitin also has a higher rate of antibiotic-associated diarrhoea and pseudomembranous colitis.

Ceftriaxone

A third-generation cephalosporin antibiotic.

Cephalosporins

Broad-spectrum antibiotics with a β-lactam ring. Cefotaxime was the first agent to be released and other members with similar structures have been grouped as first-, second- and third-generation drugs. Antibacterial activity is greatest against Gram-negative bacteria and, with few exceptions, poor against Gram-positive anaerobes and *Pseudomonas aeruginosa*. Where activity extends to these last bacteria, it is usually inferior to other agents specifically designed to act against them. Novel β-lactamase antibiotic-inactivating enzymes are beginning to restrict the use of the third-generation cephalosporins, which have been used extensively in the intravenous treatment of Gram-negative septicaemia and other severe bacterial infections.

Cephradine

A cephalosporin antibiotic, available in both oral and injectable forms, that has greater activity against Gram-positive bacteria (including *Staphylococcus aureus*) than against Gram-negative organisms.

Chloramphenicol

An orally active antibiotic with a wide range of inhibitory activity against Gram-positive, Gram-negative and anaerobic bacteria. Chloramphenicol acts by inhibiting protein synthesis. It penetrates the cerebrospinal fluid and has bactericidal activity against *Neisseria* spp. and *Haemophilus influenzae* and against some Gram-positive organisms when in higher concentrations. Chloramphenicol rarely causes an aplastic anaemia and should not be used in neonates, who may develop the potentially fatal grey baby syndrome. Its uses include topical treatment of bacterial eye infection and the treatment of bacterial meningitis.

Chloroquine

A quinolone compound used in the prophylaxis and treatment of malaria. Prophylaxis over a period of several years may result in deterioration of visual function.

Ciprofloxacin

A 4-aminoquinolone antibacterial agent with useful activity against the Enterobacteriaceae, *Pseudomonas aeruginosa*, other Gram-negative and some Gram-positive organisms. The quinolone group of antibiotics acts by preventing DNA nicking and repair during bacterial replication. Ciprofloxacin is particularly useful because of its good tissue penetration and gastrointestinal uptake. Ciprofloxacin or an equivalent antimicrobial drug may allow outpatient treatment of some Gram-negative infections that would otherwise require intravenous chemotherapy in hospital. Unfortunately, resistance resulting from mutant bacteria DNA gyrase is becoming more common, leading to more restrictive use of ciprofloxacin and related agents.

Clindamycin

A lincosamide antibiotic with activity against Gram-positive but not Gram-negative bacteria. Clindamycin often causes antibiotic-associated diarrhoea and used to be one of the most common causes of pseudomembranous colitis.

Clofazimine

An antimycobacterial agent with principal use in the treatment of lepromatous leprosy. Treatment may result in the development of a brown colour in the skin.

Co-trimoxazole

A fixed combination of the antimicrobial agents trimethoprim and sulfamethoxazole used widely in general practice for common bacterial infections. This combination acts against bacterial folate metabolism. Co-trimoxazole is one of the most common causes of the potentially severe mucocutaneous eruption known as the Stevens–Johnson syndrome. This and other forms of toxicity have led to restrictions on use of this agent in favour of the less toxic component trimethoprim. Bacterial resistance to the sulphonamide component is also very common.

Dapsone

A long-acting sulphonamide agent with bacteriostatic activity against a wide range of bacteria. Resistance can develop quickly if used as a sole agent. Principal uses include treatment of leprosy and prophylaxis of malaria.

Diaminopyrimidines

A group of antibacterial agents that act by inhibiting bacterial dihydrofolate reductase. The most commonly used agent in the group is trimethoprim, which can be used as a single agent though it has been used in combination with a sulphonamide. Trimethoprim is less likely to cause adverse effects and has better tissue penetration than the sulphonamides. It is widely used as an oral agent for treatment of urinary tract infection.

Diethylcarbamazine

An anthelmintic agent with particular use in the treatment of microfilarial infections.

Doxycycline

A tetracycline antibiotic with relatively long half-life and good tissue penetration. Uses include treatment of rickettsial infections.

Erythromycin

A macrolide antibiotic with antimicrobial activity restricted to Gram-positive bacteria, mycoplasmas, chlamydias and ureaplasmas and some Gram-negative bacteria (such as *Haemophilus influenzae*). It has no useful activity against members of the Enterobacteriaceae.

Ethambutol

An agent with antibacterial activity restricted to inhibition of *Mycobacteria* and *Nocardia* spp. Resistance develops during treatment if ethambutol is used alone. It is used in multidrug treatment of tuberculosis. Adverse effects include visual toxicity caused by a retrobulbar neuritis.

Flucloxacillin

An isoxazolyl penicillin, with resistance to staphylococcal β-lactamase. Its main use is in the treatment of infections caused by *Staphylococcus aureus*, but benzylpenicillin or phenoxymethylpenicillin is more active against β-lactamase-negative *Staphylococcus aureus*. The most important form of flucloxacillin resistance is intrinsic staphylococcal resistance (otherwise known as methicillin resistance, MRSA). Other agents in the same group of antistaphylococcal penicillins are cloxacillin, oxacillin and nafcillin.

Fluconazole

A triazole antifungal agent with useful activity against yeasts and some dimorphic species, but not against *Aspergillus* spp. Fluconazole has good tissue and cerebrospinal fluid penetration, because of its low affinity for serum proteins. Its uses include treatment of candidiasis and prevention of cryptococcal meningitis.

Flucytosine

A fluorinated pyrimidine antifungal agent with activity only against yeasts. It acts through inhibition of DNA synthesis. Resistance can develop during treatment. Flucytosine is therefore used with another antifungal agent (usually amphotericin) to treat systemic yeast infections. Depression of bone marrow function can occur as a result of flucytosine treatment.

Foscarnet

A pyrophosphate analogue (phosphonoformic acid) with antiviral activity through its ability to inhibit influenza RNA polymerase, herpes virus DNA polymerase and human immunodeficiency virus (HIV) reverse transcriptase. Foscarnet has a short half-life so must be given as an intravenous infusion. It is used in cytomegalovirus and HIV infections.

Ganciclovir

A nucleoside analogue in the same group of antiviral agents as aciclovir. Ganciclovir is phosphorylated to an active agent in infected cells. It is effective against members of the herpes virus group but, since it has an adverse effect on bone marrow, is used mainly for serious cytomegalovirus infections.

Gentamicin

An aminoglycoside antibiotic with cidal activity against a wide range of bacteria. Like other members of the group, gentamicin causes auditory and renal toxic effects. It is widely used in the treatment of systemic bacterial infection, but its use requires regular monitoring of serum concentrations.

Glycopeptides

A group of antibacterial antibiotics that includes vancomycin and teicoplanin. These agents act against cell wall formation in Gram-positive bacteria and have no useful activity against Gram-negative organisms. Glycopeptides have to be given in an intravenous infusion, and serum concentration must be monitored during use because of problems with toxicity. Their main use is in the treatment of systematic Gram-positive bacterial infections, especially in patients with penicillin allergy or with methicillin-resistant *Staphylococcus aureus* (MRSA) infection.

Griseofulvin

An orally active antifungal agent used in the treatment of dermatophyte infections.

Idoxuridine

A pyrimidine analogue that inhibits synthesis of viral DNA. Idoxuridine is toxic and insoluble in water. It is mainly used for treatment of herpes simplex infections.

Imidazoles

A group of antifungal agents that inhibit the sterol synthesis necessary for normal membrane functions in fungal cells. Their main application is in the topical treatment of dermatophyte and superficial yeast infections; however one agent (fluconazole) can be used for systemic administration.

Isoniazid

A derivative of nicotinic acid that is used in the treatment of tuberculosis. Resistance develops when isoniazid is used by itself. Adverse effects include a pyridoxine-dependent neurotoxicity.

Macrolides

A group of antibacterial antibiotics based on a macrocyclic lactone ring structure. The macrolides act against ribosomal RNA transferase in most Gram-positive and anaerobic bacteria, *Neisseria*, *Campylobacter*, *Haemophilus* spp., but not enteric Gram-negative bacilli. Important members of the group include erythromycin and its analogues. Macrolides have many uses including the treatment of respiratory tract infection, notably Legionnaires' disease and severe campylobacter infection.

Mebendazole

A benzimidazole agent that inhibits glucose uptake and microtubule formation in helminths. It is used in the treatment of intestinal helminth infections.

Methicillin

A β-lactamase-resistant penicillin that is active against most Gram-positive bacteria but is relatively less active than penicillin. Toxicity includes neutropenia, haemorrhagic cystitis and interstitial nephritis. Resistance among staphylococci (e.g. MRSA) is caused by expression of an abnormal penicillin-binding protein. Methicillin is not used in clinical practice.

Metronidazole

A nitroimidazole with useful activity against obligate anaerobes, both bacteria and protozoa. It is used to treat infections following abdominal surgery and for *Giardia lamblia* and *Entamoeba histolytica* infections.

Miconazole

An imidazole antifungal agent used to treat yeast and dermatophyte infections.

Nalidixic acid

An oral antibacterial agent related to the 4-aminoquinolone group (e.g. ciprofloxacin) that acts by inhibiting DNA gyrase. Used to treat urinary tract infections caused by enteric Gram-negative bacilli.

Nitrofurantoin

An oral agent with a wide range of antibacterial activity. Nitrofurantoin is used in the treatment and prevention of urinary tract infection. The agent is inactive in alkaline urine and should not be used to treat *Proteus* sp. infection.

Nystatin

A polyene antibiotic used to treat yeast infections. Its acts by binding sterols and disrupting membrane function.

Penicillins

A group of β-lactam antibiotics derived from benzylpenicillin. Their action is by inhibition of cross-linkage of bacterial cell wall peptidoglycan. Acquired bacterial resistance is by enzymatic hydrolysis of the β-lactam ring (β-lactamase) or by altered affinity for the target site. The parent compound benzylpenicillin is unstable to gastric acid, has a very short half-life and is prone to attack by β-lactamases. It remains the drug of choice for severe pneumococcal, meningococcal and *Streptococcus pyogenes* infections. Derivatives of benzylpenicillin have been developed for oral administration (e.g. phenoxymethylpenicillin (penicillin V)), with prolonged half-life (procaine penicillin), with resistance to staphylococcal β-lactamases (flucloxacillin), with an extended antibacterial range (ampicillin) and with activity against *Pseudomonas aeruginosa* (piperacillin). The penicillins are one of the most widely used groups of antibacterial antibiotics.

Pentamidine

A diamidine compound used to treat and prevent *Pneumocystis carinii* infection. Adverse effects are common during pentamidine therapy and include nephrotoxicity, anaemia, thrombocytopenia, neutropenia and hypoglycaemia.

Piperacillin

A ureidopenicillin antibiotic with activity against *Pseudomonas aeruginosa*, used mainly to treat severe systemic infections in hospital patients.

Polyenes

A group of amphipathic antifungal agents with a molecular structure based on macrocyclic rings. Polyenes bind sterols in the fungal cell membrane and disrupt membrane function. Notable members of the group are amphotericin and nystatin. Their uses include the treatment of systemic and superficial mycoses.

Polymyxin

A group of polypeptide antibiotics that are active against many Gram-negative bacteria but inactive against Gram-positive organisms. Polymyxins bind to the lipid A portion of lipopolysaccharides. They are not absorbed from the gastrointestinal tract. Polymyxins (e.g. colistin) have been used to attempt decontamination of the gastrointestinal tract in high-risk patients such as leukaemic and intensive-care patients.

Primaquine

An orally active compound used in treatment of malaria to prevent relapses caused by *Plasmodium vivax* or *P. ovale*.

Pyrazinamide

An antimycobacterial agent used in multidrug treatment of tuberculosis. Pyrazinamide is particularly useful against intracellular *Mycobacterium tuberculosis* and is used in most short-course regimens. Resistance may develop if the agent is used alone.

Pyrimethamine

A diaminopyrimidine agent with useful activity against *Toxoplasma* sp., *Pneumocystis carinii* and plasmodia. It is used to treat toxoplasmosis, and for malaria prophylaxis.

Quinine

An antimalarial agent used in the treatment of acute malaria, particularly when chloroquine resistance is a possibility.

Quinolones

A group of antibacterial agents (4-aminoquinolones) related to nalidixic acid that act by inhibiting the action of DNA gyrase, a topoisomerase enzyme required for cleaving and repairing bacterial DNA during growth and replication. The quinolones include ciprofloxacin, an agent with good oral uptake and tissue penetration. Antibacterial range includes most Gram-negative bacteria and many Gram-positive organisms. Quinolones are particularly useful in the treatment of hospital infections caused by *Pseudomonas aeruginosa*. Resistance is through altered DNA gyrase targets.

Rifampicin

A rifamycin antibiotic active against mycobacteria and Gram-positive cocci. Rifampicin inhibits bacterial DNA-dependent RNA polymerase. Resistant mutants develop readily during treatment if the agent is used alone. Rifampicin's main uses are in combination with other agents in the treatment of tuberculosis and some staphylococcal infections.

Silver sulfadiazine

A topical antimicrobial combination agent applied to burns to prevent bacterial infection. It has activity against *Pseudomonas* spp., but resistance may develop amongst other bacterial species during use.

Streptomycin

An aminoglycoside antibiotic with activity against a wide range of bacterial species. Streptomycin is inexpensive and, therefore, widely used in developing countries, particularly in multidrug regimens for treatment of tuberculosis.

Sulfadiazine

A sulphonamide antibiotic used topically in combination with a silver salt for burns. It is also used to prevent intracranial infection following head injury.

Sulfamethoxazole

A sulphonamide antibiotic that acts by inhibiting bacterial folate synthesis. Acquired resistance is common, as are adverse effects. Sulfamethoxazole is often used in combination with trimethoprim to treat urinary tract and other minor community-acquired infections.

Sulphonamides

A group of antibacterial agents that inhibit folate synthesis. The group includes agents with relatively short half-lives (e.g. sulfamethoxazole) and longer half-lives (e.g. dapsone). These agents are inexpensive and, therefore, widely used to treat community-acquired infections. Consequently, acquired bacterial resistance is very common. Sulphonamides are commonly associated with adverse effects including rashes and are one of the commonest causes of the ulcerative mucosal condition known as the Stevens–Johnson syndrome.

Terbinafine

An allylamine antifungal agent useful in the oral treatment of dermatophyte infections.

Tetracyclines

A group of antibiotics with useful activity bacteria and some protozoan parasites. The group includes tetracycline, oxytetracycline and doxycycline. Tetracyclines are useful in the treatment of rickettsial and other intracellular infections. Acquired resistance has developed among many bacterial species. Adverse effects include gastrointestinal upsets and deposition in teeth and cartilage of children. Tetracyclines should be avoided in children and pregnant women.

Trimethoprim

A diaminopyrimidine agent that acts by inhibiting microbial dihydrofolate reductase. Trimethoprim penetrates tissues well and is useful in the treatment of urinary tract infections.

Vancomycin

A glycopeptide antibiotic that is active against Gram-positive bacteria. It must be given by intravenous infusion and serum levels should be monitored regularly to avoid problems of toxicity. Use of vancomycin is restricted to hospital practice, where it is useful for patients with Gram-positive infections and penicillin allergy, or with severe infection with methicillin-resistant *Staphylococcus aureus* (MRSA).

Zidovudine

Also known as azidothymidine (AZT). It is an inhibitor of HIV replication through its action on reverse transcriptase. Zidovudine has many adverse effects including rashes, gastrointestinal effects, anaemia and neutropenia. Its use is mainly in the treatment of HIV infection, but some authorities claim that it postpones the onset of disease in recently infected individuals. That claim has recently been challenged by the results of prospective studies.

Index

Q indicates a topic alluded to or mentioned in a question. In some cases, actual mention of the topic may only be found in the corresponding answer. Abbreviations used: CNS, central nervous system; GI, gastrointestinal; UTI, urinary tract infection.

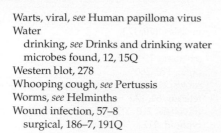